Brass Plate and
Brazen Impudence

Brass Plate and Brazen Impudence

DENTAL PRACTICE IN THE PROVINCES 1755-1855

Christine Hillam

Published for the
DEPARTMENT OF HISTORY
UNIVERSITY OF LIVERPOOL

LIVERPOOL UNIVERSITY PRESS
1991

Liverpool Historical Studies, no. 6
General editor: P.E.H. Hair

Published in Great Britain, 1991,
by the Liverpool University Press,
Senate House, PO Box 147, Liverpool L69 3BX

British Library Cataloguing in Publication Data are available

ISBN 0 85323 117 6

Printed in the European Community by
Antony Rowe Limited, Chippenham, England

For
R.A. COHEN

CONTENTS

List of illustrations   viii
Preface   ix
Acknowledgements   xi
List of abbreviations used   xii

A note on sources   1

Chapter 1 The toothdrawer and the operator: 'dentistry' before
           the eighteenth century   9

Chapter 2 The early provincial dentist: the man and his prospects 15

Chapter 3 The spread of dentistry: wider still, and wider   64

Chapter 4 Treatment   97

Chapter 5 Spurs and constraints   112

App 1 Directories examined   149
App 2 Register of provincial dentists whose names appear in
          pre-1855 trade directories, with biographical notes   153
App 3 Earliest directory evidence of resident dentists in the
          towns featuring in the register   293
App 4 Possible family connections between provincial and London
          dentists before 1855   296
App 5 Dental families established in the provinces before 1855   298

Bibliography   304

Index   323

LIST OF ILLUSTRATIONS

illus. 1   Keys, with interchangeable claws   101

illus. 2   The use of the dental key   102

illus. 3   The art of transplanting teeth, 1787   113

illus. 4   Artificial teeth as fashion accessory, 1792   114

illus. 5   Dental advertisements of 1759 and 1810   135

illus. 6   Dental advertisements of 1842 and 1853   136

PREFACE

In recent years there has been a growth in interest in the evolution of the professions and in the changes in society which allowed them to emerge. Particular attention has been directed towards medicine and especially to the socio-political aspects of its development.

Until relatively recently the dental profession has not been exposed to the same kind of scrutiny, much of the writing on the subject being concerned with individuals or with the internal significance of the reform measures of the late nineteenth and early twentieth century; little regard was paid to what the very emergence of 'dentistry' implied about the society which gave birth to it.

So normal a part of modern life is dentistry, that its existence is often assumed to be inevitable and the way in which it came to occupy its position in present-day society somehow the result of natural justice, as dentistry succeeded against all odds in coming into its own. Yet, there is a radical difference between the services provided by dentistry and the older professions of the Church, the Army, law and medicine. Life might be a more unpleasant experience without the benefits of all that is implied by modern dentistry, but the fabric of society as a whole does not fall apart through lack of them. If this is so, why should dentistry have emerged at all and what does that emergence say about a society into which it is born? Are there preconditions which must be fulfilled before dentistry can come about and further circumstances necessary before it prospers and expands?

This study of the development of dental practice over the hundred-year period 1755-1855 attempts to identify some of these prerequisites and nurturing factors. It looks at the situation in the provinces rather than that in London since, in many respects, it is here that the basic spurs and checks which interact to mould a new trade or profession are thrown into sharper relief in the absence of the advantages afforded by the capital; the most unpromising of occupations would seem likely to have a good chance of thriving in London with its greatest concentration of wealth and population. It does not purport to be a complete picture of the practice of dentistry over the period; readers are directed to the bibliography for details of the extensive literature on the scientific and technical aspects of dentistry of the time.

Throughout, 'dentistry' is used in a specific sense, conveying the meaning which led to the very coining of the word in the eighteenth century, namely the treatment of diseases of the teeth and oral tissues by preventive, restorative, prosthetic and surgical means. Although toothdrawers of many varieties enter into the tale, they are not synonymous with dentists whose story this is.

ACKNOWLEDGEMENTS

This study originated many years ago in an untidy but ever expanding collection of snippets of information on provincial dentists of the eighteenth and nineteenth centuries. That this data ever became organised was due largely to the continuing interest and encouragement of Professor R.J. Anderson of the Dental School, University of Birmingham, who rashly undertook to design a computer programme to tame it and has been unfailingly generous with his time and effort ever after. That it later formed the basis of a thesis was due to the support of Professor E.P. Hennock of the Department of History, University of Liverpool, and of the Trustees of the G.S. Veitch Fund whose grant towards travelling expenses made my research possible. Similarly, there would have been no progression from thesis to book form had it not been for the patient persistence of Professor P.E.H. Hair, also of the Department of History in the same University.

No one who researches into the history of dentistry can fail to owe a debt of gratitude to Ronald Cohen, MA, FFD, LDS, and J.A. (Archie) Donaldson, BA, FDS, for their enthusiastic support and unselfish giving of their time for exchange of ideas and material. My own indebtedness to them is very great, as it is to Dr. J.G.L. Burnby who has, over the years, passed on to me many items of dental interest encountered during her own research.

Finally, but certainly not least importantly, I have benefited enormously from the professional expertise and helpfulness of countless librarians of a good hundred collections; personal thanks are due to the staff of the library of the British Dental Association and especially to its Librarian, Miss M.A. Clennett.

Advertisements in the Menzies Campbell Collection of Newspaper Advertisements are quoted with the permission of the President and Council of the Royal College of Surgeons of England. Much of the section on education first appeared in the *British Dental Journal* (163(1987),204-207) and is reused with permission of the Editor.

Department of Clinical Dental Sciences
School of Dentistry
University of Liverpool

ABBREVIATIONS USED

ABG	*Aris's Birmingham Gazette*
Am.Jnl.Dent.Sci.	*American Journal of Dental Science*
Br.dent.J.	*British Dental Journal*
Br.J.dent.Sci.	*British Journal of Dental Science*
Bull.Hist.Dent.	*Bulletin of the History of Dentistry*
Bull.Soc.Soc.Hist.Med.	*Bulletin of the Society for the Social History of Medicine*
Caries Res.	*Caries Research*
CC	*Chester Chronicle*
Dent.Hist.	*Dental Historian*
Dent.Items	*Dental Items of Interest*
Dent.Mag.Oral Topics	*Dental Magazine and Oral Topics*
Dent.Pract.	*Dental Practitioner*
Dent.Rev.	*Dental Review*
Dent.Sur.	*Dental Surgeon*
Ec.Hist.Rev.	*Economic History Review*
J.Br.Dent.Assoc.	*Journal of the British Dental Association*
Liv M	*Liverpool Mercury*
LJ	*Leicester Journal*
LM	*Leeds Mercury*
LNJ	*Leicester and Nottingham Journal*
MCC	*Menzies Campbell Collection of Newspaper Advertisements (Royal College of Surgeons of England)*
Med.Hist.	*Medical History*
MM	*Manchester Mercury*
NJ	*Nottingham Journal*
PCC	*Prerogative Court of Canterbury*
PCY	*Prerogative Court of York*
Proc.R.Soc.Med.	*Proceedings of the Royal Society of Medicine*
Quart.J.dent.Sci.	*Quarterly Journal of Dental Science*
Trans.Inst.Brit.Geogr.	*Transactions of the Institute of British Geographers*
YC	*York Courant*

A NOTE ON SOURCES

'Dentistry' may justifiably be seen as a new phenomenon to emerge in Britain in the eighteenth century. It embraces more than toothdrawing (which, although performed surprisingly rarely before the late mediaeval period, has a long history), being a neologism coined to describe the new concept of actually attempting to repair the damage caused by caries and periodontal disease, exceedingly rare before this date. For reasons which will become clear later, the practice of dentistry did not expand on any appreciable scale until the early nineteenth century.

This relatively late emergence has implications for the researcher seeking to study the early development of this new approach to dental disease and of dental practice as a whole. 'Dentists' of the period are not to be found as a group in the kind of sources commonly taken for granted by medical historians, although a few may do so as individuals. The delay in expansion until the nineteenth century means, for example, that trainee dentists, by and large, do not appear in **apprenticeship tax records** which cease in 1811 for London and 1808 for 'country'.[1] There is no **Register** of dentists until 1879 and then it is only partial, since registration was not compulsory until 1921.[2] Dental schools and examinations,[3] professional societies[4] and the specialist press[5] are all features of the post-1855 period.

The censuses of 1841 and 1851 are useful for judging the size of the profession towards the end of the first half of the nineteenth century but are perhaps of greater value at the level of enumerators' returns than at that of the summary tables, where in 1841 dentists are found subsumed into the 527 'cuppers and dentists' in England, Wales and the Islands, with a local figure for 'dentists' available only in those areas with no cuppers. The 1851 census gives a total of 1041 dentists for the whole of Great Britain but relegates them to 'other medical men' at local level, with no possibility of retrieving the numbers of dentists in different areas. In addition, the totals given cannot be considered as accurate, for confusion arose in the reporting of occupations. The enumerators were instructed to 'insert occupations in order of their importance' and the first occupation

was generally taken for classification purposes. Dentistry was in
some cases being carried out by men who had started in another trade
and who, although now practising full-time as dentists, perhaps still
thought of themselves as, say, watchmakers or surgeons, and were
returned as such. (The 1851 *Report* (p.lxxxvii) actually states that
'the best...dentists...have the licences of surgeons, and are so
returned').   If such men declared first their trade and then their
occupation, their involvement in dentistry was lost in the process of
classification.   Even the accurate 'surgeon dentist' appears in many
cases to have been classified as 'surgeon', thus inflating the figure
for that profession and distorting the estimate of those working in
dentistry.[6]

The censuses which fall within the time span of the development
of dentistry before the middle of the nineteenth century, though
providing a wealth of information relating to individuals and an
approximate estimate of the size of the profession, strictly speaking
reflect only the state of dentistry in 1841 and 1851. The principal
sources which refer to most dentists of the whole period in their
professional capacity are **trade directories** and **newspapers**. Whilst
the latter are the more revealing about details of treatment and
patterns of practice (frequently giving information of itineraries,
charges and training), established dentists do not always advertise
their services in their home town, especially towards the end of the
period.   To rely on advertisements alone as a source for the
development of practice would present a distorted picture; they are,
perhaps, best relegated to a complementary and illuminating rôle or
used as a yardstick against which to evaluate the other major source,
trade directories.

This last type of publication first appeared on the scene in
London in 1677 with Samuel Lee's *A collection of the names of
merchants living in and about the city of London*.   It had no
successor until 1734 but thereafter directories appeared annually.

The first such provincial publication was Sketchley's 1763
directory of Birmingham but the earliest to survive is Gore's
Liverpool directory for 1766.   This was soon followed by directories
of Manchester (1772) and Bristol (1775), also towns which owed their
expansion to foreign trade.   Between 1763 and 1790 fifty provincial
directories are recorded and it is likely that others were published
which have not survived.   By the end of the century it is clear that
this form of publication was recognised as a necessary instrument of

communication, whether for purposes of trade or for the needs of visitors to the new spas and watering places.

Changes in commercial practice following the 'industrial revolution', with manufacturers seeking customers and suppliers outside their own immediate area, stimulated the production of county and national directories. By 1820, Pigot's publications covered the whole country and by the 1850s he and his successors and competitors (Slater, Kelly and White) were surveying all areas of England and Wales at frequent intervals. For this period, 'it should not be difficult for an inquirer to find a good directory of any fair-sized place in England', according to the bibliographer of provincial trade directories, Jane Norton.[7]

However, there are problems inherent in the use of individual provincial trade directories as a major source material, including the familiar fact that their coverage of the population is undoubtedly partial. Fortunately, this is probably less of a difficulty for the compilation of a list of dental practices than it is in many other circumstances, for medical men of various kinds are almost invariably included in even the most modest of publications.

More relevant is that some of the early directories are known to have disappeared, making it unwise to assume that those which survive will reveal the entire pattern of a dentist's career, particularly in the eighteenth century. (It is theoretically possible for a dentist never to appear in a surviving directory at all). Even where complete runs of directories are still extant, the methods of compilation used for individual publications[8] can make some entries dubious and others difficult to date accurately, as Norton points out.[9] These inconsistencies are compensated for to some extent where a whole series is consulted, as in the list of dentists to be found in *appendix 2.1* (where all provincial directories published up to 1855 were used). To what degree they can be ironed out can be tested by a comparison with that other major, but also incomplete, source for the names of dentists, the advertisement columns of the local newspaper.

Obligingly, early dentists had few inhibitions about advertising their services in the press, particularly at the beginning of their careers or when they were visiting other towns; indeed, it was probably essential to their professional survival at a time when the demand for dental treatment was not overwhelming. A comparative sample of the two sources (made for the purposes of the verification of the list of dental practices which forms the basis of this book), suggests that in those towns with good runs of trade directories, the trade directory is the more fruitful repository of the names of dentists in permanent practice for more than a few months than is the newspaper:

COMPLETE SEARCHES OF NEWSPAPERS		PERMANENT DENTAL PRACTICES	
TOWN	DATES	NEWSPAPERS	TRADE DIRECTORIES
Liverpool	1800–40	26	38
Birmingham	1770–1805	3	4
Bath	1800–10	4	8
		33	50

table 1: Permanent dental practices advertised in newspapers and trade directories in three towns with good runs of trade directories

In Birmingham one dentist[10] and in Liverpool three dentists[11] are found in newspapers but not in a trade directory, but their appearances there are so brief (only a few advertisements in a short space of time) that it seems likely that these were not men who set up permanent practice. In all three towns permanent dentists are found in trade directories who make no appearance in the press, although they do not necessarily take the first opportunity to enter their names.[12]

The exercise can be repeated for three towns or areas with poorer runs of trade directories (in the majority before 1855):

COMPLETE SEARCHES OF NEWSPAPERS		PERMANENT DENTAL PRACTICES	
TOWN	DATES	NEWSPAPERS	TRADE DIRECTORIES
York	1739–1810	2	1
Leicester	1769–1811	2	1
Isle of Man	1793–1840	4	2
		8	4

table 2: Permanent dental practices advertised in newspapers and trade directories in three towns with poor runs of trade directories

At first sight, it would appear that the situation here is reversed and that newspapers provide twice as many names as do the directories. One permanent practitioner who advertised in newspapers in York, Le Sec, certainly had no opportunity to appear in a trade directory during his years in the city, 1794–1801, but he was the only such individual in seventy years. Similarly, in the Isle of Man, one dentist, Archer, practised in a period deficient in directories, 1824–35, but is the only example of the phenomenon over a fifty year period. In Leicester, it is doubtful whether the extra dentist culled from the press, Clay Hextall, ever ventured into the field more than tentatively for he makes only two appearances in the press and both of those are in the same month. The same applies to the Isle of Man, where C. Thompson has but one single advertisement in the Manx newspapers.

A survey of all provincial trade directories published before 1855 produces a list of nearly 1100[13] resident dentists in 200 or so towns. If the second, more pessimistic, comparison between directories and newspaper advertisements (with one dentist being missed per town over an average of sixty years) is taken to be typical of each of the 200 towns, then a reliance on trade directories alone produces a list of nearly 85% accuracy. This estimate probably makes more than adequate allowance for the possibility that, while more than one dentist may indeed have been missed in some towns with poor runs of directories (about 170 in all), the majority of these towns were in any case often ones which other evidence suggests were unlikely to have a history of resident dentistry undiscovered for want of trade directories.[14] Bearing in mind also that the newspaper/directories comparison in *table 1* showed more dentists emerging from directories than from advertisements, then the estimate of 85% accuracy may be a conservative one.

Trade directories of the period, by their very nature, list only the principals in a practice, unlike census returns which include all those involved in the profession.[15] Thus a survey which takes them as its source charts the development of dental practice rather than the increase in the number of individual dentists. The list which appears in *appendix 2.1* contains only actual directory entries (edited for spelling where other evidence left no doubt that the same individual was being referred to), but the entries as they stand are inadequate for the purposes of examining the nature of dental practice over the period because of gaps in series of directories. For this reason, in the calculations which appear on the following pages, dummy entries have been supplied where the gap between directory entries did not exceed the average gap of five years. The cautious supply of dummy entries within a dentist's career span provides a more realistic picture of the growth of dental practice but complete accuracy cannot be attained since no deficiencies have been made good from other sources at either end of a career in the case of a dental practice in a town with poor runs of directories, in the knowledge that this could not be carried out consistently. Some of the resultant calculations therefore demonstrate the general magnitude of a parameter; where maximum precision is necessary and desirable, attention is directed only to those towns with good or complete series of directories.

NOTES AND REFERENCES

1   My own searches of 20,000 such apprenticeship records revealed no mention of dentistry. In her search of 18,040 records of Warwickshire, Joan Lane found only one dental reference, to Thomas Brown of Henley in Arden, apprenticed to his father Samuel, a surgeon, apothecary, dentist and midwife in 1828 (personal communication to R.A. Cohen). From her total survey of the apprenticeship tax records in search of medical references, J.G.L. Burnby found only four references to dentists, three of these in London, and even then dentistry is a secondary occupation in half the cases (personal communication).

2   The first *Dentists Register* of 1879 was open to those in *bona fide* practice and to those who had practised dentistry in conjunction with medicine or pharmacy. Thereafter, registration was open only to those who attained the Licence in Dental Surgery (LDS) of the Colleges of Surgeons. The use of 'dentist' and 'dental practitioner' was restricted to those on the Register but unregistered practice under some other title was unaffected.

3   The earliest dental school, the London School of Dental Surgery, was founded in 1858. The first examination for the LDS took place in 1860, but even then only a small minority of students availed themselves of the opportunity. This was especially true of dentists outside London, since after the initial opportunity to present oneself *sine curriculo*, all candidates were obliged to complete a period of hospital attendance in the capital until provincial centres were recognised later in the century.

4   The earliest of these societies, the Odontological Society of London and the College of Dentists, were not founded until 1856.

5   The dental periodical press had its hesitant beginnings in the 1840s with James Robinson's *British Quarterly Journal of Dental Science* (30 March 1843 and 30 June 1843) and *Forceps* (1844–45). They were succeeded by the *Quarterly Journal of Dental Science (Quart.J.dent.Sci.)* (1 Apr 1857–Jan 1859) and *Dental Review (Dent.Rev.)* (1859–67),supporters

of the College of Dentists, and the *British Journal of Dental Science (Br.J.dent.Sci.)* (1 July 1856-1935), which soon came to favour the Odontological Society. Whilst they yield considerable incidental information on dentistry and its practitioners in the earlier period in the provinces (as do contemporary and earlier treatises on treatment of the teeth and the records of the professional organisations of the middle of the century), they do not constitute a suitable source for a detailed study of the development of dental practice.

6   The census figures presented for Cheltenham for 1841 highlight these problems. According to the census there was only one dentist in the town in 1841, a woman over 20. The directories, on the other hand, suggest there were eight: Montague Alex and his two partners the Levasons, George Cullis, Thomas Palmer, George Shew, Somerset Tibbs and Robert Pearsall. Examination of the enumerators' returns for Cheltenham reveal that Alex and Cullis are listed as surgeons, whereas Palmer, Shew and Tibbs are returned as surgeon dentists. Only Pearsall is called a dentist. (The Levasons do not appear at their directory address which was Alex's private home). All these dentists had been listed under 'surgeon dentist' in Davies's *Cheltenham Annuaire*. Thus, presumably by recategorisation as surgeons, five men known to be practising dentists have disappeared from the national total for that trade somewhere along the journey from enumerator's pencil to statistical table. At local level, eight male dentists have become one woman.

7   For a fuller description of the development of trade directories, see the introduction in J.E. Norton, *Guide to the National and Provincial directories of England and Wales published before 1856* (1950).

8   The most successful scheme might be expected to be door-to-door visits by the compiler or a paid professional agent; those engaged on a commission basis were likely to call only at those addresses where an order for the directory was to be anticipated. Even then, however, the collector was at the mercy of weather, hostility on the part of residents and misunderstanding of local accents. Where circulars were distributed for return or advertisements placed for entries, the response must have been somewhat haphazard and the danger of misread handwriting increased. The use of ready-made lists, such as rate books, could lead to very partial results (especially in commercial premises which were sub-let) and the collection of information from servants to inaccurate trade descriptions.

9   On average, there appears to have been a time-lag of two or three months between collection of material and publication and some directories were re-issued without revision. The time of the year the survey was made is also relevant to the accuracy of the result. In a period of high mobility, annual directories were needed to keep pace with changes of address but these were rare. Most moves took place on quarter days and the best directory publishers did not attempt a compilation until January or July. Lists of alterations were issued to purchasers in an attempt to accommodate this problem, but these were essentially even more ephemeral than the directories themsleves and have not always survived.

10   Tomlinson, a surgeon to the General Hospital, who announces in a single advertisement that 'he will in future add to his other practice that of surgeon-dentist' (*Aris's Birmingham Gazette (ABG)*, 22 July

1793).

11   Haslam & Co. (Nov-Dec 1825, 4 advertisements), L'Estrange (Aug-Sept 1835; Jan, Feb, May 1836, 6 advertisements), Alexander Neibaur (Sept 1831-Jan 1832, 7 advertisements).

12   e.g. in Liverpool Samuel Berend misses two directories (1822 and 1823), James Rose four (1818, 1819, 1821 and 1822) and James Webster four (1825, 1827, 1828 and 1829) before entering their names.

13   A minimum of 1092 separate individuals.

14   As late as 1846 Robertson was able to write that the 'dentist...is generally to be found only in larger towns' (W. Robertson, *Practical observations on the teeth*, 4th edition (1846), 202). A Tavistock dentist of 1858 declared that it was impossible for him to make an adequate living by practising in that 'unfashionable town' alone (*Br.J.dent.Sci.*, 2(1858), 49).

15   Accuracy of directories and census totals apart, this is one reason for the apparent anomaly between figures from the two sources in 1841 and 1851.

CHAPTER 1: THE TOOTHDRAWER AND THE OPERATOR: "DENTISTRY" BEFORE THE EIGHTEENTH CENTURY

The word 'dentist' appears to have first entered the English language in the 1750s. This is not to say that no work in the mouth was ever performed before this period but that, although dental disease of one kind or another seems to be as old as mankind, there were few attempts before the eighteenth century to intervene to remedy the situation. A few examples have been found in Egyptian mummies of teeth wired together but there is disagreement as to whether this was intended to restore function in this world or perfection for the next. Similarly, examples survive of Etruscan and Roman artificial replacements for lost teeth but again, forensic archaeological evidence would suggest that by and large dental disease went untreated. Examination of early skulls shows carious teeth were rarely extracted.

However, by the Middle Ages a change had taken place and extraction had become more common. This was generally performed by the barbers. Their early association with minor surgical procedures is underlined by the joint duties of the *rasor et minutor* who shaved and bled the monks.[1] Albucasius complained that, despite their ignorance, barbers commonly extracted teeth. When the 10th Lateran Council of 1215 finally forbade all clergy (previously in almost total charge of the practice of all branches of medicine) to shed blood, it was the secular barbers who took on such surgical procedures as were then performed,[2] including the extraction of teeth.

In England, the Barbers' Company of London[3] was in a position by 1375 to petition for rights to control barbery and surgery in the city, notwithstanding the existence of the smaller but more select Fellowship of Surgeons, whose members practised surgery only and considered themselves superior to the barbers. The Barbers' Company's first Charter of 1462 confirms the old privileges and specifically quotes the drawing of teeth as being part of the mystery of barbery. Nearly a century later an act of 1540 united the two rival bodies into the Company of Barber-Surgeons. However, a firm distinction was now made between the two crafts of surgery and barbery; no surgeon was to practise barbery and the barbers were to be restricted in their surgical procedures to the extraction of teeth.

It would be a mistake, however, to assume that, in London at least, the barbers and barbers practising surgery were able to exercise a monopoly over the operation. The successive efforts of the Company to control the practice of barbery and surgery from the late 14th century onwards are in themselves an indication that others were by now poaching on their preserves. There are strong grounds for believing that, whilst barbers undoubtedly extracted teeth, 'the real practitioners of such dentistry as was possible were the "toothdrawers" ',[4] a separate specialist group who may be seen as the true progenitors of the modern dentist. The earliest reference to such a description yet discovered is to Peter of London, who is thus designated in a transaction of real estate in 1320.[5] It seems unlikely that he was the first of his kind, bearing in mind that the modern pattern of caries incidence had already begun to emerge by the late Middle Ages.[6] The first literary mention of a toothdrawer would appear to be in Langland's *Vision of Piers Plowman* (1377) where Glotton, on his way to mass, is involved in a brawl with, among others, toothdrawers.[7] In 1400 the pipe rolls of Henry IV record the appointment of Matthew Flint, toothdrawer, at 6d. per day for life.[8] Twenty-five years later (in 1426) one Richard Feryer, toothdrawer of Colchester, was sued for damages of £40 by Richard Jeull and his wife Joan, it being alleged that Feryer had made an assault on Joan with his forceps, lacerating her tongue and wickedly drawing blood. Feryer defended himself, claiming that he had treated Joan 'properly and according to his art'.[9]

There are two references to toothdrawers in the sixteenth century in connection with the Barber-Surgeons of London. The first is to the admittance as a brother, after payment of £1, on 10 September 1551 of John Bryckette.[10] The second individual mentioned is William Thomlyn who was granted a licence on 23 November 1557 'to drawe teethe and to make cleane teethe and no more'.[11] This would seem to mark out the toothdrawer as a group apart from the common barber who would, presumably, need no special licence to extract teeth.

In popular literature of the sixteenth century, Lindsay found other references to the toothdrawer. He appears in *Cocke Lorelles Bote* (c.1515) as one of the callings listed in the pardoner's book[12] and as a trade of everyday life in a children's book published in

1563.[13]   In a publication of 1592 entitled *Kind Hartes Dreame* the
toothdrawer is described as wearing a 'thrumde hat' and 'hanging at
it the ensignes of [his] occupation'.[14]   Elsewhere in the same work
Chettle talks of 'cousoning toothe drawers that from place to place
wander with banners full of horse teeth'; they 'haue not to do with
the means Kindhart vseth, but forsooth, by charmes they can at their
pleasure fray away the payne, which Kindhart counts little better
than witch-craft if it could doe good'.[15]   Among other contemporary
references to toothdrawers, Lindsay cites Taylor in *A toy to mock an
ape* as describing 'a fellow that wore a brooch in his hat like a
toothdrawer with a rose and crown and two letters'.[16]

It would appear that there are no surviving signboards
advertising toothdrawers, although Lindsay remarked in 1927 on a
small sign in the Odontological Collection of the Museum of the Royal
College of Surgeons of England.   Found in Devonshire, it showed a
depiction of extraction together with the motto 'Notice to quit'.[17]
She also drew attention to a sign for a doctor from Poole which
showed him operating on the mouth.[18]   This depiction would support
the contention of Burnby and others that boundaries between branches
of medicine were not as rigid as used to be supposed.[19]

Until relatively recently there was no documentary evidence
earlier than the eighteenth century[20] that blacksmiths were involved
in the extraction of teeth.   However, the will of Humphrey Baker, a
farrier in trade in the sixteenth century in Offchurch (near
Leamington Spa) shows the practice to be of long standing.   To Thomas
Jecocke of Oloughton he leaves 'my tooles which I used to draw
teeth'.[21]

It would seem, then, that while treatment of the teeth largely
involved only extraction and cleaning, its practice was in the hands
of a wide variety of people; the ordinary barber, the barber
practising surgery, the country doctor and the blacksmith - all seem
likely to have derived some of their income from the extraction of
teeth alongside the man who made a speciality of the procedure and in
consequence called himself a toothdrawer.

The seventeenth century saw the beginnings of changes in the
scope of dental treatment and the emergence of a new designation for
some of its practitioners, the 'operator for the teeth', defined in
Phillip's dictionary as 'one skilled in drawing teeth and in making
artificial ones'.   The earliest known work in English devoted
entirely to the teeth and their treatment was written by such an

operator, Charles Allen, and first published in York in 1685. Though apparently unaware of any views on anatomy and physiology other than his own, he nevertheless sets forth the feasible operations and techniques of the day, including the manufacture of artificial teeth. Allen would presumably not have published his book had there not been a potential readership for it. The foundations may already have been laid by the translation into English in 1597 of Guillemeau's *The French Chirurgerie* in which the use of artificial filling material and gold wire for the attachment of prosthetic pieces was described.

Some of these 'operators' received royal appointments[22] but it appears to be unknown what treatment they carried out in this capacity. In these days before widespread advertising, it is difficult to decide whether the making of artificial teeth was restricted to those adopting the title 'operator' or whether this was a service also offered by barbers and toothdrawers who chose to retain the old designations for some reason. It is equally unclear whether the operators were principally a phenomenon of the practice of dentistry in London or whether they appeared in the provinces in any numbers.

What is certainly true is that treatment of the teeth was beginning to draw other trades into its ambit. Guillemeau had recommended that metal work in prostheses should be sent out to a goldsmith. By the end of the seventeenth century the early London newspapers carried occasional advertisements for such tradesmen who made artificial teeth:[23]

> Mr. Pilleau a French Goldsmith living in St. Martin's Lane...does give Notice, That by an Experience of 18 Years, he has found out a way to make and set Artificial Teeth in so firm a manner, that one may chew with them...Any Operator for the Teeth may buy some ready made by him at a reasonable price.

A year later Pilleau's advertisement omits any reference to supplying operators and it may be surmised that he was by this time fully occupied with dealing direct with patients.

However, it seems likely that the provision of artificial teeth remained a minor part of the practice of treatment available. The unfortunate Mrs. Samuel Pepys repeatedly had teeth drawn by eminent toothdrawers and barber-surgeons during her short life,[24] but there appears to be no mention in her husband's diary of their replacement by artificial ones, although the couple were certainly in an economic position to be able to afford them. The bulk of dental treatment carried out still remained limited to extraction and cleaning, traditionally at the hands of the barber or specialist toothdrawer, and even then was still a rarity in the population at large. It was the eighteenth century which was to see the emergence of the modern concept of 'dentistry'.

NOTES AND REFERENCES

1   B.W. Weinberger, *History of Dentistry* (1948), I, 234.
2   J. Dobson and R.M Walker, *Barbers and Barber-Surgeons of London* (1979), 7.
3   The earliest reference to the Company is in 1308 when Richard le Barbour was admitted as Master before the Court of Aldermen (*ibid.,* 9).
4   L. Lindsay, 'Notes on the history of dentistry in England up to the beginning of the nineteenth century', *Br.dent.J.,* 48(1927), 268.
5   J.A. Donaldson, 'Peter de London, toothdrawer', *Br.dent.J.,* 119(1965), 147-148.
6   W.J. Moore and M.E. Corbett, 'The distribution of dental caries in ancient British populations. II Iron age, Romano-British and Mediaeval periods', *Caries Res.,* 7(1973), 139-153.
7   'peeled tooth drawers' -quoted by L. Lindsay, *A short history of dentistry* (1933), 30.
8   Quoted by Lindsay 1933, 30-31.
9   Quoted by Lindsay 1933, 31-32.
10   S. Young, *Annals of the Barber-Surgeons* (1890), 270. Six years later (26 Aug 1557) 'it was ordered that Mrs. Dawson, the widow of one Bryckette -a tooth drawer- shall pay no quarteryge to the hawse nor hange oute any signe or cloth with teethe as she heartofore hath done' (*ibid.,* 177).
11   *ibid.,* 178.
12   'also mathewe tothe drawer of London' (Wynkyn de Worde, *Cocke Lorelles Bote,* p.5 in *Ancient poetical tracts of the 16th century* (1843), Percy Society, VI).
13   *Dives Pragmaticus* (1563); quoted by Lindsay 1927, 269.
14   H. Chettle, *Kind-Hartes Dreame* (1592), p.11 in *Early English poetry, ballads and popular literature of the middle ages* (1841), Percy Society, V.
15   *ibid.,* 28.
16   Taylor, *A toy to mock an ape,* quoted by Lindsay 1927, 268.
17   L. Lindsay, 'The London dentist of the 18th century', *Dent.Surg.,* 24(1927), 179. No trace remains of this unique dentist's signboard and it is not mentioned in any of the catalogues of the Musuem. It is considered that Lilian Lindsay may have been mistaken in its location (communication (1984) from the curator of the Hunterian Musuem, Miss E. Allen).
18   Lindsay 1927a; the original sign was damaged in 1941 but a coloured copy hangs in the entrance hall of the College.

19   e.g. J.G.L. Burnby, 'A study of the English apothecary from 1660-1760' (unpublished PhD. thesis, University of London, 1979), 107.

20   Prints of the 18th century frequently show blacksmiths acting as toothdrawers, albeit in comic circumstances. Parson Woodforde called in a farrier to extract a tooth for him in 1776 and a dentist from Tavistock identifies blacksmiths as 'rival key manipulators' as late as 1858 ('Suaviter et fortiter', 'Quackery and country practice', *Br.J.dent.Sci.,* 2(1858), 49).

21   Reported by R.A. Cohen, *Lindsay Club Newsletter,* 10(1984), 11. The will, made in 1610, in located in Lichfield Record Office.

22   e.g. Thomas Middleton, Peter de la Roche, George Gosling, John Persimore and Dr. Clark (L. Lindsay, 'The London dentist of the 17th century', *Br.dent.J.,* 80(1946), 75-80).

23   *Postman,* 30 Jan 1696, the earliest such advertisement yet reported. Quoted by W.H. Dolamore, 'Some old advertisements', *Br.dent.J.,* 45(1924), 185.

24   11 Mar 1660, a front tooth removed by Peter de la Roche; 18 May 1669, a tooth removed by Robert Leeson; 1667, a surgeon had declined to extract a tooth, apparently a common attitude among surgeons who, like Wiseman (1676), recommended recourse to a toothdrawer (Lindsay 1946, 75-80).

CHAPTER 2: THE EARLY PROVINCIAL DENTIST: THE MAN AND HIS PROSPECTS

In 1728 there was published in Paris Pierre Fauchard's *Le chirurgien-dentiste*, one of the most influential books in its field. This (with the second edition of 1746) brought together all that was best from the worlds of the operator, the toothdrawer, the anatomist and the craftsman, describing as it did all aspects of disease in the mouth and giving full details with case histories and illustrations of how to deal with it. There are chapters on scaling the teeth, filing them free of caries, filling cavities, cauterisation, moving teeth for orthodontic purposes, extraction and the manufacture of a variety of artificial appliances to replace lost teeth and the tissues of the palate. This represented a new departure. References to the teeth and their treatment can be found scattered in the writings of anatomists, surgeons, operators and others from the sixteenth century (particularly on the Continent) but never before had every aspect of the field been fully expounded in a single work, with so little regard to the commercial risk of revealing trade secrets.

Fauchard's book stimulated rival productions, both at home and abroad as his ideas and techniques became more widely disseminated. Nevertheless, available sources suggest that the numbers of dental operators remained very low all over Europe until the middle of the eighteenth century when a modest upsurge occurred. In the first quarter of the century, London had been home to Pilleau, the French silversmith, and to Rutter and Watts (members of a long-lived practice in Raquet Court which survived into the late nineteenth century). Thereafter, the city had been host to such men as Gamaliel Voice (in the 1720s and 30s), M. Milpentine (1732), Lemaire (1740), surgeon-dentist to the Duke of Artois, and Paul Jullion from Paris (1750s).[1] Not until the 1760s and 70s is there evidence of the presence of dentists in any numbers, and many of those (such as Bellejean, Ruspini, Van Butchell, Hemet, Landymiey, Talma, Martiniani, Scardovi and Dumergue) were of foreign origin.[2]

Even then it would seem that demand for treatment was not overwhelming, for by the middle of the eighteenth century, there is newspaper evidence of dental practitioners from London paying visits

to provincial towns. The earliest such visits yet discovered date
from 1752 when Bartholomew Ruspini, originally from Bergamo, lodged
at the 'Black Swan' in York. From this base he offered to 'destroy
all kinds of scurvy in the mouth and gums' using a small brush, a
'spunge' and the dried roots of mallows. He had already cured
several persons in Manchester and no payment was required until after
the cure was performed.[3] On his 1753 visit, Ruspini was competing
with Annibal Toscan, born in Parma and with many years' practice in
Italy, Paris and most other principal parts of Europe. More
immediately, Toscan had arrived from Oxford. Among his
accomplishments was the ability to give instant relief for toothache
and to fasten loose teeth; he drew teeth and fitted artificial ones.
Advice given in his chambers attracted the fee of 5s., but 'he
attends any person at their house in town' for 1 gn., would travel
two miles for two guineas and further for proportionately higher
fees.[4]

The following year, Thomas Steele, a native and freeman of York,
calling himself 'Operator for the Teeth', arrived for the summer from
Paris, where he had been educated under Mons. Du Verdière and Mons.
Capperon, 'surgeon dentists to the King of France'. He was able to
offer all the operations practised by his preceptors including the
application of a powder which set an ivory lustre on the teeth and
nourished the gums and the fibres of the mouth.[5]

Exotic connections continued to feature as a recommendation: Mr.
Gason drew attention to the fact that he was a former pupil of Signor
Palermo, 'dentrificator in London'. In York he proposed to scale
teeth, cure scurvy of the gums 'as is now practised by the most able
artists of the profession in Paris and London', and fix artificial
teeth.[6]

These mid-century visitors reflect the growing interest in care
of the teeth in the provinces. As early as 1724 William Prior of
Newcastle, a maker and seller of musical instruments, declares that
'he also makes and sells artificial teeth so neatly as not to be
discovered from natural ones.'[7] In the same town, Dr. Lucas was
selling his 'chemical preparation for killing the toothache without
drawing'. However, neither of these two gentlemen offered the full
range of operations on the teeth which might be considered
'dentistry' and Boyes found no truly dental references in the
Newcastle press until the visit of Michael Whitlock to the town in
1760.[8] The same may be said of York, where there are occasional

earlier advertisements for toothache cures[9] but no references to
dentists until Ruspini's visit of 1752. In Birmingham, too, an
isolated reference is found in 1741 to a maker of artificial teeth[10]
but the true visiting dentist makes his first appearance in the 1750s
in the person of Mr. Foy of London.[11] Travelling around the West
Midlands, he included Stafford and Wolverhampton on his itineraries.

All in all, then, whilst isolated examples can be found in the
early eighteenth century of instrument and appliance makers including
artificial teeth among their repertoire of products, it would seem
that travelling dentists, offering the full range of operations on
the mouth, did not appear in the provinces as visitors until the
early 1750s. These visiting dentists became increasingly common with
time.[12] In addition, the end of the eighteenth century saw the
appearance in a small number of provincial towns (16) of resident
dentists, most of whom themselves travelled to other towns for part
of the year, swelling the numbers of visitors.

Despite this apparent upsurge in interest in care and treatment
of the teeth, the numbers of dentists in the eighteenth century were
never more than exceedingly modest. Trade directories suggest that
even by 1800 there were probably no more than twenty in the provinces
with perhaps twice that number in London.[13] But once it had emerged,
dentistry continued to make its presence felt. During the first half
of the nineteenth century it grew at a remarkable rate; by 1855 there
were about five hundred dental practices in the provinces and nearly
three hundred and fifty in London. This rapid expansion raises many
questions: where did these new dentists come from and what kind of
men were they, was dentistry a universal phenomenon, why did the
upsurge occur when it did and not in the seventeenth century...? The
remaining sections of this book will attempt to supply some tentative
answers to these and other hitherto unexamined questions.

2.1 Trade origins

Of the forty or so first generation resident dentists in the
provinces identified in trade directories, a quarter came from
London[14] or abroad.[15] Many of the remainder can be identified as
local traders who added the practice of dentistry to their
repertoire:

DENTIST	TOWN	PREVIOUS/OTHER TRADE*
Thomas Brewer	Bath	apothecary/druggist
Goldstone (2)	Bath	apothecary/druggist
Thomas Clarke	Birmingham	victualler
William Nailer	Birmingham	toothdrawer
Joseph Parsley	Bristol	barber-surgeon
James Blair	Leicester	hairdresser/perfumer/toyman
Thomas Twyford	Lichfield	perfumer/toyman
William Perry	Liverpool	surgeon
Edward Alsop	Manchester	barber/perfumer
Thomas Faulkner	Manchester	fustian cutter, toothdrawer
Benjamin Wildsmith	Manchester	perruke maker
George Bott sen.	Nottingham	wool sorter, toothdrawer/bleeder, patent medicine vendor
Robert Wooffendale	Sheffield/Liverpool	apothecary/druggist
Tearne (2)	Worcester	surgeon

* information from trade directories and newspaper advertisements

table 1:   Previous trades of some eighteenth century provincial dentists

It seems likely that many of the remaining thirteen were also local tradesmen before adopting dentistry as their calling, especially in those cases where they bear names distinctive to their towns, as did Birch Hesketh in Liverpool and John Ormrod in Manchester.

New recruits continued to enter the practice of dentistry from these diverse origins throughout the period up to the middle of the nineteenth century as demand outstripped the supply of those who could be properly trained by practising dentists. They ranged from those with some surgical or para-medical training[16] who acquired the necessary technical skills to those who approached dentistry from the other direction, starting out, say, as jewellers[17] or watchmakers[18] and adding a veneer of surgical knowledge to their range. While some moved completely and decisively over from one trade to the other, for others the transition was gradual and, in some cases, never completed.

The available data suggests that for at least 20% of those in

practice in the provinces before 1855, dentistry remained a second
string to their bow or an occupation which they tried for only a few
years.[19] The majority of these would appear to have been medically
connected:

1 medical men	2 paramedical	3 chemist/ druggist	4 cosmetic	5 mechanical	6 misc.
91(43%)	36(17%)	69(32%)	7(3%)	6(3%)	5(2%)

1 -physicians, apothecaries, surgeons[20]
2 -cuppers(18), bleeders(7), aurists(5), chiropodists(3),
  medical electrician(1), bone setter(1), toothdrawer(1)
3 -pharmaceutical chemists(18), chemists and druggists(46),
  patent medicine dealers(3), herbalists(2)
4 -perfumers(4), hairdressers/perruke makers(3)
5 -instrument makers(2), jewellers(3), watchmaker(1)
6 -musician(1), materials manufacturer(1),fustian cutter(1)
  bricklayers(2)

table 2: The distribution of second trades among 214 pre-
1855 provincial dentists

Although those in a medical field (groups 1, 2 and 3) form 92%
of those practising another trade, they constitute only 17% of the
total number of dentists in the provinces before 1855. It is
commonly assumed that country doctors removed teeth on occasion, but
as yet no evidence has emerged from doctors' account books or diaries
of this period of their involvement in anything more complex. James
Robinson's statement in 1844 that 'other operations of dental surgery
form an important part of their [country surgeons'] practice, and
their judgement is frequently taxed to regulate the teeth and perform
all the duties of the dentist'[21] seems more likely to be a
description of the few doctors who turned permanently to dentistry,
having given up medicine, rather than of the medical profession as a
whole.

Evidence of a formal professional education is available for 43
of these 91 medical men (*table 3* overleaf). It would seem that only
4% of all provincial dentists before 1855 (in total nearly 1100) had
a formal medical training. If the 'doubtful surgeons' are deducted
from the 48 'possibly unqualified', this last group is reduced to a
more realistic twenty-one. Ten of these are recorded in a variety of

Licence of the Society of Apothecaries (LSA) only	19
Membership of the Royal College of Surgeons (MRCS) only	13
LSA/MRCS (including one with MB, one with MD)	7
MD only	2
apprenticeship only	2
possibly unqualified (including 27 doubtful surgeons)	48

table 3: Qualifications of the 91 medical men practising
dentistry

sources as practising openly as medical men in the eighteenth century
and the first decade of the nineteenth. They may well have served an
apprenticeship which is not recorded in the tax records, perhaps
because it was served to a member of the family and no premium paid.
The remaining eleven began practice as dentists in 1816 (1), the
1820s (9) and the 1830s (1). These may have served a surgical
apprenticeship after the end of the apprenticeship tax (1811),
although if they were acting as apothecaries/general practitioners
after the passing of the 1815 Apothecaries Act, they were doing so
illegally. The official closing of this field to them may have led
them into dentistry.

Discounting the 'doubtful surgeons', over 40% of the medical men
trying dentistry before 1850 advertise as such for less than five
years and it may reasonably be assumed that they continued to
practise general medicine as their basic profession. However, from
the 1830s, some dentists, for instance, John Gray, are known to have
qualified as Members of the Royal College of Surgeons with the
deliberate intention of practising only as dentists.[22] James Orrock
of Leicester is a provincial example of this trend and is included in
those 13 in *table 3* who were qualified MRCS only. Such men continued
to be found in medical lists compiled on the basis of qualifications
rather than of occupation and so appear to be medical men practising
dentistry.

Quite apart from 'doctors' who practised dentistry, a number of
early nineteenth century dentists appear to spring from medical
families. A comparison between the surnames of those in purely
dental practice before 1855, those who feature in the 1847 *Medical
Directory* and the list of those who obtained the LSA before 1852,
yields more than 20 unusual names in the same locations.[23] It may be

that members of medical families were moving into dentistry in modest numbers in the first half of the nineteenth century. As requirements for medical practice[24] became more demanding of time and money, perhaps in an overcrowded medical world dentistry had its appeal to impecunious medical fathers when faced with the placing of their sons. References to those who were originally destined for medicine (such as C.S. Bate) in this period, may also conceal academic failure.

As regards chemists and druggists, from the beginning of the nineteenth century they appear to have taken over from the toothdrawer as extractors for the common man and from the 1840s some began to practise dentistry. This does not,however, make all chemists and druggists 'dentists', any more than medical men would have considered or advertised themselves as such on the grounds that they extracted half a dozen teeth a year. Advertisements for dentistry by chemists and druggists[25] suggest that those who called themselves 'dentist' offered the full range of dental treatment. Faced with such competition, it would be surprising if other chemists and druggists in a town did not retaliate with their own advertisements in the same vein if they really had the same service to offer.

Of all the groups practising dentistry in conjunction with another trade, chemists and druggists appear to have been most likely to persist; 65% were still practising dentistry after five years and 45% still associated with dentistry after more than 20 years, a length of dental career attained by only 23% of the medical men.

The numbers of these 'multitraders' increased with time but they formed a progressively smaller proportion of the new practices being established, lending weight to the contention that the numbers of full-time dentists rose sharply as the century progressed. In the first decade of the nineteenth century 45% of new practices were set up by such men; in the period 1850-55 only 13%.[26]

2.2 Education for dentistry

Such diverse trade origins were matched by equally diverse professional education, for its quality, quantity and even necessity were not legally regulated in any way. As James Robinson remarked in 1844, 'a brass plate and brazen impudence [were] all the diplomas necessary'.[27] Dentists could be found who had learned all they knew in a few weeks, whilst others had followed a formal apprenticeship. Yet others had been employed for variable lengths of time as 'assistants' and learned on the job.

For those who moved over to dentistry from another trade, 'training' frequently consisted in a brief initiatory period with a dentist already in practice, after which the new practitioner might feel free to advertise his services to the public. The period of instruction was usually a brief one. James Blair of Leicester can have spent no more than a few months in 1787 (at the age of forty) learning the business from George Bott of Nottingham;[28] nor can his son-in-law, William Robertson of Birmingham, who acquired his dental instruction from Thomas Faulkner of Manchester in 1821 (at the age of twenty-seven).[29]   George Bott himself claimed to have learned his dental skills 'under one of the most celebrated dentists in England' in the last two months of 1777, aged twenty-nine. After he had trained his widowed daughter-in-law, Sophia (aged thirty-eight), for an equally brief period, he declared her:[30]

> as being fully capable of performing any operation on the teeth and gums. She can put in artificial teeth from one to a complete set, to appear perfectly natural and be easy and comfortable to the wearer.

Although such short periods of initiation might be commonplace, it is clear that, even in the eighteenth century, they were not considered desirable by the leading figures in the field. Robert Wooffendale (1742–1828) based his whole career on the claim that he had been instructed by Thomas Berdmore, surgeon-dentist in ordinary to the King. So incensed by this was Berdmore, that he placed the following advertisement in the *York Courant* on 26 January 1773:

> MR. BERDMORE is very sorry the Imprudence of Mr. Wooffendale obliges him, in his own Vindication, to take the least notice of him in a News Paper. Mr. Berdmore wishes not to prejudice the young Man in the Opinion of such as may be inclined to employ him, but he cannot suffer the Sanction of his Name to be disingenuously imposed upon them. Mr. Wooffendale some Years ago was taken from a Druggist's Shop (to which Business he was brought up) by Mr. Berdmore, at a Salary of 25 l. per Ann. and at the Expiration of seven Years was to have been admitted to a small share of his Business; and in order to secure his Services, as it was supposed he might then be competently qualified in the Profession, he was bound in a Bond of 1000 l. not to practise in London; but either not liking the Confinement, or proposing some greater Advantage, he thought it fit to remove himself to America in less than six

Months, during which Time he was employed in cutting Bone [ivory], and other trifling Offices. This is the plain State of the Matter. And now whether Mr. Wooffendale be, as he professes, amply qualified as a Dentist or not, Mr. Berdmore neither knows nor concerns himself. If he is, Mr. Berdmore only desires it may be understood that he cannot be so from any Instructions received under him.

Clearly, Berdmore considered that less than six months' training did not provide an adequate education for a dentist. Undeterred, Wooffendale continued to use his former master's name for the rest of his life, winning for himself in the process the probably undeserved title of the first trained dentist in America.[31]

Wooffendale was not alone in citing a well-known dentist as his trainer: Twyford informed clients that he had spent 'some time' with George Bott jun.;[32] E. King, about to operate in Kent in 1834, included among his credentials the fact that he used to be with Cartwright, the prominent London dentist;[33] James Karran was 'late Pupil and Assistant to Mr. William SMITH, 39, Bold St., and from the Medical School of the Royal Institution, Liverpool'.[34] None saw fit to give details of the length of their training.

As demand grew, the provision of brief training courses became a business side-line for some dentists. Robinson stated in 1844:[35]

We know of one man who prepares dental practitioners with more than railroad speed - who has the unblushing effrontery to promise to fit them for the profession in one month- to teach them the whole art and science of dentism, both surgical and mechanical, in 26 days; and this, not requiring their constant attendance, but two hours twice or three times a week. After this elaborate preparation, which is in some instances extended to the enormous period of three months, he gives his pupils certificates of competence; surely he must mean incompetence, and ushers them into the world as perfect dentists - certificates of competence, the competence of 48 hours' study.

This allocation of time seems almost excessive when one reads a handbill for a 'Mr. Henry' visiting Glasgow in 1844 to deliver a

private course of demonstrations of dental surgery and mechanics which will convey a rapid but comprehensive knowledge of the art, and qualify Medical Practitioners, Students, Chemists, etc. to undertake all the duties of the Dentist.

This was to take place on 3 January between four and five in the afternoon, the fees being 2 guineas for surgical instruction and 3 guineas for initiation into the mechanical side of dentistry.[36]

However, if a Carlisle correspondent of 1858 is to be believed, many dentists of the 1850s did not even go thus far to equip themselves for practice. He knew some[37]

> who never spent a shilling on instruction in the art before commencing its practice; whose present proficiency, such as it is, has been obtained at the expense of their patients and who could no more pass such an ordeal as the College has now set up [an examination] than they could jump over Mont Blanc.

A small number of London businesses operated a kind of franchise system. For the payment of a few pounds, these firms undertook to tell the aspiring dentist 'how to stop a tooth, acquaint him with some of the technical phrases, and show him how to take an impression in wax'. Having ventured on to the road, the initiate[38]

> gets his credulous customer, takes a mould of his mouth, and sends it to his instructor, the wholesale tooth manufacturer, who sets to work, makes the artificial teeth.... it is forwarded to the new dentist, crammed in the mouth of the patient for better or worse, and, after a few days' suffering, disappointment, and waste of money, it is thrown by.

De Loude omits to name these 'three or four extensive working dentists' who he claims indulged in these practices but prime candidates for such a description were the notorious Mallan family[39] for whom Abraham Moseley operated a practice in Bristol. Moseley had received his professional education from John Mallan:[40]

> whether he was instructed by the great man himself, or by the workmen employed, we will not stay to inquire; certain it is that he made such progress in his professional acquirements, that after a short probation, he travelled for the *firm* under the name of Mallan, at that time (seven years since) in the zenith of its popularity. Whether he was paid a fixed salary or received a share of the profits, we do not know.... he still practises under the name of Mallan and Sons, who, however, we have every reason to believe, have nothing whatsoever to do with the business more than giving it the very questionable advantage of their name.

Often mentioned by *Forceps* in the same breath as the Mallans were the Le Drays,[41] the Moggridges and the Joneses, all disreputable London dentists in the 1830s and 1840s who may well have been the remaining 'working dentists'. However, in each of these cases, another factor has to be borne in mind. A recurrent theme in comments on dentistry of the period is the presence of 'foreign Jewish adventurers' in London. Purland, Gray and *Forceps* lose no opportunity to point out Jewish dentists, usually to the latters' disadvantage. It was the misfortune of ethical Jewish practitioners that some of the greatest scoundrels in London dentistry, Le Dray, Mallan and Jones, were also Jewish. Their known malpractice tarnished the reputations not only of their co-religionists but also of the whole dental profession, particularly in the capital, to which most comments about empiricism refer. It is difficult to assess how much of this comment was based on fact and how much arose from anti-semitic feeling.

Provincial dentists did not escape scot free from James Robinson's acerbic pen in this vexed matter of training 'courses'. He calls Sinclair of Brighton[42]

> the prince of cheap dentists....who it is said *qualifies* more young men for the profession in *six* months in his own particular way, than any other mechanical dentist in England.

He also quotes the case of the dentist from Canterbury[43] 'one of the numerous class "who have seen better days" ', who gave mechanical instruction to Edward King and 'at the same time supplied him with a practical advertisement in the shape of various specimens of ready made dentistry'.[44]

Not that a swift training led inevitably to a poor practitioner. John Tomes, arguably the most prominent dentist of the nineteenth century, was still working to acquire the rudiments of mechanical dentistry only three weeks before he put up his brass plate in Mortimer Street. He, however, had the advantage of a medical education and a number of years' special study of the teeth; he also fully expected to employ a mechanic: 'I shall never do much of that sort of work myself'.[45] A brief initiation was no drawback either to William Robertson of Birmingham who made a major contribution to the understanding of the mechanism of caries in his *Practical treatise on the teeth* of 1835.

A substantial proportion of early dentists probably entered the profession after a short period with a practising dentist, although their numbers cannot now be ascertained.

Side by side with the dentists trained by these questionable methods were those who served an apprenticeship (of three to five years) to a practising dentist. The quality of their training

depended very much on their master since there was no external body
during this period to regulate or monitor training. There was also
little in the way of serious dental literature to help the student in
his studies.   Such trainees were likely to emerge from their
apprenticeship without any systematic knowledge of the surgical side
of dentistry, according to Tomes, but even he admitted that 'it
cannot be denied that they more than held their own against those
whose surgical education was complete before they thought of dental
practice'.[46]

The 'regularly trained' dentist is exemplified by Thomas
Sheffield of Exeter (1804–84), the eldest of three brothers educated
for the profession by their father, Thomas Sheffield of Carlisle.[47]
He, in turn, took on other young men as apprentices,[48] among them
A.J. Woodhouse (1824–1906) who recalled the time he spent with
Sheffield in the early 1840s in an address to the annual meeting of
the British Dental Association in 1896:[49]

> I had the good fortune to be placed with Mr. Thomas Sheffield of
> Exeter, who was in the fore-front of the best practitioners of his
> day.... My articles bound me to Mr. Sheffield for four years, in
> them he undertook to teach me 'the art, mystery, and professional
> employment of a dentist,' and I promised to 'serve him faithfully
> and keep his secrets....'
>
> The mode of instructing me that Mr. Sheffield adopted was to work
> with me at the bench and occasionally to take me into his surgery,
> where I saw him operate. I was also at his side when he saw the
> gratis patients who came to him each morning at nine o'clock to be
> relieved of pain.   I did all his mechanical work during my
> apprenticeship, and after about three months he gave the care of
> the gratis patients into my hands, and I well remember when I went
> down alone to extract my first tooth, which I am happy to say I
> accomplished successfully. From that time I selected from among
> the cleanest of these poor people those who needed teeth stopped,
> and attended to them. Mr. Sheffield used to examine the teeth
> when I had prepared them, and afterwards when the filling was
> completed, but he soon left me to my own devices, except when any
> great difficulty arose, when he always came to my help. After
> about a year or so, he left me in charge of his private patients
> when he went for his holiday....
>
> We, at Exeter, made most of our own instruments, for those to be
> bought were very indifferent; we even made our own forceps,
> carefully adjusting them to the teeth for which they were to be
> used.... In my early days we got our gold leaf and tin from local
> gold-beaters.... I had sometimes to go to their workshop and wait
> while it was beaten.....

Clearly, Woodhouse's apprenticeship was not confined to mechanical work; from an early stage in his training he was treating patients and working unsupervised, first on the non-paying patients and progressing to be in full charge on occasions after only a year.

It is noticeable that he makes no mention of any theoretical instruction received from Sheffield; it may be that he considered it too obvious to remark upon. James Orrock, however, who after one year of medical studies in Edinburgh, joined his father's former pupil, William Williamson, in Leicester to learn mechanical dentistry, certainly had ample opportunities to acquire a good surgical knowledge, attending as he did Leicester Dispensary to study operations there.[50] 'Senex', who began his apprenticeship to a London dentist in 1855, similarly had opportunities to attend lectures at St. George's Hospital where his preceptor was dental surgeon.[51]

The earliest reference yet found to dentistry being taught in the context of an apprenticeship dates from 1720, when William Norman of Stepney, 'perruke maker and operator of teeth', took as apprentice Moses Burch for a period of seven years at a premium of £8.[52] (The majority of the small number of eighteenth century references to dentistry in apprenticeship records which have yet been siscovered involve masters who practised dentistry only as a subsidiary activity to their main trade of surgeon, apothecary or hairdresser). The earliest apprenticeship to a full-time dentist would currently appear to be that offered by Robert Spence in his notice in the *Edinburgh Advertiser* for 22 September 1789:[53]

> Wanted, An Apprentice to a Genteel Profession – a young lad of a mechanical genius. For particulars inquire at Mr. Spence, dentist, James's Court, Edinburgh.

In provincial England also, the available evidence points to the end of the eighteenth century as the beginning of purely dental apprenticeships. By this date the first generation of provincial dentists were putting their sons to the profession. Bearing in mind the necessity to ensure that sons made a worthwhile contribution to the family fortunes and reputation, it seems likely that they at least received an adequate training, probably by apprenticeship. Two of the earliest examples of second generation dentists are to be found in George Bott jun. and Robert Shew. Bott declared himself to the inhabitants of Birmingham as one who had been 'from the age of

fourteen [in 1786] under the instruction of his father'.[54]   Robert
Shew, also practising in Birmingham but in the early 1800s, was the
son of George Shew of Bath, a dentist there from the last decade of
the eighteenth century.

By the period 1830–50, 13% of all dentists in provincial
practice and 23% of those in practice for over five years were
offshoots of such families.   As these made their presence
increasingly felt, so it is likely that the incidence of dentists who
had served an apprenticeship also rose.   Apprenticeships were not,
however, confined to dental families.   Peter Flint, who toured the
Midlands and the north of England in 1802, stated himself to have
been apprenticed to George Bott of Nottingham.[55]   Newspapers carry
occasional advertisements for pupils[56] and obituaries in the early
dental press (starting in 1856) provide further instances.[57]   Robert
Were Fox of Exeter is noted as one who not only instructed his own
sons but also trained many well-known practitioners.[58]   Census
returns also reveal the presence of dental apprentices.[59]

No precise figures are available for the number of dentists who
served a dental apprenticeship before the middle of the nineteenth
century since their agreements mostly post-date the tax on
apprenticeships[60] and the survival of the actual indentures is a
matter of pure chance.   It may be conjectured, however, on the
available evidence, that about one quarter of all dentists up to this
date and nearly half those who made dentistry their career entered
the profession by this route.

Also setting up practice alongside the briefly initiated and the
'regularly educated' were former assistants.   Some of these had
clearly been fully trained, especially if they were members of dental
families.   George Frederick Fox and Richard Lloyd were but two of the
many who acted in this capacity for their fathers before branching
out alone or carrying on the family business under their own name.
However, that there were others who had not been formally trained is
clear from the opposition they met with from writers of the early
nineteenth century lamenting the current state of the profession.
This 'untrained' group may have comprised those who could not afford
to commit themselves to an apprenticeship of five years or who,
having trained for some other trade such as watchmaking or instrument
making,[61] became employed by a dentist to carry out his mechanical
work in the first instance.   William Henry Barron of Birmingham
advertised for such an individual:[62]

PARTNERSHIP
A single man, without incumbrance, in the profession of Surgeon-
Dentist and Cupper, is about taking a house in Town, suitable to
the purpose, and wishes to meet with some respectable person
desirous to be instructed and to gain a thorough knowledge of the
profession; if acquainted with any light mechanical work, it may
be accomplished in a very short time.

Some of these may well have soon broken away and started up for
themselves as a 'surgeon-dentist', as Snell complains, whilst having
experience only of constructing prosthetic appliances and no
knowledge of surgical and operative procedures. However, there is
ample evidence to suggest that many assistants were involved in the
clinical work of the practice where they were employed. John
Cherriman specifically says that during his period as an assistant to
Mr. Reale, he practised 'as an operator as well as a mechanic'.[63]
Joseph King of York is reported to have been assistant to Benjamin
Hornor before entering into partnership with him; it seems unlikely
that Hornor would have entered into such an agreement with a
mechanic.[64] Robinson states that Sale had been an assistant to
Maclean,[65] John Durance George to the famous Cartwright[66] and Edward
King to William Lukyn of Oxford.[67] King was rather too successful
for his master's good:

he soon made the big-wigs of the University understand that he was
a very talented individual, and a much superior man to the
gentleman whom he had done the honour of selecting as an employer,
and managed matters so well that eventually they justly
transferred their august patronage from Mr. Lukyn to himself...
Our hero... set up in the *teeth* of his old master... He had
forgotten the trifling circumstance of having signed a bond...
restricting him from practising in the locality of the High-
street... That he could not practise in his own name was clear...
he sent, therefore, for his old tutor from London, and advertised
him in all the local papers as a pupil of Spence and Ruspini...
Mr. King gradually absorbed all the practice of the district till
his *ci-devant* master, having tried all other moves unsuccessfully,
moved off, and left the coast clear...

Not all assistantships were so short. Newspaper and directory
advertisements would have one believe that many new dentists had been
'assistants' to others for lengthy periods before starting their own
practices. In 1841 James Edwards presents himself to the inhabitants
of Bath as one who had 'Twenty years' experience in all branches of
his Profession, under Mr. Prew, of Bath, and Mr. FEATHERSTONE, of

Albermarle Street, London'.[68] T.P. Payne had been 'for upwards of Thirteen years the principal Assistant and Designer to Mr. C. Bromley' before opening his own practice in Southampton in 1845[69] whilst James Robertson of Bath branches out on his own with an advertisement declaring him to be 'Successor and Assistant to the late Mr. Prew, and Principal Assistant to the late Mr. Parkinson'.[70]

If these claims can be taken at their face value, then an extensive period spent in a position analogous to that of the modern solicitor's clerk seems likely to have equipped assistants for dental practice as well as, if not better than, a formal apprenticeship.

The early nineteenth century ideal

Confronted with this diversity of approaches to dentistry and the unsatisfactory situation which resulted, writers of the early part of the nineteenth century expounded their views on what did constitute an adequate preparation for the practice of dentistry. There was general agreement that dentistry 'is both an art and a science: an art that requires great mechanical skill, and a science demanding much mental cultivation'.[71] It has its surgical and mechanical aspects, and the majority of its practitioners were deficient in their knowledge of one or other, if not both. Those who approached dentistry via some degree of surgical training[72] followed by a brief period of instruction from a dentist were considered as unprepared as those who started from the mechnical end of the spectrum and had but the scantiest grasp of the medical aspects of their operations. Those whose only insight into dentistry had been gained in a few weeks' instruction were considered to be the most dangerous of all, both to their patients and to the reputation of the conscientious members of the profession.

Most writers would have supported Robinson in his assertion that[73]

> the *handicraft* of the profession can only be acquired by perseverance, attention, and *practice* at the workbench of a professor; and consequently a probation, varying as to time, from three to five years, either as an apprentice or as a pupil, is essential to the formation of a perfect dentist.

A partial dissenter from this view was John Gray who considered that the correct training for the mechanical side of dentistry was not, in fact, to be had at the hands of a dental mechanic:[74]

A boy at the age of twelve years with such a development of
faculties as clearly indicates a 'mechanical genius', should be
placed in a clockmaker's shop till the age of seventeen; if the
work carried on in the shop be of a general or mixed nature, which
is commonly the case, and if men be employed, so much the better,
provided the principal part of the work done be clockmaking. From
the age of seventeen to nineteen or twenty he should be employed
at watch work, either repairing or finishing, in order to 'fine
down his hand', so that he may never afterwards experience any
difficulty with work on account of its minuteness.

Having now, it is presumed, acquired mechanical knowledge and
manual dexterity, he may commence the making of artificial teeth
under the best instructor he can procure; and if the education of
the dental preceptor has not been equal to that of the pupil, the
latter will soon surpass the master.

This mechanical education must be the first step

for, it has been observed, that he who is not an expert mechanic
at the age of twenty, will never afterwards be able to acquire the
mechanical dexterity that is necessary for the fabrication of
artificial teeth; whereas, in the acquirement of surgical
knowledge, so much more serious thought and riper judgement are
requisite, that the student reaps comparatively but little benefit
from his studies before that age. Hence a mechanic may become a
surgeon, but he who is first a surgeon can never afterwards become
a mechanic.

Where Robinson and Gray differed fundamentally was on the
question of the acquisition of surgical knowledge. Gray was a
proponent of the view that all dentists should be Members of the
Royal College of Surgeons, like himself:

If the surgical is intended to be added to the mechanical
education, his anatomical and other surgical studies may be
commenced simultaneously with those of the dentist, without
prejudice to either, for they will assist rather than retard each
other... At the age of twenty-five his surgical knowledge may be
so complete as to procure his admission as a member of the
College; and, when a few years of experience in the actual
practice of his profession have given him the ease and confidence
attendant on ability, he will be able to look back with
satisfaction on the progressive steps by which he gained his
knowledge and present eminence.

A young man of genius and sufficient enthusiasm for the task, may,
by his own exertions, acquire the above education, including the
surgical part, without assistance from parents or friends. I
mention this for the encouragement of merit, knowing it to have
been achieved with comparative ease. Similar spirits may aspire

to the same honour.

Whether Gray actually planned his own progression from watchmaker to dentist in this way is open to question.

Robinson, however, shared the view of Spence Bate that 'the College of Surgeons is no college for dentists'.[75]   In reply to a surgeon correspondent to *Forceps* he stated[76]

> as for passing the examination of the College of Surgeons for the express purpose of being considered qualified to practise Dental Surgery, it is an infamous fraud upon the public. The examiners never test the *learning* of their candidates upon the subject, for the simple reason that they themselves are as ignorant upon all matters relating to the teeth (with a very few exceptions) as those who possess their diploma, and afterwards tack the initials to their name and practise as dentists.

If a relevant surgical education was not to be acquired from an orthodox medical education, then other channels must be devised.   In 1839 a dentist correspondent to the *Lancet* had expressed the hope that it would not be long before an examination in dentistry was instituted.[77]   Two years later, J.L. Levison pressed for a 'faculty of surgeon–dentists' to be set up by the profession to examine prospective dentists[78] but Robinson appears to be the first to set out in detail what he considered to be a suitable scheme for the theoretical training of dental practitioners:[79]

> The curriculum of education should be fixed on a liberal scale - it should not be such as would ensure mere capability, but should embrace anatomy, physiology, pathology and surgery, as far as these sciences are in the most remote degree connected with Dental Surgery in its more extended sense. The principles of mechanics should be studied, not as applied to the dental art *alone*, but in their broad and fundamental principles, and to this should be added an acquaintance with geometry and mathematics; and while chemistry, as affording a wide field for energy and research, should not be omitted, a knowledge of the French and German languages would be found of the greatest advantage.
>
> Modelling, and other processes involved in the practice of the mechanical part of the art, and which would form a necessary part of the instruction, would of course come under the department of the private teacher. To superior minds, many other studies, such as comparative anatomy, etc., would necessarily suggest themselves, and which, though not essential to the practice of Dental Surgery, mark the man of education and science.
>
> This course of education might be carried out by the establishment

> of normal schools on the one hand, and lectureships and a *dental,*
> similar to the ophthalmic institution, on the other - a dispensary
> devoted to the teeth, and *open to all,* where the student might
> acquire a knowledge and experience in the different diseases and
> imperfections of the teeth and gums - the imperfections of the
> palate, and every branch of Dental Surgery; tracing their
> symptoms, watching the different modes of treatment, and learning
> to remedy, mechanically, those imperfections in which curative
> means are of no avail.

Support grew for the institution of special dental schools but unhappily the profession did not find itself in agreement as to how this might be brought about. Two rival groups emerged, one (the Odontological Society) pressing for an examination in dentistry to be held by the Royal College of Surgeons, the other (the College of Dentists) for an independent qualification to be awarded by itself. Both set up their own dental schools and hospitals to prepare students. Partly through lack of action on the part of the College of Surgeons but also through the disunity in the dental profession, with 'respectable' dentists unwilling to ally themselves with less ethical practitioners, these seeds of reform in the education of dentists did not come to fruition until 1860, the year of the first examination for the Licence in Dental Surgery of the Royal College of Surgeons. Not until 1921 was a full academic training and examination compulsory for all those starting out on the practice of dentistry.

2.3 Empiricism

The 1820s saw the beginning of a substantial increase in the number of those offering their services as dentists. Several writers of the 1830s and 1840s felt they knew precisely where the expansion was taking place: among the ranks of 'empirics', of whom there had been a 'recent unexampled increase',[80] the 'imposters who call themselves surgeon-dentists'.[81] Accusations of empiricism were liberally made both by those whose genuine concern was with the state of the profession, like James Robinson, and by those more motivated by self-interest than they would have their readers believe, like John Gray. Both categories of writer, for their different purposes, tried to reveal the parlous condition of dentistry to the public at large, the one in an attempt to protect the patient and the other to establish himself in the public eye as a practitioner superior to the majority.

That perjorative accusations were not new is to be seen from such advertisements as the following, placed by Mr. Restieaux on a visit to Leicester in 1785:[82]

> his character as a Dentist will, he is confident, be sufficiently announced, by the Inspection of those credential Letters which he has in his Possession, not only from the most eminent Physicians and Surgeons at Norwich, (where he has resided nine years,) but also from Nottingham, and every other Place in which he has practised. -- These he hopes will make a characteristic Difference between him and Itinerant Empirics.

Accusations of the early nineteenth century focus on the dubious and ill-founded treatments offered by some dentists of the time. The *Lancet* devotes nearly three columns to J.L. Levison's[83] 'Exposure of Quackeries in Dental Surgery', in which he condemns all the new filling materials being currently advertised as ineffective and, on occasion, injurious to health.[84]   These he states to be the 'wonderful discoveries' of

> a set of persons who have yclept themselves "surgeon dentists", under the supposition that it was the most lucrative part of the medical profession; and many of these men have commenced with no other pretension to public favour, than a determination of gulling by some extraordinary novelty; thus, in lieu of anatomical and physiological knowledge, they possessed the advantage of ignorance and impudence... if they cannot "rub" the people out of the money, they will "plug" it from them.

In the same journal, J.K.M.[85] relates the sorry tale of an itinerant dentist who extracted from an eight year old girl four permanent incisors which were erupting before the deciduous teeth; he[86]

> assured the parent of the unfortunate child that her daughter had a double row of teeth, and that he had frequently met with similar occurrences... This person at that time advertised as dentist to the King of Holland; he is now one of the leading advertising London dentists, and I believe in the receipt of a considerable income, though I need not say rejoicing in a very different name from the one he assumed four years ago.

Alfred Hill, chronicler of the dental reform movement, looked back at some of these exposers of malpractice with a quizzical eye:[87]

> they draw over their own ink-stained fingers the whitest of kid
> gloves, and with lifted shoulders and outstretched arms implore
> the deluded, but patiently enduring, outside world to remember
> that they are the only individuals capable of taking care of its
> interests, so far as the teeth are concerned, at the least, and
> how delighted they will be to become the fortunate deliverers of
> the prey from the spoiler.

Certainly, in this period of expansion (a classic scenario for accusations of 'empiricism')[88] these writers of pious tracts had every reason to align themselves on the side of the angels against the hordes of the 'quack', the man who made the self-righteous feel their reputations and very livelihoods were so threatened by association in the public imagination. Nevertheless, there can be no doubt that malpractice of one kind or another was a reality, even though no contemporary commentator attempts to quantify the problem or to name more than a very few of the perpetrators of 'charlatanism'. Any retrospective attempt to do so is bound to be speculative, for quackery is largely in the eye of the eholder at a specific moment in time. It centres on three main areas: the quack is inadequately trained and hence ignorant, he is incompetent and he is unprincipled in his dealings with his patients. Any one or any combination of these elements may be enough to attract accusations of empiricism from the outraged or the xenophobic. Each of them may spring from subjective self-interest and each can be a rationalisation or justification for the unspoken objection, the fear of the intruder. The incomer disturbs the market; while there is felt to be a surplus of demand, the incompetent or unethical can be ignored and left to find their own level. When there is a sudden increase in supply, ranks are closed and 'quackery' used as a discriminator. Dentists of the early nineteenth century did not welcome the increase in the numbers of practitioners as a sign of growing demand for their services and of the long overdue spread of relief of suffering to wider sections of the population; rather they saw it as a dilution and a threat. The accusation of 'inadequate' training came largely from those who had served an apprenticeship and considered the ground was being cut away from beneath their feet when a rival who had picked up dentistry in a short 'course' or as a mechanic set up so easily in opposition, undermining aspirations to professionalism. (This argument conveniently ignored the fact that many a respected figure had entered dentistry by precisely this route and that, as we have seen, minimal education in the secrets of dentistry did not automatically make for a poor dentist). There was a tendency for 'inadequate training' to mean training which was not the same as that which the writer had himself received. As for 'incompetence', this was not unknown to emanate from the surgeries of the well-established; it certainly cannot be assumed to be restricted, for example, to those who used the new filling materials so decried by Levison. Nor can it have been true that all who used them were *ipso facto* incompetent; rather they presented a threat to the mystique and territory of old guard in that the treatment they offered was faster, cheaper and called for less skill. Similarly, sharp practice (often a matter of opinion) was no monopoly of the newcomer any more than was newspaper advertising, for there is ample evidence of apparently reputable dentists spending some of their time visiting other towns and hence needing to alert potential patients of their arrival.[89]

We have seen that it is not possible to arrive at a cut and dried picture of the dental 'quack' of the early nineteenth century for use as a tool in retrospective identification. It was not so much a particular group of individuals which appeared as a threat to the wearers of the white kid gloves as quackish practices, which might be found among the old established as well as the newcomers and for which the detailed evidence is now lacking. One can, however, hazard a guess at the numbers of those who combined in their persons both poor training and incompetence and who probably formed the main body of those against whom accusations of empiricism were made. These are the dentists who were in practice for only a short period. The most likely reason for abandoning a profession (particularly in the competetive commercial climate of the times) is lack of success; a man who has invested time and money in a lengthy training to acquire a skill does not give up lightly after only a few years. We will see that these 'short-term dentists' formed a substantial and increasing proportion of those in practice in the first four decades of the nineteenth century. It can be argued that it is these who seem likely to constitute the core of the 'pretenders' and 'imposters' of whom there had been 'a recent unexampled increase' in the eyes of Gray.

2.4 Careers in dentistry

Because brief experience of dentistry had become associated with incompetence in the public mind at an early stage, many dentists were at great pains to establish their credentials by reference to the length of time they claimed to have been in practice. Thomas Faulkner of Manchester, faced with competition in the form of the visiting James Blair in 1796, reminds the inhabitants of the city that he has been a 'practical resident for 20 years'.[90] (He continued to be so for a further twenty-three years). In the same way, Mr. Whitlock, on a visit to Birmingham in 1768 reassures his potential clients that he has 'above 35 years Experience'.[91] Similar statements are to be found in nineteenth century advertisements: Quintin B. Hair, on a visit to Kent from London, stresses that, although he may only attend one or two days a week, he has been in practice twenty-three years and has been visiting Tunbridge Wells for the last twenty-one.[92] Venturing north to Liverpool from London in 1833, a member of the Crawcour family claims that the firm has been in existence for nearly a century,[93] although he not unnaturally omits to remind his readers of the reputation for charlatanry it had acquired in the process.[94]

All over the country, in fact, dentists were attempting to disassociate themselves, by reference to their lengthy experience, from the fly-by-night empiric, that 'class of itinerant quack that infect the country everywhere'.[95] Nor were their claims necessarily inflated, for despite the undoubted presence of the 'short-term dentists'[96] remarked on earlier, there is ample evidence that those who survived the first few years often remained in practice for considerable periods of time,[97] as is shown by individual cases: an obituary for Sophia Bott of Birmingham (1768–1859)[98] states that she practised in the town for nearly forty years; James Lewis Cafferata of Sunderland (1797–1870) was declared to have been a dentist there for forty-five years[99] and Leopold Dreschfeld of Manchester (1822–97) to have practised fifty years in that city.[100]

Few of these cases are particularly unusual among those who survived the first five years in their chosen profession, as is demonstrated by the career lengths of large numbers of pre-1855 provincial dentists. The most accurate overall picture available is probably to be obtained in towns where the principal sources (trade directories) are virtually complete, such as the developing cities of

Bristol, Liverpool and Birmingham and the smaller (but perhaps more fashion-conscious) communities of Bath, Cheltenham and Exeter.[101] Between them these towns saw 273 dentists (25% of the national total) set up practice before 1855. The mean practice length of this group emerges as 16 years, the median as 11 years. There are, however, variations with date, depending on when the practices were started:

STARTING DATE	NO.PRACTICES	MEAN LENGTH	MEDIAN LENGTH
18th century	28	12 years	6 years
1800s	12	32 years	36 years
1810s	16	18 years	15 years
1820s	39	17 years	9 years
1830s	68	17 years	12 years
1840s	64	17 years	11 years
1850–55	46	10 years	4 years

table 4: Mean and median lengths of 273 practices started at different dates before 1855

A substantial proportion (22%) appear to have been in practice for only one year. Whilst they constituted under 10% of the practices started before 1820, after this date they formed about 20% of new practices. In the period 1850–55, they rose to 35% thus reducing the overall mean and median lengths. Those who dropped out before the end of five years amount to 38%. Again, the incidence tends to increase throughout the nineteenth century:

STARTING DATE	PRACTICES OF 5 YEARS OR LESS DURATION AS % OF TOTAL NO. OF PRACTICES FOUNDED IN THE DECADE IN THE 6 TOWNS
18th century	38%
1800s	8%
1810s	19%
1820s	33%
1830s	44%
1840s	36%
1850–55	52%

table 5: Practices of 5 years' or less expressed as a percentage of the total number of practices founded at different dates in the 6 towns

If it is true, as suggested earlier, that a short practice is indicative of lack of training, then *table 5* would show that an increasingly high proportion of the new practices in the nineteenth century were set up by those who were untrained. By the early 1850s, over half the new dentists may have fallen into this category.

The intake of those who went on to practise for more than five years, who might be termed 'career dentists' (as opposed to 'short-term' ones) scarcely increased from 1830 onwards and with time came to form a smaller proportion of the new practices:

STARTING DATE	NO. PRACTICES OF MORE THAN 5 YEARS DURATION	AS % OF NEW PRACTICES FOUNDED IN THE DECADE
18th century	17	62%
1800s	11	92%
1810s	13	8P%
1820s	26	67%
1830s	38	56%
1840s	41	64%
1850-55	22	48%

table 6: Dentists in practice for more than 5 years

The career dentists founded practices which lasted, on average, 24 years (median length 22 years). This figure reflects the fact that many had no doubt spent some time as assistants before setting up their own practices[102] or had taken to dentistry later in life. For those who survived the first ten years of practice (about 50%), the average rises to 30 years (median 29 years). When added to the mean age at starting independent practice, this produces a mean retirement age of sixty for half the dentists in practice in the six provincial towns before 1855.

There is some tendency for the mean and median lengths of the practices of career dentists to decrease with time.[103] Whether this is due to increased competition as time went on, forcing some dentists out of practice, or whether it is an indication that so much money was to be made from the middle of the century that it was feasible to retire early, is impossible to say.

Contained within the mean length of practice for career dentists of 24 years are practices varying in duration from six to sixty-five

years.[104]   Some of the very long practices recorded in the
directories (over 50 years) may possibly be trading names of other
members of the family or no longer operated by the original founder.
However, a number of the thirteen are still described in probate
documents as 'dentist', despite having reached the age of eighty.

There are some interesting differences between the two groups of
towns.   The cities of Bristol, Liverpool and Birmingham have larger
proportions of practices lasting under 5 years (44% of the practices
there) than do the smaller communities (Bath, Cheltenham and Exeter)
with 27%. The reverse is true for practices lasting on average 11–15
years and 16–20 years, which form a higher proportion of the
practices started in the towns (13% and 11%) than in the cities (6%
and 4%).   It may be that the larger proportion of 'short-term'
dentists in the cities reflects a greater scope for the transient
opportunist there, with the constant supply of new potential clients.

2.5 Family involvement

One of the most striking aspects of dental practice in its early
development is the extent to which it became the province of whole
families, as sons, sons-in-law, nephews and grandsons were channelled
into the family business.

Some such families have been the subjects of extended studies.
Stoy directed his attention to the Clarke family of Nottingham and
Belfast, with its three generations of dentists.[105] Perhaps the most
thorough study in this fild has been Richards's work on the Fox
family. The founding father of this last dynasty, Robert Were Fox of
Exeter (1792-1872), though born into 'ample means',[106] met with
misfortune in his thirties and was forced to start again, this time
in dentistry. His choice of second career may have been influenced
by members of his wife's family, the Prideaux, who included several
dentists among their number. He trained five of his sons as
dentists: Robert Were of Bristol (1816-59), Charles Prideaux (1820-
76), George Frederick of Gloucester (1822-76), Sylvanus Bevan (1825-
1912) and Octavius Annesley of Brighton (1829-1920). Octavius's
daughter married the dentist Charles Peckover and two of their sons,
Lancelot Eric Charles and Hugh Douglas (still in practice in the
1960s) followed their father into dentistry. George Frederick's

three sons (Walter Henry (1854-1942), Ernest William (1859-1939) and Charles Herbert (1861-1939)) all became dentists as did his grandson Frederick Neidhart (1881-1923, son of Walter Henry) and great-grandson, George Anthony (b. 1935 and still in practice). Over five generations, the descendants of Robert Were Fox have included thirteen dentists among their number.[107]

This family continuity is evident throughout the period before 1855. In a newspaper advertisement George Bott jun. (1772-1804) draws attention to the fact that he has been 'carefully instructed by his Father, in every Branch of the Profession, for several Years past'.[108] Arman Talma reminds his readers that he is the 'son and pupil of Mr. Talma, Dentist'.[109] James Robertson (1817-67), setting up practice in Worcester in 1840, uses his father's name as a recommendation[110] as does Mr. Evatt of Leeds, 'successor to his late Father, who had for nearly Fifty Years been patronized by many of the Nobility, and most respectable Gentry'.[111]

Over a third of the obituaries in the dental press for dentists who began practice before 1855 mention other dental members of the deceased's family. One learns that Thomas Gill Palmer of Cheltenham (1811-75) was in partnership first with his brother James Edwin Palmer in Peterborough and then with his own son Gasgoigne.[112] Thomas Sheffield of Exeter (1804-84) emerges as the son of a Carlisle dentist of the same name and the brother of two others, John (1821-74) and Isaac (1816-81).[113] James Robertson of Bath (1811-64) is revealed as the nephew of William Imrie of Savile Row.[114] Probate records are also informative on this head. It is not unusual to find dentist sons named as executors, as in the case of Ephraim Mosely (d. 1873) (who assigned this duty to three of his sons, Benjamin Ephraim, Alexander and Alfred Isaiah)[115] and James Lewis Cafferata of Sunderland (1797-1870) whose son Philip was one of his executors.[116] Dentist brothers also make an appearance in this capacity[117] as do nephews upon occasion.[118]

Continuity of surname is the most obvious sign of a dental family, although clearly care has to be exercised before making a firm identification. For this and other reasons, the number of such dynasties identified before 1855 is open to underestimation. Inevitably omitted by the use of surname identification alone are the undoubted cases of family influence in choice of career on grandsons, nephews and even sons-in-law not bearing the family name. The family and business connections of James Blair (1747-1817) of Leicester,

Chester and Liverpool exemplify some of these instances.   Blair's daughter, Jane, married her cousin, William Robertson of Birmingham (1794-1870), also a dentist, whose two sons, James (1817-67) and Henry (1826-53), followed their father into dentistry.   The entry into the profession of a great-grandson of Blair's[119] seems more than co-incidental, especially since close contact was maintained between the different branches of cousins.   It seems likely that it was family influence which led Robertson into dentistry in the first place.   Thus Blair's influence can be seen extending to a nephew and son-in-law, two grandsons and a great-grandson, only one of whom bore his surname.

James Blair's last partner in Liverpool was Thomas Whitfield Lloyd (1783-1861) who founded his own practice after his agreement with Blair's widow had expired.   This concern was carried on by two of his sons, Richard (1817-68) and James Blair (1825-96);   the eldest son, Thomas Bridge (1808-45) had his own practice in Manchester. James Blair Lloyd took into the practice his sister's son, Edward James Montagu Phillips (1852-1918) whose dental career embraced hospital and university teaching as well as the family general practice.   Here again, is a case of family continuity prosecuted through the female line.

There are also a few known instances of family members being involved in a dental practice without ever appearing in trade directories as dentists.   It seems unlikely that Thomas Prew (brother of James Prew of Bath) who is described as a dentist only in the 1851 census[120] is an isolated case.

Some of the provincial dentists in practice before 1855 were undoubtedly either offshoots of London practices or the founders of dynasties which continued in the capital rather than in the provinces.   Over forty of such instances can be identified from trade directories alone (*appendix 4*) with some confidence, although there is need for further detailed genealogical research in some cases to establish the links with certainty.   In a number of cases, the connection is supported by other evidence, as in the instance of Christopher Shew, who advertised in the London press that he had studied with his uncle in Bath,[121] and Joseph Hart of Bristol, who assures his clients that[122]

the best material...is obtained by Mr. Hart, through the medium of his brother (Mr. A.S. Hart, Dentist, Lownde's Terrace, near Hyde

Park Corner) with whom he is constantly communicating.

Many of the dentists in provincial practice went on to found their own dynasties after 1855, as can be seen from their obituaries[123] and from the appearance of familiar names in early *Dentists Registers*. Obituaries for dentists in practice from the middle of the nineteenth century frequently mention a dental father, as in the case of Nathaniel Tracey of Ipswich (1830–1902), the son of John Tracy (in practice in the town from 1839–74) and whose own son, Hugh, carried on the family tradition.[124] Probate records also reveal second generation dentists who had not entered into practice by 1855.[125] Thus, it may be seen that if the families of all pre-1855 dental practitioners were examined in detail, the number of dental dynasties might well prove to be considerably in excess of those so far identified.

Counting only those dynasties which had already been established in the provinces by 1855, then 110 dental families can be identified, comprising 317 individual practitioners (29% of the total number before 1855) (*appendix 5*). On average, just over 18% of dentists with their own practices between 1800 and 1855 came from dental families, in that they had a father, uncle, brother or other close relative who was also a dentist.[126] This probably understates the real situation among the profession as a whole, as it discounts the qualified assistants who worked anonymously in family practices.[127] By comparison, fewer than 10% of present-day dentists appear to come from families with a dental tradition and only about 2% to be the children of dentists.[128]

Using post-1855 trade directories and the *Dentists Registers* from 1879 onwards, it is possible to examine the length of association with dentistry of the 110 family groups which can be identified with some certainty. The mean length for the whole group is 64 years (range 1–138 years) with a median length of association with dentistry of 41 years (*table 8* overleaf). It would seem that the later the dynasty was founded, the shorter the links with the profession. This may perhaps be a reflection of greater social mobility in the later period, with dentistry being the springboard for entry into other professions, particularly general medicine, as individual cases suggest. The Blair, Fox and Lloyd families cited earlier all have medically qualified members in the late nineteenth and the twentieth centuries and this is by no means a rare phenomenon

in other dental families.   Insufficient work has yet been done on
this aspect to establish its prevalence.

date of founding of 1st practice	no. of families	mean length	median length
pre-1800	12	61 yrs (15-106)	56 yrs
1800-29	38	53 yrs (1-157)	42 yrs
1830-55	60	36 yrs (1-138)	30 yrs

table 8:   The mean and median lengths of association with
dentistry of 110 families in the provinces before
1855

Thirty-six of the families were still active in dentistry at the
time of the first *Register* of 1879.   Twenty of them survived into the
twentieth century, although half of these had disappeared by the
beginning of the First War and another six by 1939.   Members of the
Jones family (of Cambridge and Suffolk) and the Rose family (of
Liverpool) were still in provincial practice in the 1950s after an
association with dentistry of over 130 years.   A member of the Little
family (originally of Plymouth in the 1830s) was on the *Dentists
Register* until 1967.   A descendant of Robert Were Fox of Exeter is
still in practice, although not in the provinces.

The introduction of legislation in 1878 probably brought about
the demise of some dental families.   Whilst a dentist in *bona fide*
practice before this date was eligible for inclusion on the *Register*,
subsequent entry, with its right to the use of the title 'dentist'
(and similarly legally defined designations), was restricted to those
who had followed a prescribed course of training culminating in an
academic examination.   There seem likely to have been cases where a
son, who would in the normal course of things have been introduced
into dentistry in the 1880s, was either reluctant to or incapable of
tackling the intellectual hurdle of examination in order to carry on
the family business with the same status as his father had achieved
merely by the good fortune of already being a dentist when the Act
came into force.   It is probably also true that only those dentists
in lucrative practice could afford to invest time and money in the
formal education of their sons;   if these resources were available,
they were, perhaps, considered by some to be better expended on
training for some more prestigious profession, such as medicine,

especially as the training period was no longer than that for dentistry and the clinical hospital experience could be gained in the provinces.

2.6 Income, wealth and social standing

Income

> I have made up my mind to become a dentist...Kiernan when I told him my resolution, said my fortune was made. ...My fresh plan will carry me to good fortune or great poverty; the first I hope, the second I doubt.
> (John Tomes to his friend Harris, 3 January 1840. Quoted by Cope, 1961, 10)

> Bell tells me that it will be my lot to make not less than £200 the first year, and go on doubling it.
> (Tomes to Harris, January 1840, *ibid*, p.11)

The *Lancet* claimed that in London of 1846 'the receipts of many dentists in good practice range from 1,000 l. to 5,000 l. a year'.[129] It was estimated that even if the average income of dentists without membership of the Royal College of Surgeons was put at only £300, then £60,000 was being diverted from what the editor considered its legitimate destination, namely the pockets of the Members. 'This amount is the property of the profession, though neglect has suffered it to pass into other and more active hands'.[130]

Although these estimates cannot automatically be assumed to be applicable to the provinces, it is clear that a substantial income from dentistry was not a purely London phenomenon. In 1800 George Bott of Nottingham was described by a cleric as 'a man very eminent in his profession and carrying it on to a very considerable extent as to emolument'.[131] Bott left an estate valued at nearly £10,000 in 1820.[132] We shall see that he was not the only one to amass a considerable fortune from the practice of dentistry during the period.

It might be difficult for some to establish themselves in the first instance,[133] but a substantial income awaited the successful. A 'respectable and increasing' dental practice, established twelve years in the north of England and declared to gross over £600 annually, was offered for sale in 1856. 'Sum required for goodwill, fixtures of house, and portion of furniture, nearly £400, for the payment of which accommodation would be offered'.[134]   An old established Yorkshire practice, grossing £700–£800 p.a. was offered for exchange, preferably with a similar one in London.[135]

This might be compared with the income attainable by the general medical practitioner of the early nineteenth century.   From an examination of the incomes recorded for Bristol doctors, Loudon found a range of £50 to (exceptionally) £1,000.[136] He considered that the majority of provincial practitioners were likely to earn under £200[137] and quoted Hudson as saying that in 1842 a 'moderate general practitioner in London' earned £300–£400 a year, whereas in the provinces his income amounted only to £150–£200.[138]

The most detailed picture of the income of a provincial dentist in the early part of the nineteenth century is to be found in the surviving account and cash books of James Prew.[139]   Having begun as an assistant to Joseph Sigmond of Bath in his late twenties, Prew entered into a brief partnership with Stephen Baker, dentist and cupper of 2, Charles St, Bath in 1823.   The following year he began practice at the same address under his own name.   By 1829 he had taken over Sigmond's old practice address of 8, Edgar's Buildings. By 1830 he had begun a branch practice in Bristol in rented accommodation at 58, Park St.   In 1840 and 1841 money is recorded as being spent on fitting out 57, Park St as a dental practice.   Prew's will (made in May 1842) makes it clear that he owned this house, although the 1841 census shows it as occupied by his dentist son-in-law George Salusbury [sic] Williams, with whom he seems to have had some kind of financial arrangement.   (Between October 1841 and August 1842, for example, Prew received £680 from him).   Williams practised from this address in his own name from 1843–53.   Prew left the house and its effects to his own son James, still a minor at the time of his father's death in 1846.   In addition to his property ventures in Bristol, Prew was a man of varied business involvements.   He owned and rented out property in Burnham on Sea (where his wife appears to have lived until 1845), was on the committee of the Burnham Dock and Branch Railway and borrowed money in substantial amounts to finance property development.   As early as 1838 he notes the receipt of £300 from a partnership concern, but no details are given.[140]

Prew's income from his professional work was substantial, placing him comfortably within Musgrove's definition of middle class professional men:[141]

year	Bath	Bristol	total
1830	no surviving accounts	£ 342.17.9	£ 342.17.9.
1831	no surviving accounts	£ 275.11.6	£ 275.11.6.
1832	no surviving accounts	£ 419. 8.0.	£ 419. 8.0.
1833	no surviving accounts	£ 539. 0.0.	£ 539. 0.0.
1834	no surviving accounts	£ 746. 8.6.	£ 746. 8.6.
1835	no surviving accounts	£ 631. 6.4.	£ 631. 6.4.
1836	£ 850. 2.0.	£ 808. 5.0.	£1658. 7.0.
1837	£ 777. 2.6.	£ 740. 3.0.	£1517. 5.6.
1838	£ 772. 4.0.	£ 604. 5.0.	£1376. 9.0.
1839	£1147. 1.0.	£ 924. 7.6.	£2071. 8.6.
1840	£ 858.10.6.	£ 914.16.0.	£1773. 6.6.
1841	£ 894.12.6.	£ 400.16.6.*	£1295. 9.0.
1842			£1148. 9.0.

* appears to be a sum paid by Williams as part of the financial
agreement between the two

table 9: James Prew's practice income, 1830-42[142]

Unfortunately, Prew's account books make little systematic
record of his expenses. For 1830 and part of 1831 there is some
mention of outgoings,[143] listing his weekly travelling expenses to
Bristol (between 8s.6d. and 11s.), the quarterly rent of 13 guineas
for 58, Park St and the occasional advertisement (£1.4s.0d. a time).
A few bills for materials have survived from 1843 and 1844, but no
mention is made of the wages of assistants or mechanics, although
other evidence makes it clear that he had such employees.[144] Some
rough estimate may, however, be attempted of Prew's professional
expenses on the basis of the evidence available:

item of expenditure	£
rent of 58, Park St, Bristol [145]	55
wages of assistant, 52 x 3 guineas[146]	164
travelling to Bristol, 100 journeys @ 10s.	50
advertising	5
materials teeth[147]	30
gold, ivory, etc[148]	100
income tax[149]	20
	£ 374

table 10: Rough estimate of Prew's annual professional
expenses at Bath and the branch practice at 58
Park St, Bristol, 1830-42

This estimate presumes that Prew employed only one assistant or mechanic at a time and discounts other travelling expenses he undoubtedly incurred, especially to Burnham.   His professional expenses were thus probably nearer £400 p.a., accounting for between 20% of his gross takings in his best year (1839) and 35% in his worst (1842).   This would nevertheless always leave him with a net income far in excess of that of the average provincial medical practitioner of the day.

Wealth at death

A discussion in the   Registrar General's   *22nd Annual Report* of 1861 notes that a large proportion of surgeons and medical men left property in 1858.   Of those 300 whose estates had been valued for probate in that year, 127 had left over £1,000 (including three who had estates of over £50,000 and twenty who left in excess of £10,000).   It was unknown how many left no personal property, 'but the number of such cases cannot have been considerable'.[150]   Bearing in mind the potentially higher incomes which were to be made from dentistry, it might be expected that these comments would be even more applicable to dentists and this, in fact, seems to be the case.

Not that all early dentists were able to leave the substantial fortune of a Thomas Berdmore (over £40,000 in 1785).   When James Lewis Cafferata of Sunderland died in 1870, leaving less than £100, his widow experienced severe financial hardship.   By 1879 she was in receipt of £50 raised by appeal by the editor of the *British Journal of Dental Science* who urged the cause of setting up a benevolent fund for those falling on hard times.[151]   Even during his lifetime, Peter Michel of Bath was reduced to destitution in 1809 when fire broke out in his house in Orange Grove.   He was rescued by public subscriptions collected through the circulating libraries, each of which was acknowledged in the local press.[152]   However, despite these and other sad exceptions, a comparison between the estates of early nineteenth century dentists and medical men dying in 1858, does indeed show dentists as a whole maintaining their greater prosperity even in death.[153]

The values of 119 estates of provincial dentists in practice for more than ten years before 1855 range from £13[154] to £70,000.[155]   The median values show those who started practice in the 1840s as a prosperous generation within the profession:

sample	median probate value
gross sample	£ 1,500-2,000
'1840s dentists'	£ 2,500-3,000
wills proved in 1860s (28)	£ 1,000-1,500
wills proved in 1870s (32)	£ 1,500-2,000
wills proved in 1880s (24)	£ 1,500-2,000
wills proved in 1890s (12)	£ 3,255

table 11: Median probate values

They were also more likely to accumulate very large sums (£10,000–£50,000) than the group as a whole:

sample	probate values						
	hundreds			thousands			
	under 1	1-5	5-10	1-5	5-10	10-50	over 50
gross sample	10%	19%	12%	31%	9%	18.5%	0.5%
1840s dentists	8%	22%	10%	27%	6%	25.0%	2.0%

table 12: Distribution of probate values

By comparison with the 'medical men' with wills proved in 1858, the samples of pre-1855 dentists appear to have been worth more on death and considerably more likely to leave over £10,000:[156]

probate value[157]	medical men	gross sample	1840s dentists
under £ 100	12%	10%	8%
over £ 1,000	42%	59%	60%
over £ 10,000	7%	19%	27%
over £ 50,000	1%	0.5%	2%
average value	£ 3,139	£ 5,874	£ 7,390
median value	£ 600-1,000	£ 1,500-2,000	£ 2,500-3,000

table 13: A comparison between the probate values of the estates of the gross sample of pre-1855 dentists, the 1840s dentists and medical men dying in 1858

Whilst it may be said that the '1840s dentists' derived much of their income from the period after 1858, it is also true to say that they entered dentistry aware that dentists were already more likely to accumulate wealth than their counterparts in medicine;[158]   the average value of the 70 probates granted for dentists in the gross sample who began practice before the 1840s stands at £4,714, 50% more than the average for medical men dying in 1858.

Socio-economic standing

> Dentist: an artizan, who confines himself to the extraction of teeth and to several operations required by their defects, redundancies, accidents or disorders.   ...The head surgeons in London deem this branch of their art beneath notice and generally decline interfering in it.[159]
> (A. Rees, *Cyclopaedia* (London, 1819))

> Treatises on teeth appear at least one a quarter; and dentistry, as we find it called, is growing into a profession which numbers nearly as many members as surgery. Great rogues many of them are.
> (*Tait's Edinburgh Magazine*, 5(1838), p.197)

> The assertion is frequently made that if a man failed in every other business he would be sure to succeed as a coal merchant or a dentist.
> (*Br.J.dent.Sci.*, 2(1858-59), p.28)

From such damning comments as these, it is generally considered that dentists in the early period enjoyed only a 'lowly status'[160] and 'were clearly held in no high esteem'.[161]   'It would seem that [dentistry] tended to suffer from public ill-repute'.[162]

Indeed, some of the most derogatory statements about the practice of dentistry emanated from dentists themselves who, like De Loude, saw dentistry being brought into disrepute by the quacks of whom they were every bit as contemptuous as were the medical establishment, and from equally mixed motives, as we have seen.

There is, however, good reason for believing that it was individuals who were held in contempt in the early nineteenth century, not the profession as a whole. Whilst decrying quackery, the *Lancet* was quite prepared to accept non-medically qualified dentists as correspondents, not only on political issues but on clinical matters as well. Social and professional interaction between medical men and 'unqualified' dentists was by no means a rarity, as individual cases testify.

In society at large, those dentists who were frequent advertisers and who maintained a showroom in the manner of the present-day optician would probably always be tainted with the nineteenth century designation of trader and be relegated to their appropriate social rank. The tale was told of how Gladstone, having enjoyed an entertaining conversation with a fellow traveller to London, invited him to visit him and suggested they exchange cards. His companion had only business cards with him. 'Mr. G., upon perceiving that it was a dentist he had been entertained by, immediately gave him the positive cut, taking no further notice of him'.[163] As Peterson states, 'the essence of quackery was tradesmanship'.[164] In this, dentists were probably regarded in no different light to the surgeon-apothecary who kept a shop for the sale of drugs and toiletries. In an age which viewed the whole medical profession with a sceptical eye, unethical dentists may have attracted no greater opprobrium than avaricious physicians or incompetent surgeons.

Certainly dentists as individuals were not regarded as social pariahs by other professional men; they are to be found among the members of literary and philosophical societies,[165] organisers of charities,[166] governors of hospitals,[167] members of masonic lodges[168] and involved in local politics.[169]

The socio-economic standing of dentists as a whole is not easy to assess but Brown's work on the medical men of Bristol provides a useful starting point. In his study of the profession in the city in 1851, Brown considered size of household and the number of living-in servants kept as key indicators of socio-economic status.[170] He found the practitioners of medicine,[171] to whom he added dentists as a point of comparison, fell into distinct groups, each with its own socio-economic characteristics (*table 14* overleaf). From Brown's figures a clear gradation can be seen among the purely medical men (from physicians down to unqualified surgeon)[172] in the features which might be thought the best indicators of socio-economic status (mean size of household, mean number of resident servants, household sharing a house, extended or multiple family). On this basis, dentists rank above the unqualified surgeons in the first two respects and above the qualified surgeons without hospital appointments (the general practitioners) in regard to extended families. In their higher degree of multi-occupancy of houses, they resemble the chemists and druggists more closely than the medical

group	no[1].	socio-economic characteristics									
		A	B	C 1	C 2	C 3	D	E	F	G
physicians with hosp.appointment	15	45	7/93	100	---	---	8.86	3.21	7	43
surgeons with hosp.appointment	27	41	65/35	92	4	4	7.08	2.96	4	25
qual.surgeons without hosp. appointment	73	40	61/39	77	20	3	5.67	1.64	2	16
unqualified 'surgeons'	23	47	35/65	65	10	25	3.92	1.15	15	8
herbalists	13	37	45/55	64	9	27	2.71	----	57	14
chemists/druggists MPS	41	37	58/42	89	8	3	5.12	1.29	6	18
chemists/druggists non-MPS	70	35	69/31	72	23	5	3.91	0.65	22	17
dentists	19	36	47/53	82	12	6	5.50	1.36	21	21

[1] all sources: the remaining detail extracted from census returns

A mean age
B percentage born locally/not locally
C position in household 1-head 2-kin of head 3-lodger/visitor
   (expressed as percentage)
D mean size of household
E mean number of servants, if head
F percentage living in shared house
G percentage living in extended/multiple family group

table 14: Socio-economic characteristics of medical and dental practitioners in Bristol in 1851 (after Brown)

men. When compared with the pharmaceutical practitioners, dentists have most in common with the qualified chemist and druggist. It might perhaps be deduced that it was of greater importance for a dentist to have premises in a good trading position than to have sole occupancy of his house.

When Brown's criteria are applied to other provincial dentists, a similar situation obtains, except that there is less multi-occupancy and the mean number of servants is lower in each of the towns examined:

group	no.	socio-economic characteristics							
		A	B	C 1	2	3	D	E	F	G
dentists	45	39	40/60	76	18	6	5.5	0.9	6	21

table 15: Analysis of 1851 census data available for dentists in Birmingham, Bath, York and Leeds (after Brown)

Again it would seem that dentists in 1851 occupied a socio-economic position on a par with that of the qualified surgeon or chemist and druggist, although likely to keep fewer servants. In towns where there was pressure on fashionable accommodation, he was perhaps more willing to occupy shared premises for the sake of a good trading address.

NOTES AND REFERENCES

1   T. Purland, *Dental memoranda [Purland scrapbook]*, MS 63518, Wellcome Institute, e.g. 69, 71, 71v.
2   *ibid..* See also D.W. Wright, 'London dentists in the 18th century', *Dent.Hist.*, 12(1986), 8-16.
3   *York Courant (YC)*, 19 May 1752. The earliest advertisement for Ruspini yet found. Menzies Campbell dismissed the unsubstantiated statement by Boggis (F.W. Boggis, 'The Chevalier Ruspini, dental surgeon to George IV', *Br.dent.J.*, 42(1921), 336-338) that Ruspini had come to England in 1750, being convinced from his own lengthy research that he had not done so until 1759. Campbell considered that Ruspini's first advertisement in England was to be found in the *Bath Journal*, 16 Apr 1759. The life of Bartholomew Ruspini, dentist to George IV and founder of the Royal Cumberland Freemason School for Girls, was extensively examined by Campbell in *Dent.Mag.Oral Top.*, 70(1953), 402-422.
4   *YC*, 15 May 1753.
5   *ibid.*, 4 June 1754.
6   *ibid.*, 11 May 1756.
7   J. Boyes, 'Medicine and dentistry in Newcastle upon Tyne in the

18th century', *Proc.R.Soc.Med.*, 50(1957), 230.

8   When visiting York in 1769, Whitlock claimed above 35 years experience in 'all capital places in Gt. Britain and the Universities of Oxford and Cambridge where he has attended six years' (*YC*, 10 Oct 1769) but no trace has yet been found of him in the 1730s.

9   e.g. *YC*, 9 Sept 1740, Powell's Tincture; 2 July 1742 *et seq.*, Greenough's Tincture.

10   Robert Law, instructed for 14 years by 'that ingenious Mechanick John Dappe of London', and a maker of a wide variety of orthopaedic and prosthetic appliances, including artificial teeth (*ABG*, 15 Nov 1741, *Menzies Campbell Collection (MCC)* 25).

11   *ABG*, 26 Dec 1757 and 12 Feb 1759.

12   Liverpool was still receiving visitors in the 1830s at the rate of 2.2 per year (range 1-5) despite the presence of never fewer than 16 resident dentists in the same decade.

13   see introduction for a discussion of trade directories as a source material.

14   e.g. Thomas Weale of Liverpool; Charlton of Bath; Goldstone of Bath; George Arthur Manne[r][?] of Nottingham.

15   e.g. Andrew Restieaux of Norwich and Arman Talma of Chester from France; Bartholomew Ruspini of Bath from Italy; Hemet Hart and Mr. & Mrs. Sedmon of Bristol, Joseph Sigmond of Exeter and Bath, all from Germany.

16   Of these, John Watts, the founder of the Raquet Court practice in 1702, is presumably an example. He was Master of the Barber-Surgeons Company from 1732-36 (L. Lindsay, 'The London dentist of the 18th century', *Dent.Surg.*, 24(1927), 181). However, it must be borne in mind that by this period the Company had become very mixed in its membership and no longer restricted to barber-surgeons (J.G.L. Burnby, *A study of the English apothecary from 1660-1760* (1983), 15).

17   A tradition which has only recently died out; see obituary for James Johnston Davidson (1884-1981), (*Br.dent.J.*, 151(1981), 70.

18   e.g. John Gray began as a watchmaker (*Forceps*, 1(1844-45), 12) and Brophy as a jeweller (*ibid.*, 159).

19   Estimate based on information from trade directories (which probably understate the degree of multioccupation) and on the following records: P.J. and R.V. Wallis, *18th century medics; subscriptions, licences and apprenticeships* (1985); *London and provincial medical directory* (1847); S.F. Simmons, *Medical register* (1779, 1780, 1783); Royal College of Surgeons of London, *List of members of the Royal College of Surgeons in London* (1805, 1825, 1835, 1845); Society of Apothecaries, *A list of persons who have obtained certificates of their fitness and qualification to practise as apothecaries from Aug.1 1815 to July 31 1840* (1840); *ibid...from Aug.1 1840 to July 31 1852* (1852); Pharmaceutical Society of Great Britain, *Register of Pharmaceutical Chemists and Chemists and Druggists* (1869); General Medical Council, *Dentists Register* (1879). A search of the membership records of the Pharmaceutical Society (founded 1841) would perhaps yield further names, but the names of the majority of such traders are not to be found collected together until the first Register of 1869. Until this date, membership of the Society had been voluntary.

    The picture is hence still possibly incomplete for want of records of non-medical traders and for chemists and druggists who ceased business before 1869.

20   Medical men are here grouped together since it is known that most were general practitioners, whatever their original background. In addition, many were described differently on different occasions; the same man may appear sometimes as a surgeon, elsewhere as an apothecary and in places as a physician. Included in this category are 27 dentists also described as surgeons (usually on only one occasion) who may not in fact have been so. Most of these potentially 'doubtful surgeons' derive from an 1839 directory published by Robson (Norton 101), which bears 'the marks of hasty and slipshod compilation'. 'Surgeon-dentist' appears to have been taken to mean 'surgeon, dentist'.

21   *Forceps*, 1(1844-45), 17.

22   Dental students of a later generation were advised to take the MRCS in addition to the LDS, if possible, to obtain a 'deeper insight into the mysteries of science' (*Br.J.dent.Sci.*, 15(1872), 412).

23   Aldridge, Bird, Blackmore, Buckell, Church, Corey, Dunsford, Gantherry, Goldstone, Hopton, Hugo, Meears, Messenger, Middleton, Nathan, Nelson, Nowell, Oxley, Rothwell, Sayles, Stuart, Waller, Windsor.

24   The LSA required 5 years apprenticeship to an apothecary followed by time spent in a hospital; the would-be MRCS was required to spend a similar period of preparation and attendance at lectures.

25   e.g. James Eno of Newcastle upon Tyne and J.B. Dixon of Hanley.

26   Percentage of new practices set up in the provinces by multitraders:

18th cent.	1800s	1810s	1820s	1830s	1840s	1850-55
41%	45%	41%	22%	13%	13%	15%

27   *Forceps*, 1(1844-45), 62.

28   C. Hillam, 'James Blair (1747-1817), provincial dentist', *Med.Hist.*, 22(1978), 44-70.

29   R.A. Cohen, E.A. Marsland and C. Hillam, 'William Robertson of Birmingham, 1794-1870', *Br.Dent.J.*, 142(1977), 64-69 and 99-102.

30   *ABG*, 15 Dec 1806.

31   e.g. *Williamson's Liverpool Advertiser*, 16 May 1791. He continues to be hailed as the first trained dentist in America and is considered the father of American dental literature on the basis of his *Practical Treatise*, written, in fact, in Liverpool.

32   *ABG*, 9 Mar 1795.

33   *Kentish Gazette*, 15 July 1834.

34   *Manx Sun*, 7 June 1845.

35   *Forceps*, 1(1844-45), 105.

36   'Henry' is identified by Purland as D.W. Jobson of 38, Albemarle St, Piccadilly (*Purland Scrapbook*, 127v).

37   *Br.J.dent.Sci.*, 2(1858), 81.

38   L.C. De Loude, *Surgical, operative and mechanical dentistry* (1840), 141. His book was prefaced by a list of respectable subscribers and dedicated to his pupils. Like Gray, he was anxious to establish himself as a professional oasis of sanity in a naughty world of empiricism. By exposing the iniquities of their confrères, their own virtues shone more brightly.

39   This firm had become established in Great Russell St in 1826 as
Mallan & Son and by the early 1830s had acquired another branch in
Halfmoon St, apparently operated by the son, John. The patriarch of the
family, Van der Molen, came from Holland. James Michael Mallan first
appears on the scene in 1838 at 10, Ludgate Hill. He disappears
temporarily in 1843 and 1844 although other Mallans continue, albeit at
somewhat movable addresses, until 1848. James's absence is explained in
articles in *Forceps*, 1(1844-45), 6 & 36. Following a court case brought
by a Mrs. Poulcard for inadequate work, Mallan thought it 'advisable to
pay the United States a professional visit'. However, advance publicity
from the dental profession in England had 'prevented the empirical
vagabond from gaining a foothold in any other place than New York, where
he was reduced to the alternatives of either flight or starvation'.
After 2 years in the city, he returned to London in 1844 and a warning
of his imminent arrival appeared in the *American Journal of Dental
Science*.
         This was not James Mallan's only encounter with the law. In 1858
he appeared before Bloomsbury Crown Court accused of fraud. The defence
stated that the prosecution had no right to refer to their client's past
misfortunes, nor to state that he had been constantly before the police
courts, and sailing under assumed names for the purpose of fraud. It
was true that their client had changed his name, but it was because the
Times had refused to publish his advertisements in his own name; ...that
he had from private speculation been compelled to emigrate to America,
and upon his return had taken the benefit of the Insolvent Debtor's Act,
but that was from private speculation and was not an issue in this case.
The defendant admitted that he had passed by the names of James,
Cartwright and Cartwright & Davis but denied that he had been before the
police magistrates or had refunded any moneys obtained by him
(*Br.J.dent.Sci.*, 2(1858), 125).
         When he reappeared on the London scene in 1844, it was as Michael
James & Co. of 58, Fleet St. He continued to practise under his own and
other names until 1885.

40   *Forceps*, 1(1844-45), 52.
41   Identified in 1835 by Purland as the trading name of John Jordan,
'the quack doctor of Houndsditch' (*Purland scrapbook*, 104).
42   *Forceps*, 1(1844-45), 171.
43   Possibly Henry Jones.
44   *Forceps*, 1(1844-45), 98.
45   In a letter to a friend (Z. Cope, *Sir John Tomes, pioneer of
British dentistry* (1961), 11).
46   *ibid*, 15.
47   John and Isaac practised in London, Isaac becoming the President of
the Odontological Society in 1873.
48   Including Henry Campion (1828-1904) whose obituary described
Sheffield as one 'who in the middle of the last century made such a name
for himself as a dental practitioner in the West of England'
(*Br.dent.J.*, 25(1904), 837).
49   *J.Br.Dent.Assoc.*, 18(1897), 21-31.
50   B. Webber, *James Orrock, R.I.: painter, connoisseur, collector*,
vol.1, (1903), 9.
51   'Senex', 'A reminiscence of dentistry in the old days: a fortunate
dental student, 1855', *Br.J.dent.Sci.*, 63(1920), 6-12.   'Senex'

described in detail the techniques he learned as an apprentice.
52   I.R./1/8 Nov. 1720; reference supplied by Dr. J.G.L. Burnby.
53   *MCC* 903.
54   *ABG*, 22 July 1793.
55   e.g. *Chester Chronicle (CC)*, 26 Mar 1802; *Nottingham Journal (NJ)*, 25 May 1802; *Lancaster Gazette*, 27 Mar 1802. Apprenticed 7 Apr 1798 for 4 yrs 9 days (Wallis 1985).
56   e.g. Jones in *Kentish Observer*, 26 June 1834.
57   e.g. Thomas Gill Palmer (trained by Parmly and Charles Bromley, c.1827: *Br.J.dent.Sci*, 18(1875), 685); Richard White (by James Robinson c.1835: *J.Br.Dent.Assoc.*, 13(1892), 625); Samuel Lee Rymer (by W. Perkins, c.1849: *Br.J.dent.Sci.*, 52(1909), 334).
58   *Br.J.dent.Sci.*, 15(1872), 487.
59   e.g. James Boucher apprenticed to Thomas C. Parson, Bristol, 1851 (HO 107/1951(2)435); George Fox to Robert Fox, Bristol, 1841 (HO 107/371); Frederick Morgan, Bath, 1841 (HO 107/969); William Winckworth to father John, Bath, 1841 (HO 107/969); William Moore, 'About to be apprenticed' to James Edwards, Bath, 1851 (HO 107/194).
60   The registers of agreements cease in 1811 in London and 1808 for 'country'.
61   Thomas Whitfield Lloyd, assistant and successor to James Blair in Liverpool, had been trained as a cutler and instrument maker.
62   *ABG*, 26 Aug 1822.
63   *Forceps*, 2(1845), 194.
64   *J.Br.Dent.Assoc.*, 15(1894), 810.
65   *Forceps*, 1(1844-45), 123.
66   *ibid.*, 2(1845), 56.
67   *ibid.*, 1(1844-45), 98.
68   H. Silverthorne, *Bath directory* (1841).
69   Forbes and Knibb, *Post Office Directory of Southampton* (1849).
70   F.N. Erith, *Bath Annual Directory* (1850).
71   De Loude 1840, 140-141.
72   Little or no attention was paid to the teeth in the training of a surgeon at the beginning of the 19th century. Extractions at hospitals were normally performed by unsupervised and uninstructed students before the appointment of dentists to these establishments.
73   *Forceps*, 1(1844-45), 106.
74   J. Gray, *Dental practice*, (1837), 5. This unexpected advice becomes less surprising when one reads (*Forceps*, 1(1844-45), 12) that this was the path Gray had himself taken into dentistry. He had begun as a watchmaker in Aberdeen at the beginning of the century before coming to London to ply his trade. Here he began to produce artificial teeth for a fellow Scot who had turned dentist. Starting up for himself as a dentist, 'he soon found to his cost, that unless he could tack the mysterious letters MRCS, etc., etc., to his name, he had better have remained a journeyman watchmaker'. In 1812 he presented himself successfully for the examination of the Royal College of Surgeons. His subsequent *Dental practice* was distributed with the author's compliments to 'those who were likely to express their gratitude by sending him patients'. *Forceps* branded him a 'genteel advertiser'.
75   C. Spence Bate, 'On the education of dentists', *Lancet* (1846), 230-231.
76   *Forceps*, 1(1844-45), 99.

77   J.B., 'Quack dentists', *Lancet* (1839), 383-384.
78   J.L. Levison, 'Suggestions for a faculty of dental-surgeons', *Lancet* (1840-41), 898.
79   'On the education of dentists', *Forceps*, 1(1844-45), 105.
80   Gray 1837, vii.
81   *Lancet* (1839), 383.
82   *Leicester and Nottingham Journal (LNJ)*, 27 Aug 1789.
83   In practice in Birmingham, London and elsewhere.
84   *Lancet* (1830), 764.
85   Possibly Joseph Kinnaird Murphy, in practice in Sheffield in 1846.
86   *Lancet* (1839), 112.
87   A. Hill, *The history of the reform movement in the dental profession in Great Britain* (1877), 14.
88   cf I. Loudon, 'The vile race of quacks...', in W.F. Bynum and R. Porter (eds.), *Medical fringe and medical orthodoxy, 1750-1850* (1987), 108.
89   e.g. James Robertson, trained by his father William, who visited Worcester from Birmingham (*Worcester Herald*, 23 Jan 1841).
90   *Manchester Mercury (MM)*, 9 Aug 1796.
91   *ABG*, 11 April 1768.
92   J. Colbran, *Handbook and directory for Tunbridge Wells* (1850).
93   *Liverpool Mercury (Liv M)*, 18 Jan 1833.
94   J.M. Campbell, *Dentistry then and now* (1981), 265-268.
95   as 71.
96   Of all the practices started in the provinces before 1850, 32% survived only one year and 42% no more than five. The principal may, of course, have been an assistant for some time before setting up his own independent practice.
97   One dentist who began practice in the provinces in the 1820s appears on the first *Dentists Register* of 1879. Also in this list are 7% of those who founded practices in the 1830s (14), 19% of those beginning in the 1840s (68) and 23% from the 1850s (83).
98   *Br.J.dent.Sci.*, 3(1859-60), 82.
99   *ibid.*, 13(1870), 241.
100   *J.Brit.Dent.Assoc.*, 18(1897), 730.
101   A combination of trade directories up to 1879 and the *Dentists Registers* from 1879 onwards, where applicable, make it possible to chart the practice careers of all the dentists active there before 1855.
102   The mean age for starting independent practice of 174 dentists whose dates of birth are known (16% of the national sample) is 30 years (median 29). This varies little with decade or length of practice.
103   e.g. from a mean length of 28 years for practices founded in the 1830s to 19 years for those set up in the period 1850-55.
104

			practice founded						
A	B	C	18th c.	1800s	1810s	1820s	1830s	1840s	1850s
6-10	34	12.5%	7	1	3	7	3	7	6
11-15	22	8.0%	1	-	3	1	3	9	5
16-20	16	5.9%	1	1	-	1	5	6	2
21-25	22	8.0%	3	1	1	5	6	3	3
26-30	19	6.9%	2	1	3	5	5	-	2

A	B	C							
31-35	12	4.4%	2	-	1	1	4	2	2
36-40	16	5.9%	-	5	1	2	4	4	-
41-45	7	2.6%	1	-	1	2	2	1	-
46-50	7	2.6%	-	-	1	2	3	-	1
51-55	9	3.3%	-	-	-	1	3	5	-
56-60	3	1.1%	-	2	-	-	-	-	1
61-65	1	0.3%	-	-	-	-	-	1	-

A length of practice in years
B number of practices
C % of sample of 273

table 7:   Chronological distribution of practices of more than 5 years duration in the 6 towns.

105   P.J. Stoy, 'Early dentistry in Belfast', *Br.dent.J.*, 120(1966), 258.
106   obit., *Br.J.dent.Sci.*, 15(1872), 487.
107   N.D. Richards, 'Destiny or dynasty', *Bull.Soc.Soc.Hist.Med.*, 16(1975), 11-12, supplemented by personal communication from Dr. Richards.
108   *ABG*, 3 Jan 1791.
109   *Williamson's Liverpool Advertiser*, 3 Sept 1792.
110   *Worcester Herald*, 19 Sept 1840.
111   Charlton & Archdeacon, *Directory of Leeds* (1849).
112   *Br.J.dent.Sci.*, 18(1875), 685.
113   *J.Brit.Dent.Assoc.*, 5(1884), 697.
114   *Dent.Rev.*, 6(1864), 196.
115   *Calendar of Probate*, 1874.
116   *ibid.*, 1870.
117   e.g. Edward Downing for his brother Richard of Newcastle upon Tyne (*ibid.*, 1861) and Simeon Mosely for Charles Mosely of Preston (*ibid.*, 1861).
118   e.g. William Fort of Preston acted as executor for his uncle William Titterington of Lancaster in 1857 (Lancashire Record Office Wills, R470).
119   James Blair of Uttoxeter (1847-84).
120   1851 census of Bath, HO 107/970.
121   *Morning Herald*, 3 June 1824 (*NCC* 450).
122   Mathews, *Bristol directory* (1839).
123   One of the most prolific was Richard White of Norwich (1819-92), a number of whose 12 children became dentists (*J.Br.Dent.Assoc.*, 13(1892), 625).
124   *J.Brit.Dent.Assoc.*, 23(1902), 401.
125   e.g. John Brooks Bridgman acted as executor for his father, William Kencely Bridgman (1812-84), in practice in Norwich from 1845 until at least 1864; Thomas Edward King, son of Joseph King of York (1808-94) in practice 1837-86.
126   1800s:18%; 1810s:13%; 1820s:19%; 1830s:21%; 1840s:21%; 1850-55:18%.
127   This makes for an interesting comparison with Zwanberg's study of Suffolk apothecaries in which he found 29% between 1815 and 1858 apprenticed to close relatives (D. Van Zwanberg, 'The training and

careers of those apprenticed to apothecaries in Suffolk, 1815-58',
Med.Hist. 27(1983), 139-150). Similarly, from the records of the
Apothecaries' Society between 1817 and 1889, Peterson found 26% of
apprentices trained by relatives (M.J. Peterson, *The medical profession
in mid-Victorian London* (1978), 42).

128   Based on a survey carried out in February 1985 among all staff and
students of the Liverpool Dental Hospital and School; size of
sample:368; response rate: 44%.

129   Samuel Cartwright (1789-1864) is reported to have earned £10,000 a
year (L. Lindsay, 'Personalities of the past, IX', *Br.dent.J.*, 98(1955),
259).

130   These were precisely the same arguments used by the apothecaries in
face of encroachment by the chemists and druggists in the 1790s (S.W.F.
Holloway, 'The apothecaries' Act, 1815: a reinterpretation', *Med.Hist.*
10(1966), 109).

131   *Times*, 19 December 1800.

132   Prerogative Court of York, *Calendar of Probate*, (1820).

133   An anonymous dentist of 1857 looked back to his early days in
practice: 'I had been two months, with my name and profession displayed
on the door, and I had not seen one patient in that time, save my
landlady, for whom I had made a gratuitous repair to one of the vilest
silver pieces I ever saw'. (*Br.J.dent.Sci.*, 1(1856-57), 204).

134   *Br.J.dent.Sci.*, 1(1856-57), 32.

135   *ibid.*, 197.

136   I.L. Loudon, 'A doctor's cashbook: the economy of general practice
in the 1830s', *Med.Hist.*, 27(1983), 259. (Information from *Bristol
Royal Infirmary: biographical memoirs,* Bristol Record Office).

137   *ibid.*, 261.

138   J.C. Hudson, *The parents' handbook -or guide to the choice of
employments, professions, etc.* (1842).

139   Account books (1830-46) of James Prew (MS 5208-5214), Wellcome
Library.

140   The Bristol rate books are at variance with this account, in that
they show Prew only as the occupier of 57, Park St. from 1841/2 to
1845/6. However, the books appear to have been carelessly kept at these
dates. (For example, the name of the owner of 57, Park St. is spelled
in three different ways in seven years although clearly referring to the
same person). All this time Prew continued to have entries in some
directories in his own name at 58, Park St., although his business cards
(e.g. an 1842 example in the *Purland Scrapbook*) gives 57, Park St. as
his Bristol address on Wednesdays and Saturdays.

141   F. Musgrove, 'Middle-class education and employment in the 19th
century', *Ec.Hist.Rev.*, 12(1959-60), 99-111.

142   The account-keeping deteriorates after 1842. From 1843-45, Prew
appears to have himself earned an annual average of about £730 but was
clearly in receipt of other money from Bristol, presumably from his
arrangement with Williams.

143   e.g. £71.9.11. in connection with Bristol in 1830.

144   Both James Edwards and James Robertson, Prew's successor, had been
employed by him. There is also a dentist named Thomas Prew living in
Bath in 1841 with a 20 yr old dentist in his household. This may be the
source of his partnership interest of £300 mentioned in 1838.

145   The cost of his Bath premises are excluded as a normal living

expense.

146 2-3 gns. is cited as a typical mechanic's/assistant's wage in 1844 (*Forceps*, 1(1844-45), 111).

147 Based on the number fitted in 1843 at 1s.6d. each.

148 Based on surviving bills in MS 5214.

149 Bill paid Jan. 1844 for previous half year: £9.3.9. If all this tax was paid under schedule B rate of 3½d in the £ in 1842 (E.R.A. Seligman, *The income tax* (1914), 133), then Prew had a taxable income of £630 for the second half of 1843.

150 Registrar General, *Report of the 1861 Census* (1861), 174-181. This opinion cannot be tested since 1858 was the first year of medical registration and from sources available it is not possible to say how many medical men died in that year. 'Personal estate' : 'cash, shares, goodwill, leases, carriages, wine, furniture, plate, books, pictures, jewels, proceeds of real and leasehold estate directed to be sold' (xlvi). Debts were also included.

151 *Br.J.dent.Sci.*, 22(1879), 294.

152 e.g. *Bath Chronicle*, 2 March 1809.

153 The number of dentists dying in any one year in the 19th century is too small to form the basis for a year by year comparison between their estates and those of the medical profession as a whole, but some idea of the wealth to be accumulated from the practice of dentistry can be obtained from an examination of the probate valuation of the estates of samples of the provincial practitioners who were active before 1855. Although these dentists died over a long period, it was nevertheless one which saw 'almost no alteration in the general level of prices' (J. Burnett, *A history of the cost of living* (1969), 196). Only the 262 dentists who were in practice for more than 10 years before 1855 are included in the comparison on the premise that for these practitioners it can reasonably be assumed that the practice of dentistry was the basis of their wealth.

  Many of the 262 died during the period before 1858, when a will might be proved in a variety of ecclesiastical courts of which there were about 300. A will was proved in that court which had jurisdiction over the geographical area in which the effects were to be found. First recourse was had to the archdeaconery court; if property was left in more that one archdeaconery, the will was proved in the consistory court, if in more than one diocese, in the provincial court. This theoretical hierarchy was not always observed and many wills went straight to the Prerogative Court of Canterbury (PCC). Bearing in mind that not all records have survived, it will be seen that it is difficult to make a definite statement about probate status of individuals who died before 1858, especially when it is not known where they might have owned property.

  Attention is thus focused on those known to have died after this date, in the period of civil probate, when it can be said with certainty whether or not probate was granted on an estate. Those who clearly died after 1858 numbered 141 (53%) and complete searches were made for grants of probate for this group. When the date of death was not known, a lifespan of 85 years was allowed, assuming that a dentist's first directory entry appeared when he was aged 20. In other cases a date of birth was known from census records. All but a very few dentists should have been detected in this way, since most began their own practices at a later age and evidence (based on the known lifespans of nearly 200 dentists) suggests an average age at death of 70 (median 72). In addition, definite statements about probate status can be made about a further 48 provincial dentists, 19 of whom had a final directory entry before 1858 but died after this date. Twenty-nine had wills proved in ecclesiastical courts. This brings the total of those about whom there is probate evidence (positive and negative) to 189, 72% of the total of 262 'ten year dentists'. These constitute the 'gross sample'.

A more homogeneous sample is formed by those 82 who began their own practices in the 1840s, a decade when contemporary commentators pointed out financial expectations as one of the attractions of the practice of dentistry. It is possible to make definite statements on probate status about all but 4 of this group and to make some assessment of whether their hopes were fulfilled. These are the '1840s dentists'.

In the gross sample of 189, grants of probate are found for 119 (63%). An almost identical proportion (60%) is found in the smaller sample of 82 '1840s dentists'. In the population at large only one in ten of those dying in 1858 left wills (Registrar General's *22nd Annual Report* (1861), xlvi). Absence of a grant of probate among the remaining 40% does not necessarily imply poverty, but it does indicate a lack of assets in the form of property interests, shares and other repositories for surplus capital which might require legal formality for transfer on death. It should also be pointed out that assets might have been disposed of before death (to set up a s n in business or provide a dowry for a daughter), but there does not seem to be any reason to believe that dentists were more likely to have done this than other comparable economic groups in society.

154   William Lambert of East Grinstead, d. 1887.

155   Richard Lloyd of Liverpool, d. 1868.

156   Rubinstein considers that until 1870, anyone leaving £10,000 can be designated 'very prosperous'. The 'rich' might expect to leave £50,000. Between 1870 and the First War, these amounts were typical of, respectively, a successful small businessman and a factory owner or banker (W.D. Rubinstein, *Men of Property* (1981), 121).

157   The points of comparison given in the 1861 *Census Report* discussion of the Registrar General's *22nd Annual Report.* The break-down of values in the actual *Report* (House of Commons Papers, 1861, XVIII.545, 174 *et seq.*) does not allow for direct comparison with Table 13.

158   It is unfortunate that the Registrar General's *Report* does not make any estimate of those medical men on whose estates no probate was granted. It may be that a higher proportion had grants of probate than did dentists but this seems unlikely, bearing in mind the poor financial prospects of the average provincial doctor before 1855 identified by Dr. Loudon (note 137).

159   It should be pointed out that the 'head surgeons' in London were very much a group apart who probably had a similar attitude towards the country surgeon-apothecary with his involvement in midwifery. The Royal College's neglect of instruction in anything connected with the treatment of the teeth whilst at the same time complaining that, as a profession, they were being robbed of the fees consequent on dentistry, has already been noted. The medical hierarchy were frequently vociferous towards all those they considered 'unqualified', whichever branch of medicine they trespassed on and even where, as in dentistry,

an orthodox medical training was not appropriate to its practice.
160   Campbell 1981, 237.
161   N.D. Richards, 'Dentistry in the 1840s', *Med.Hist.*, 12(1968), 139.
162   *ibid.*
163   *An.Jnl.Dent.Sci.*, 9(1859), 350. The writer of this article, a visiting American, attributed to the majority of dentists a very discreditable reputation. However, his views on dentistry appear to have been based only on observations in London and on information obtained from the leaders of the reforming movements who might be expected to present a gloomy picture of the situation.
164   Peterson 1978, 258.
165   e.g. William Robertson in Birmingham and Felix Yaniewicz in Liverpool. Yaniewicz was secretary of his society and gave the first demonstration of inhalation anaesthesia in the city to a medical audience.
166   e.g. George Bott's 'Bott's Benevolent Society'.
167   George Bott was a visitor and governor of Nottingham General Hospital and director of the Vaccine Institute in the town.
168   Bartholomew Ruspini was a member of a Bristol lodge, a founder member of a London lodge and co-founder, with the Prince of Wales (to whom he was dentist and personal friend) of Lodge no. 259. He founded what is today the Royal Masonic Institution for Girls.
169   e.g. Norman King in Exeter and Edwin Wade, who became the Lord Mayor of York.
170   P.S. Brown, 'The providers of medical treatment in mid-nineteenth century Bristol', *Med.Hist.*, 24(1980), 297-314.
171   Chemists and druggists were included since it was known from contemporary sources that many practised medicine in Bristol.
172   i.e. without either LSA or MRCS. Some of the 23 were known to have been in practice before 1815.

CHAPTER 3: THE SPREAD OF DENTISTRY: WIDER STILL, AND WIDER

3.1 Growth in the numbers of provincial dentists in the early nineteenth century

Contemporary estimates of the number of dentists in provincial practice in the first half of the nineteenth century are hard to come by.[1] Samuel Lee Rymer, writing in December 1856, declared, 'I believe there are about 900 dentists in the country'.[2] However, it is unclear what he means by 'the country' and just whom he includes in the term 'dentist'. It seems likely that the latter embraces at least assistants, who were eligible for membership of the College of Dentists (in connection with which Rymer made his observations). Alfred Hill, who was secretary to the College at this period and whose task it was to write to every 'dentist' in the 'country', put the figure for Great Britain, in retrospect, at 1300–1400 in 1857;[3] this would suggest that Rymer's figures refer only to England.[4]

A number of nineteenth century writers comment on the substantial increase in the number of dentists between 1800 and their own day. John Gray looks back to the end of the eighteenth century 'when ... dentists were scarcely known, except for a few tooth-extracting barbers'.[5] Now, he says, there are up to 120 in London alone.[6] John Tomes observed in 1877:[7]

> In London, at the commencement of the century, there were not, I believe, a dozen Dentists, now there are about 500. In Edinburgh there were not four, now there are over forty; and in the provincial towns they had no existence. Now there are in Gt. Britain nearly 2,000, without counting those in Ireland.

One might dispute Tomes's impression that there were no dentists at all in the provinces at the beginning of the century, but he was certainly correct in his observations on the remarkable increase in numbers over the century.

Although these contemporary commentators did not attempt to present any evidence for their assertions, their subjective impressions (which might be expected to be influenced to some extent by self-interest) are borne out by trade directory evidence.[8] The expansion can be charted in a number of ways. *Figure 1* (overleaf) shows the actual numbers of provincial practices recorded in trade directories for individual years up to 1855 (including dummy entries). Numbers are seen to remain very low for much of the period, not regularly exceeding 20 until 1810 and not reaching 50 until 1822. The hundred mark was passed in 1834, with a further 100 by 1844. In 1855, there were just over 500. Between 1810 and 1855 the number of practices at any one date doubles about every ten years. The expansion in London over the same period (1810–55) was slower; whereas between these dates the number of provincial practices at any one time increased about 20 fold, in London the number of practices increased by a factor of only 9.[9]

It would be a mistake, however, to assume that the profile demonstrated in *figure 1* was achieved by the simple addition of more dentists to an existing and continuing pool. The number of new practices was considerably in excess of the numerical gain apparent between 1800 and 1850:

all practices		new practices			
year	no.	decade	no.	increase over previous decade	% increase over previous decade
1800	20	1800s	20		
		1810s	32	12	60%
		1820s	101	69	215%
		1830s	200	99	98%
1850	360	1840s	366	166	
			719		

table 1: Comparison between the number of practices in 1800 and 1850 and the number of new practices in the intervening decades

Provincial dentistry appears to have had no difficulty in attracting new recruits, particularly in the 1820s.

If one considers the number of dentists in practice at some time in a decade rather than at specific sequential dates, again the 1820s is revealed as the period of greatest expansion in terms of percentage increase over the previous decade:

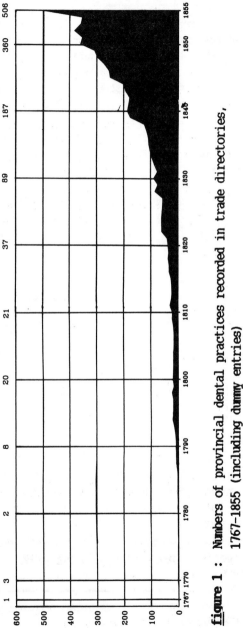

figure 1 : Numbers of provincial dental practices recorded in trade directories, 1767–1855 (including dummy entries)

decade	no. of practices at some time in decade	increase over previous decade	% increase over previous decade
1800s	34		
1810s	54	20	59%
1820s	149	95	176%
1830s	272	123	83%
1840s	534	262	96%

table 2: The numbers of practices at some time in the decades 1800-1850

The fact that the number of new practices set up is over twice that of the gain over the period 1800-50 (see *table 1*), suggests a high rate of turnover among early dentists. Indeed, in each decade the considerable proportion of incomers is partially offset by the high rate of drop-out from the profession:

DECADE	INCOMERS		OUTGOERS	
	number	as % of total no. of practices in decade	number	as % of total no. of practices in decade
1800s	20	59%	12	35%
1810s	32	59%	19	35%
1820s	101	68%	64	43%
1830s	200	74%	114	42%
1840s	366	69%	234	44%

table 3: Movement into and out of dental practice in the provinces 1800-50

Whilst it might be no surprise to find that, in an expanding profession, six to seven out of every ten practitioners in each decade were new recruits, a drop-out rate of four in every ten is another reminder of the unregulated state of dentistry at the time, with anyone who chose able to give this new form of treatment a try for a brief period.

The survival rate from one decade to the next was consequently low with, on average, only 54% of the practices in one decade likely to be still in operation in the next:

survival from	to	% of practices surviving
1800s	1810s	64%
1810s	1820s	59%
1820s	1830s	45%
1830s	1840s	56%
1840s	1850-55	47%

table 4: Survival rates of practices from one decade to the next

Clearly, many early practices were short-lived. Directory entries reveal that, of all the practices started before 1850, 32% survived only one year and 42% no more than five. This phenomenon appears to have become somewhat more prevalent with time:

decade	% of practices at some time in the decade lasting	
	no more than 1 year	no more than 5 years
1800s	15%	21%
1810s	14%	22%
1820s	21%	29%
1830s	25%	33%
1840s	23%	30%

table 5: % of practices of no more than 1 year or no more than 5 years' duration

Once again it is the 1820s (already identified as the beginning of trends towards expansion in terms of new recruits and the number of practices at some time in the decade and as a time of increased drop-out from the embryonic profession), which emerges as the pivotal decade.

3.2 Geographical expansion

We have already seen that between 1810 and 1855 the number of dental practices doubled approximately every ten years. However,

this overall rate of expansion conceals wide variations. In over
half the places where dentistry was established (54%) no expansion[10]
took place at all before 1855. This is particularly true of those
places which first saw a resident dentist in the 1840s and early
1850s. Whilst 80% of towns with a first dentist between 1810 and
1839 showed expansion, this rate dropped to 43% for those places
whose first dentist appeared in the 1840s and 2% where the same
phenomenon occurred in the period 1850–55.

This is not entirely surprising when one examines the pattern of
expansion in the towns which do show growth. It appears that there
was often a considerable delay before expansion took place. *Table 6*
shows the length of this period of delay decreasing somewhat with
time:

towns showing expansion		period of delay before expansion		
no.	decade of 1st app- earance of dentist	median length	range	mean length
2	1800s	13 yrs	13-19 yrs	16 yrs
7	1810s	12 yrs	4-30 yrs	15 yrs
15	1820s	18 yrs	9-32 yrs	19.4 yrs
22	1830s	9 yrs	6-16 yrs	9.9 yrs
25	1840s	6 yrs	1-14 yrs	7 yrs
1	1850-55	2 yrs		2 yrs

table 6: Median and mean lengths of the period of delay
before expansion, 1800-1855

Even with the gradual reduction in the average length of time
before expansion was likely to take place, most of the towns which
first saw dental practices in the late 1840s and early 1850s were
still in the initial stage of non-expansion by 1855. Continuous
expansion was, in fact, a rarity. More typical were decades of
growth alternating with decades of stability. The 'expanding' towns
were in a minority and even then only a proportion showed active
growth in any one decade (*table 7* overleaf).

Figure 1 shows the number of provincial dental practices
doubling every ten years from 1810. In the majority of places with
dental practices over this period, however, the rate of growth was
slower than this. Dental practice was expanding into more places

towns showing expansion	1800s	1810s	1820s	1830s	1840s	1850-55
as % of total no. of towns with dental practices	20%	19%	35%	39%	40%	34%
% in active phase of expansion	14%	19%	39%	41%	61%	66%

table 7: Proportion of 'expanding' towns showing active growth of dentistry in any one decade

rather than expanding at an even rate in all towns which acquired a resident dentist. *Table 8* confirms the impression of nineteenth century observers that, whereas very few places had resident dentists in 1800, by the middle of the century they were to be found in most towns:

decade	no. of towns with dental practices
1800s	10
1810s	21
1820s	40
1830s	61
1840s	126
1850-55	165

table 8: The number of towns with dental practices

In all, 204 towns show directory evidence of resident dental practice before 1855 (see *appendix 3*). Many towns make only a brief appearance in the list. Included in the proportion of towns where dentistry did not expand are those where it actually disappeared, such as Macclesfield and Braintree, which are recorded as having dentists only in the 1830s. The pattern of increase in the numbers of places over the period was not a simple one of more towns being progressively added to the list; as new towns acquired dentists, so others lost them. There was a turnover in places as well as in personnel.

From the second decade of the nineteenth century approximately half the places which saw new practices had not had a dental practice before:

DECADE	TOWNS WITH NEW PRACTICES			
	previous evidence of dental practice ('old' towns)	no evidence of previous dental practice ('new' towns)	total	'new' towns as % of total
1800s	5	2	7	29%
1810s	8	9	17	53%
1820s	19	16	35	46%
1830s	25	27	52	51%
1840s	53	60	111	53%
1850-55	79	54	133	41%

table 9: Towns with new practices

The number of new dental practices over this same period, however, does not show the same distribution; new dentists continued to favour the established towns as their location:

DECADE	NEW DENTAL PRACTICES			
	in 'old' towns	in 'new' towns	total	% started in 'new' towns
1800s	18	2	20	10%
1810s	20	12	32	38%
1820s	78	23	101	23%
1830s	141	60	200	30%
1840s	278	89	366	24%
1850-55	292	72	364	20%

table 10: The location of new dental practices, 1800-55

This must, in part, be due to the growing number of family practices in the 'old' towns, with sons succeeding their fathers.

To summarise, the numbers of both dental practices and towns where they were located increased rapidly during the first half of the nineteenth century. The expansion of dentistry in individual places was, however, uneven, with 54% of the towns showing no growth at all and continuous expansion in any one place being a rare phenomenon. From about 1810 around half the towns with new practices were those which had not previously seen a resident dentist, but at the same time between 60% and 80% of the new practices were being located in towns where dentistry had already become established.

3.3 The choice of location for dental practices

Only sixteen places show directory evidence for a resident dentist in the eighteenth century. The earliest entries into the field are to be found in Liverpool (first dentist 1767), Birmingham (1770), Manchester (1781), Norwich (1783), Bath and Bristol (both 1787) and Worcester (1788). During the last decade of the century, nine other places were added to the list, some of them (like Hull, Chester and Exeter) old established ports and commercial centres, others (like Leicester and Nottingham) rapidly expanding manufacturing towns. The remaining towns to acquire a resident dentist in the 1790s (Lichfield, Leominster, Stamford and Windsor) were small towns with populations of under 5,000 in 1801.[11]

The first decade of the nineteenth century saw only two new places with dentists (Leeds and Halifax) and the 1810s nine,[12] again including a few (Stonehouse, Burton and Romsey) with populations of under 5,000. The number of places with dentists doubled in the 1820s and included sixteen towns which had previously had no dentist.[13] Again the list includes places with very small populations (Leamington Spa and Weymouth, both with little over 2,000 permanent inhabitants). In the 1830s, dentistry reached 27 additional places.[14] In the 1840s there were 60 new places[15] and in the period 1850-54, 54.[16]

By the 1840s, as noted earlier, over half the places which saw a new practice set up had never had a dentist before. By the middle of the century, most major towns had their resident dentist and others which had not yet reached this stage had a branch practice.[17]

It can be argued that the expansion of dentistry is closely linked with the spread of ideas of 'fashion' and with an urban culture. If this is true, it is no surprise to find the earliest resident dentists in the provinces in such developing cities as Liverpool, Bristol, Manchester and Birmingham, with their merchant and professional classes. That these cities also had large populations appears to be almost incidental; some very sizeable towns had to wait a long time before they saw a permanent practitioner of dentistry in their midst, whilst around them much smaller places had their own dentists. Bradford is a case in point. Its population had to reach nearly 34,000 before a dentist set up practice there, although Halifax had its own dentist in 1816 when its population numbered only about 11,000.[18] Stoke on Trent is an even more extreme instance. This town had no dentist until the inhabitants totalled about 89,000 in 1854 whereas neighbouring Stafford had acquired a dentist four years previously with a population of only 12,000. Some of the very large manufacturing towns of Lancashire still had no dentist of their own by 1855. Clearly, size of population was not enough to attract a dentist. If social attitude was the principal initial determinant, as can be argued, it is equally to be expected that dentists should appear in those towns which were developing into fashionable spas and resorts as the concept of the holiday gained ground over this same period. Bath had been host to visiting dentists during the season for some time before any became resident and continued to be so thereafter, as demand increased.[19] The same can be said of Brighton (first resident dentist in 1818), Leamington Spa (1822), Weymouth (1828), Cheltenham (1830), Tunbridge Wells (1839), Scarborough (1841), Eastbourne (1845), Lewes (1845), Margate (1849), Lyme Regis (1855) and Malvern (1855).

Yet the majority of places which saw resident dentists before 1855 can scarcely be cast in the rôle of centres of fashionable ideas; they are neither the large cities in which were concentrated the burgeoning middle classes in pursuit of gentility nor the holiday towns to which these same groups resorted. Some of the earliest towns to produce dentists were small, even by contemporary standards: Lichfield (pop. c. 4,000), Leominster (c. 3,000), Stamford (c. 4,000) and Windsor (c. 4,000). This phenomenon is repeated throughout the period, with Romsey acquiring a dentist in 1811 with a population of about 4,000, North Shields in 1828 (pop. c. 6,000), Braintree in 1839 (pop. c. 3,500), New Alresford in 1848 (pop. c. 1,500) and Tetsworth in 1854 (pop. c. 500). Undoubtedly, each of these small towns could provide a dentist with a certain number of potential socially emulative clients and their surrounding dependent hinterlands with a few more, but the supply can never have rivalled the markets

available to the city dentist.   Nevertheless, these towns were the
locations for resident dentists.

Some of the explanation for the location of dental practices in
small towns may lie in the distribution of individual wealth in the
provinces.   From their examination of assessed tax records for the
late 1840s,[20] Phillips and Walton postulated[21] that individual wealth
was to be found on a greater scale in towns with small populations.
Towns with between 2,500 and 10,000 inhabitants returned twice as
much tax per head (£0.22) as those with 50–100,000 (£0.12).   Whilst
the larger centres of population yielded the highest amounts of tax,
the total per head decreased with an increase in the size of the
population.   This was especially so in the new industrial towns where
increased size was due to an influx of those unlikely to be liable
for assessed taxes.   (Commercial centres and ports were less affected
by this phenomenon).   The two exceptions to this trend were London
(£0.42 per head) and the watering places, 'towns which purposefully
encourage ostentation and magnificence', and where one might also
expect to find dentists.   (Bath returned £0.59 per head and
Cheltenham £0.57).

Outside these towns (the spas and old commercial centres), the
dentist in search of a sizeable wealthy population would look to a
county town or old manufacturing centre (such as Norwich) rather than
to a new expanding industrial town (such as Stoke on Trent), where
the core of those who both wanted and could afford his services was
too small numerically to make practice viable.

However, a concentration of wealth does not appear to have been
the only factor.   The Tavistock practitioner of the 1850s states that
if he were forced to remain at home in what he considers 'an
unfashionable town of some 8,000 or 10,000 inhabitants', then he
could not earn an adequate living, 'unless one's stamina could be
maintained on Scotch diet, porridge and salt'.   He is 'one of those
who prefer a country practice to one in the town, and therefore
regularly visit two small places'.[22]   Dental practice based on a town
of the type and size of Tavistock clearly obliged the dentist to go
out to find his patients, as countless examples show.   Even city
dentists, with their better supply of patients, travelled to some
extent[23] and indeed it may be that this opportunity for variety was
part of the attraction of dentistry for some of its practitioners.
Certainly, 'Suaviter et Fortiter' enjoyed his way of life and chose
it deliberately, having no intention of moving to the city where

patients might be expected to be more easily come by. Perhaps the same may be said for those who equally deliberately chose to practise from such unexpected places as Spilsby[24] and Fakenham[25] (both of which had populations of about 2,000 at the time of their first dentist); they may simply have preferred the life-style attendant on 'country practice', a view shared with the rural surgeon-apothecary, another practitioner who spent much of his time on the road. It should also be remembered that a tradesman who turned to dentistry as a new line of business would probably have remained in his native town where he was known to his potential patients and on whose likely demand for his services he had probably based his decision.

The presence of dentists in unlikely places has its parallels to some extent in the location of provincial newspaper presses in the eighteenth century. Cranfield came to the conclusion that this had less to do with the size of population of a town than with the presence of an individual who was prepared to undertake the risk of production for minimal returns.[26] High circulations were achieved by an efficient distribution system over a wide area. Of the growth of the provinical press, Cranfield states, 'the tendency was not only for the number of newspapers to increase steadily, but also for them to be produced in a steadily-growing number of different towns...in this period the human factor was undoubtedly the decisive one'.[27]

Even in modern times, when setting up in dentistry involves a very high financial outlay and commercial considerations might be expected to be paramount, personal motives play a surprisingly large part in the choice of location of practice. Robinson found that nearly 54% of a representative sample of practitioners had located their practices where they did for no other reason than that they already had family connections in the town.[28] In the early part of the nineteenth century, when there were such differences in amenities and in the social and economic life between city and small town and when a degree of itinerancy was accepted as part of the practice of dentistry, wherever a dentist was based, a practitioner might choose the life-style which suited him best within his area of operation. As long as 'there is in this country, plenty of scope for dental practice, thus rendering close competition equally ungenerous and unnecessary',[29] then commercial pressures seem to have been of secondary importance to personal preference in the location of new dental practices.

3.4 Dental practice/population ratios

The rate at which dentistry expanded in the early nineteenth century resulted in a dramatic improvement in the dental practice/population ratio in the country as a whole, from approximately 1:205,000 in 1801 to 1:28,000 in 1851:

	population of England and Wales[81]	DENTAL PRACTICES[80] provincial	London	total	dental practice/ population ratio in England and Wales
1801	9,060,993	19	25(1805)	44	1:205,931
1811	10,322,592	30	35	65	1:158,809
1821	12,105,614	41	69(1820)	110	1:110,051
1831	13,994,460	75	136(1832)	211	1: 66,324
1841	15,929,492	182	165	347	1: 45,906
1851	17,982,849	351	290	641	1: 28,054

table 11: The dental practice/population ratio in England and Wales between 1801 and 1851

Dentist (as opposed to practice) /population ratios are more difficult to assess because of the unknown number of journeyman assistants.   However, even if one allots one assistant to each practice, the dentist/population ratios remain low as late as 1851 (1:11,000–14,000) compared with the modern United Kingdom figure (1:3,000–4,000).[32] The overall figures given in *table 11* conceal the very different ratios for London and the provinces:

date	dental practice/population ratio London	provinces
1801	1:38,354	1:426,427
1811	1:32,537	1:306,125
1821	1:19,984	1:261,626
1831	1:12,169	1:164,526
1841	1:11,808	1: 76,819
1851	1: 8,145	1: 44,503

table 12: The dental practice/population ratios in London and the provinces between 1801 and 1851

Even by 1851, despite a dramatic improvement in the ratio, the provinces as a whole had still not achieved the dental practice/population ratio reached by London at the beginning of the century. These ratios, however, should be accepted with a degree of caution since the census definitions do not necessarily correspond with spheres of influence; the capital serviced a larger population than that designated 'London'. The same *caveat* must be applied to any attempts to determine the ratio for individual towns in the provinces. It is almost impossible to delineate the boundaries of spheres of influence; newspapers bearing advertisements for dentists circulated anything up to forty miles away from the towns of printing, affording the potential patient more choice than might at first be suspected. Some dentists were prepared to supply artificial teeth by post (having sent the patient a block of wax to bite on to provide the basis for an impression), which confuses the issue further. In addition, dentists regularly paid visits to towns which one might not normally consider as dependent on their home town. Thomas Whitfield Lloyd, for example, continued to visit Shrewsbury from Liverpool for twenty years for the good reason that a clientèle had been built up there by his former partner, James Blair, many years before when he was operating out of Chester at the beginning of the nineteenth century.

As we have seen, dentists of this period can be thought of as belonging to a whole area rather than to a particular town or even county, whilst having their home in the urban area from which they derived most of their patients. If most of a city dentist's patients probably came from the town itself, it might be thought that the dental practice/population ratios of different towns might be compared. When such a comparison is made, it is possible to demonstrate that Leeds and Sheffield have worse ratios for most of the period compared with Birmingham, Liverpool and Manchester and that Exeter and Bristol were consistently better served:

	dental practice/population ratios (000s)					
	1801	1811	1821	1831	1841	1851
Leeds	-	1:63	1:42	1:31	1:19	1:12
Sheffield	-	1:53	1:33	1:31	1:19	1:14
Birmingham	1:37	1:43	1:27	1:29	1:16	1:16
Liverpool	1:26	1:31	1:30	1:24	1:15	1:16
Manchester	1:23	1:26	1:36	1:20	1:16	1:16
Exeter	1:17	1:19	1: 8	1: 7	1: 6	1: 4
Bristol	1:15	1:14	1:21	1:15	1:14	1: 9

table 13: Dental practice/population ratios in 7 towns, 1801-51

One might build on this a hypothesis that Lancashire had a better supply of dental services than Yorkshire and that the southwest of England was substantially better off than the north and the midlands.   However, although this may have been the case, the argument would be flawed by the fact that the ratios are calculated on the basis of the gross populations. Dentistry in the nineteenth century was not a service in the modern sense but was aimed at only a section of society, those with the money and inclination to devote to the care of the teeth. The proportion of the population which this group formed in individual places is uncertain. It could well be that their numbers were very low in Sheffield, for example, and high in Exeter. As both towns had approximately the same number of dental practices from 1811-51, this would make the target population of Sheffield better served for dental treatment than the same group in Exeter, with its apparently more favourable ratios.

3.5 The mobility of provincial dentists

Part of the pattern of expansion of dentistry into the provinces is attributable to mobility. For some dentists it was a move for training, for others a subsequent uprooting to set up their own practice and for a smaller number quite radical changes of practice location, sometimes with some frequency. Even those trained in family firms are seen setting up their own practices in another town. For a few, their greatest dislocation was their initial move to England.

Some of the earliest dentists were from abroad. Advertisements appear in the eighteenth century London press for a host of foreign practitioners[33] and the tradition continued to some extent into the nineteenth century.[34]   Similarly, some of the earliest visiting dentists in the provinces were of foreign origin[35] and the presence of practitioners from abroad is still observable in the nineteenth century.[36]

A number of these foreign dentists ultimately set up permanent practice in the provinces. Mr. and Mrs. Sedmond are to be found in Bristol in 1797-98 and Ruspini practised in Bath for a number of years before moving to London in 1766. Arman Talma based himself in Chester for several years whilst Joseph Sigmond, originally from Germany, settled in Exeter in 1786 before moving to Bath.[37]

Restieaux of Norwich and Hull seems likely to have been French, as does Peter Michel of Bath.[38]

The more northerly areas also attracted foreign dentists into permanent practice there, but usually in the nineteenth century. Manchester was the destination of the Richerauds (from Paris) and Eleazer Gidney, an American dentist, whose time in the city spanned twenty-five years. The Berend brothers from Hanover arrived in Liverpool in 1823.[39] Samuel remained in the city until 1860 whilst Louis moved on to Manchester in 1835 where he was in practice until 1858.[40] Another German dentist in the north-west was Leopold Dreschfeld, a former revolutionary activist from Bavaria who settled in Manchester in 1852.[41] Leeds saw Antoine Bernasconi 'Chevalier de la Barre...Parisian dentist...surgeon-dentist to the King of France'.[42]

The frequency with which exotic origins are claimed, especially in the eighteenth century, shows that a certain prestige and even mystique was attached to the foreign practitioner and that experience abroad was valuable currency in the search for patients. (Even as late as 1844, it was stated in *Forceps*: 'The reputation of having studied abroad [is] a passport to immediate practice').[43] It did not take long for English dentists to see the usefulness of a foreign connection. Thomas Steele, on a visit to his home town of York, claims to have just come from Paris for the summer. In the nineteenth century, Farthing of Southampton claims experience in New York[44] and De Loude, who elsewhere poured scorn on the empirics travelling the country as 'signor' or 'monsieur' described himself as[45]

Member of Felix Mérités, Amsterdam and Teilers Museum, Haarlem... Medical Electricity on French and La Baume system.

Even a remote foreign connection appears to have been seen as enough: Dinsdale of Newcastle boasts of a Paris branch[46] and Eskell of Leeds offers 'all the modern Improvements of Paris and Berlin'.[47]

We have seen already that family links promoted a certain degree of interchange of personnel between the provinces and London. Directory and newspaper evidence also identifies the moves to and from London of a number of individual provincial dentists. In some cases, the record is of visits made by London dentists to the provinces; Foy, Grimaldi, Ruspini and the Crawcours made frequent such excursions outside the capital in the eighteenth century, a tradition continued into the nineteenth.[48]

For other London dentists, the move from the capital was of a permanent nature:

NAME	DIRECTORY ENTRIES	
	LONDON	PROVINCES*
Clark, Andrew	1822-52	Brighton, 1851-55
Cornwall, Augustus	1846-52	Reading, 1852-54
Dash, James	1854	Brighton, 1854-55
Ferguson, Ralph H.	1842	Stockton, 1847-48
Fox, Charles Prideaux	1843	Torquay, 1844
Garner, Joseph Samuel	1840	Boston, 1849-50
Gedge, William Edward	1850-51	Torquay, 1852
Hepburn, Duncan	1850-53	Nottingham, 1853-55
Leigh, Edward Philip	1854	Ipswich, 1855
Lukyn, William	1840-44	Leamington, 1845-50
Rogers, Thomas	1838-40	Leicester, 1842-46
Rose, Robert	1826-36	Liverpool, 1837-48
Rose, John Frederick	1850	Liverpool, 1851-55
Stanbury, Nicholas	1849-51	Brighton, 1851-54
Styer, Abraham	1838-42	Northampton, 1845-52
Tibbs, Somerset	1836-38	Cheltenham, 1839-53

* the terminal dates do not necessarily indicate the end of a dentist's provincial practice

table 14:   Examples of London dentists who moved permanently to the provinces(from a comparison between pre-1855 London and provincial trade directory entries)

In addition to those for whose move to the provinces there is corroborating evidence, many other dentists claimed experience in the capital:

NAME	LOCATION OF PROVINICIAL PRACTICE	SOURCE FOR CLAIM TO EXPERIENCE IN LONDON
Alex, J.	Cheltenham	*Cheltenham Chronicle*, 3 Oct 1822 (MCC 9)
Aranson, Pasco	Liverpool Birmingham	*Liverpool Chronicle*, 15 Apr 1807
Cordon	Liverpool	*Liverpool Mercury*, 21 June 1833
Edwards, James	Bath	H. Silverthorne, *Bath directory* (1841)
Farthing, John	Southampton	Forbes & Knibb, *Southampton*

		directory (1847)
Hunt, William	Yeovil	*Br.dent.J.*, 26(1905), 638
Law, Robert	Birmingham	*Aris's Birmingham Gazette*, 15 Nov 1741
Manne, George	Bath etc.	*Bath Journal*, 28 Jan 1822 (MCC 394)
Moor	Oxford	*Leicester Journal*, 12 Nov 1790
Mummery, John R	Dover	*J.Br.Dent.Assoc.*, 6(1885), 53
Palmer, Thomas G	Peterborough	*Br.J.dent.Sci.*, 18(1875), 685
Parkinson, George T.	Bath	*Dent.Rec.*, 10(1890), 281
Robertson, James	Bath	*Dent.Rev.*, 6(1864), 196
Rogers, Thomas	Southampton	Forbes & Knibb, *Southampton directory* (1851)
Rogers	Northampton	*Northampton Herald*, 22 Jan 1842 (MCC 754)
Rymer, Samuel Lee	Croydon	*Br.J.dent.Sci.*, 52(1909), 334
Simpson, John	Liverpool	*Liverpool Mercury*, 15 Nov 1833
Talma, Arman	Chester	*Liverpool Advertiser*, 3 Sept 1792*
Taylor, Thomas	Liverpool	*Liverpool Mercury*, 27 Apr 1832
Turner	Liverpool	*Liverpool Mercury*,2 Jan 1824
Weale, Thomas	Liverpool	*Liverpool Advertiser*, 25 Apr 1791*
White, Richard	Norwich	*J.Br.Dent.Assoc.*, 13(1892), 625
Woolfryes, Henry	Northampton	*Northampton Herald*, 2 Nov 1844 (MCC 765)

* references supplied by A.R. Allan, Assistant Archivist, University of Liverpool

table 15: Examples of provincial dentists who claimed experience in London or for whom such experience can be deduced

However, the flow of dentists was not all in one direction. A number of provincial practitioners are shown by trade directories to have moved to London:

NAME	PROVINCES	LONDON*
Bayley, William Henry	Brighton, 1822-24	1826-36
Bew, Charles	Brighton, 1818-40	1840-45
Drury, Alexander Rupert	Halifax, 1850	1853-55
Fielding, Frederick William	Croydon, 1845	1854-55

Fisher, Frederick	Brighton, 1844-46	1846
Gabriel, Lyon	Hull/Liverpool, 1840-47	1849-55
Hart, Abraham Septimus	Bristol, 1822-29	1832-55
Haslam, Simeon	Hertford, 1850	1855
Hoskins, Francis	Nottingham, 1847-48	1853-55
Jarritt	Richmond, 1851	1851-55
Lowe	Ryde, 1839-48	1849-55
Lukyn, William	Oxford, 1829-40?	1840-44
Medwin, Aaron	Greenwich, 1845-51	1853
Merryweather, J.	Newcastle, 1844	1848-54
Middleton, Thomas P.	Manchester, 1845-51	1855
Prideaux, Thomas Sims	Southampton, 1843-49	1853
Saunders, Josiah	Cambridge, 1846	1848-55

*   the terminal dates do not necessarily indicate the end of a
      dentist's London practice

table 16: Examples of provincial dentists who moved permanently to
London (from a comparison between pre-1855 London and
provincial trade directory entries).

Examples can also be found of dentists who began practice in the
provinces and who, on moving to London, retained their provincial
practice, presumably to be operated by another member of the family
or by a manager:

NAME	PROVINCES*	LONDON*
Albert, Edward	Manchester, 1848-52	1849-55
Jones, Henry	Kent, 1831-55	1833-55
		(Jones & Bell)
Clark, Ebenezer	Brighton, 1839-55	1848-55
Hair, Quintin Burns	Kent, 1839-55	1841-55
Harrington, George Fellowes	Portsmouth, 1848-55	1855
Levason, Lewis	Leamington/Chester/	1852-53
	Aylesbury, 1828-53	

*   the terminal dates do not necessarily indicate the end of practice

table 17: Examples of dentists who moved to London but retained their
provincial interests

Newspaper and obituary evidence points to London dentists who
trained in the provinces but who, not having their own practices
there, do not appear in provincial trade directories. Christopher
Shew (trained by his uncle George in Bath)[49] belongs to this category
as does Isaac Sheffield (trained by his brother Thomas in Exeter).[50]
His brother John, on the other hand, after a brief partnership with

their father in Carlisle, moved to London to work for Isaac in the capacity of assistant and hence without London directory entries of his own. The well-known London dentist Felix Weiss was also trained in the provinces, being apprenticed to Felix Yaniewicz of Liverpool.

Experience in London established itself at an early date in the provincial imagination as an indicator of expertise and sophistication. Few opportunities were lost to emphasise a London connection, however remote. When T.D. Kidd visited Liverpool in 1828, although an established dentist in Edinburgh it was the fact that he had previously been an assistant to J.P. Clark of London that he chose to stress.[51] Dinsdale of Newcastle claimed a London branch, although no such name occurs in contemporary directories for the capital and no other dentist appears to have practised at that address.[52] Wood of Brighton thought it sufficient recommendation that he visited London monthly[53] whilst Montague Alex of Cheltenham reassured his patients that his 'system of practice combines all the improved methods adopted in London'.[54]

The evidence available makes it difficult to calculate with accuracy the number of provincial dentists who may have had practice experience in London at some time in their careers. If those who can be identified as having a foot in both camps (*tables 14-17*) are augmented with just one representative from each of the forty families who appear to have practised in both London and the provinces, then it can be speculated that a minimum of 1 in 10 provincial dentists had experience of practising in London at some time in their lives. It seems likely that this proportion would be higher if career details were known of all provincial and London dentists of the period.

Moves within the provinces

For a number of dentists, the move came when they wished to set up their own practice after serving as an apprentice or assistant. Like Wooffendale some were probably bound by a restrictive clause in their agreement with their former principal which prevented them from setting up within a certain distance of his practice. There are many known examples of dentists training in one town but opening their own practice in another,[55] although the evidence is too incomplete to form the basis of a meaningful analysis. More directly quantifiable are the moves made by established dentists which are detectable in trade directory entries.

In the period before 1855, 67 individual dentists (6% of the total) moved the location of their practices to elsewhere in the provinces, 22% of these more than once; the number of instances of such mobility total 86. The actual number of moves of this kind increases with time but the incidence of mobility among established dentists remains virtually the same throughout the period:

decade	1 dentists in practice at some time	2 instances of mobility	2 as % of 1
pre-1800	44	2	5%
1800s	34	2	6%
1810s	54	3	6%
1820s	149	6	4%
1830s	272	13	5%
1840s	534	33	6%
1850-55	671	27	4%

table 18: Incidence of mobility within the provinces of established dentists before 1855

It would appear that, once they had set up practice, an average of only 5% of dentists made a further move.

A total of 58 towns were involved in this mobility, although some feature more prominently than others:

town	instances of mobilty	losses	gains	net effect
Liverpool	18	11	7	-4
Manchester	13	7	6	-1
Birmingham	11	5	6	+1
Exeter	9	4	5	+1
Leeds	8	4	4	no change
Hull	8	4	4	no change
Nottingham	6	4	2	-2
Leamington	5	2	3	+1
Halifax	5	2	3	+1
Bath	5	2	3	+1
Southampton	5	3	2	-1
Cheltenham	5	2	3	+1

table 19: Net effect of intra-provincial mobility of established dentists on towns affected by 5 or more instances of mobility

No major patterns in the exchange of personnel can be discerned (e.g. from cities to small towns or *vice versa*). Those who uprooted themselves cannot be cast in the rôle of pioneers, since only 7 of the 67 then settled in a town which had previously seen no resident dentist. However, a degree of geographical limitation can be seen in the origins and destinations of dentists moving to and from Liverpool, Manchester and Birmingham, the towns most affected by this intra-provincial mobility. All the arrivals and nearly all the departures (9/11) involving Liverpool were to and from the north of England and the midlands. Similarly, incomers to Manchester all came from the north, all but one of them from Liverpool. Five out of seven of the city's losses were again relatively local. None of the dentists attracted to Birmingham came from south of the city.[56]

Taken together, the available evidence for mobility[57] points to about 15% of the dentists in provincial practice before 1855 as having moved in pursuance of their profession, either before or after setting up their own practices. This seems likely to be the minimum estimate since more instances of mobility would undoubtedly come to light were career details available for all 1100.

3.6 Branch practices

The expanding profession of dentistry reached some towns through the agency of branch practices. Regular visits to another place several times a year were a common feature of early practice and by the mid-1850s it is clear that some of these visits had become more frequent, presumably in response to an increase in demand for treatment. Our Tavistock dentist of 1858 points out that he regularly visits two small places and that many of his fellow members of the College of Dentists have for many years visited one day a week 'in some pretty place to treat families who cannot conveniently travel to see them'. Robinson remarks that 'as provincial towns are not usually sufficiently populous to support exclusively dental practitioners who may happen to settle in them, these gentlemen visit the neighbouring localities'.[58]

Such a regular commitment can be considered as constituting a branch practice.

Provincial directory entries reveal 115 such branches[59] in the form of second addresses contemporary with those for home bases. It seems almost inevitable that this is an understatement of the real situation, since fuller advertisements in the same directories can sometimes be found which cite branches not mentioned in the main entries. The London firm of Jones and Bell, whose main entry in Phippen's 1850 directory of Maidstone gives only their address in that town, also placed a full page advertisement in the same publication which reveals that the firm attended Canterbury two days a week and Ramsgate a further one day a week. Similarly, another London dentist, George Levason, has an entry for his Aylesbury branch but in addition an advertisement which shows that he attends monthly at Newport Pagnell, Stoney Stratford, Winslow and Thame.[60] The Cambridge dentist Henry Lyon keeps the information that he attends Ely on Thursdays for his advertisement.[61]

Table 20 shows the growth in the number of branches declared in directory entries up to 1855:[62]

date	no. of branches	branches as % of dental addresses	% of dentists with branches
pre-1830	4 (6% of total)	2%	2%
1830s	13 (8% of total)	5%	3%
1840s	43 (35% of total)	8%	6%
1850-55	73 (51% of total)	11%	7%

table 20: The growth of branch practices as revealed in trade directory entries

It will be seen that the incidence of branches increases, both in absolute numbers and in the proportion they form of the number of dental addresses in individual decades. The percentage of dentists with branch practices also appears to rise over the period. The figures reflect the move away from the twice or thrice yearly visits of about a week to a number of places (a feature of provincial dentistry in the eighteenth and early nineteenth centuries) towards the establishment, by the middle of the century, of more regularly attended branch practices nearer to hand. Were the directory advertisements, which appear mostly in the 1840s and 1850s, to be included, the change would be even more striking.

It is a reasonable assumption that the increase in the number of branches reflects the increase both in demand for dental treatment and in dental manpower. That demand was not yet satisfied is shown by the location of the branches. While 33 were indeed opened in places which had not seen a dental practice before,[63] over twice as many were established in towns which already had resident dentists[64] but where there was still plenty of scope for the newcomer.

Most branches were probably manned by the principal himself but in other cases it is clear that sons were sent out to the branches. An advertisement for Messrs. (Daniel) Nightingale of Newcastle upon Tyne concludes with the statement that[65]

Mr. Charles Nightingale may be consulted EVERY WEDNESDAY, AND EVERY EVENING, at his residence, EAST PERCY STREET, NORTH SHIELDS.

Some branches were operated by managers, as in the case of Abraham Mosely, working a practice in Bristol for the Mallan family. Somerset Tibbs had been employed by the firm in the same capacity before opening his own practice in Cheltenham in 1839, fortunately severing his connection with the Mallans before their activities came to the attention of the courts.[66] A newspaper advertisement for the family in the Liverpool press of 1832 states that 'one of the firm' will be in attendance, further evidence for their use of managers.[67]

Advertisements reveal that most branches were operated on a part-time basis, usually for one or two days a week. Thus Jardine of Leeds visits his branch at Huddersfield on Wednesdays and that at Bradford on Thursdays.[68] Hair of London spends every Friday and Saturday in Tunbridge Wells[69] and Manne of Hull every Wednesday in Louth.[70] Other branches were in operation only monthly: Moore of Plymouth went to Teignmouth on the first Monday of each month and Mason of Exeter to Chard on the first Monday and Lyme Regis and Axminster on the first Tuesday.[71] James Robertson of Birmingham was somewhat unusual in operating a branch in Worcester for two weeks every month,[72] as was F.A. Sayles of Lincoln, whose Retford branch was open only between April and October.[73] Other dentists responded to fluctuating demand in the manner of Samuel Brown of Henley whose Leamington branch was active in the social season.[74]

The most detailed record to survive of the operation of a branch practice in the early part of the nineteenth century is to be found in the account books of James Prew (kept between 1830 and 1846) discussed earlier. Here it is seen that as much money was to be made in the Bristol branch as in the home base in Bath.[75] Clearly, a

branch practice was not a sideline for such a man as Prew. Whereas
the eighteenth century dentist such as James Blair or George Bott may
have kept his fingers in other commercial pies to supplement his
income from dentistry, his nineteenth century counterpart was opening
branch practices to supply this deficiency.

Provincially based branches

Trade directories alone reveal 74 branches based on provincial
practices. Nearly one third (31%) are found to be within ten miles
of base and a further 24% between 11 and 20 miles away:

distance from main practice	number of branches	% of the sample of 74
0-10 miles	23	31%
11-20 miles	18	24%
21-30 miles	16	22%
31-40 miles	5	7%
41-50 miles	10	13%
over 50 miles	2	3%

table 21: Geographical distribution of provincially
based branches recorded in trade directories

The branches furthest distant from the main practice are to be
found concentrated in the 1840s and 1850s:

decade[a]	distance of branch from initiating practice in miles					
	0-10	11-20	21-30	31-40	41-50	over 50
pre-1830	-	2	1	1	-	-
1830s	2	2	1	-	1	-
1840s	10	4	7	2	3	-
1850-55	11	10	7	2	6	2

[a] median distance in 1830s:12 miles; all other decades: 20 miles

table 22: Distribution of branches by date and distance from
initiating practice

To some extent this can be attributed to the greater ease of
transport in these decades. However, also characteristic of this

period are increases in the incidence of family concerns and of non-familial partnerships, albeit somewhat short-lived. Of those branches located more than 20 miles from the initiating practice, nearly 40% are started by dental families and may well have been operated by the principal's son or brother. A further 20% are part of a partnership concern and may have been operated full-time by the second member of the firm.

Branches based on a London practice

A small number of ordinary London dentists had branches outside the capital, particularly in Brighton.[76] However, the overwhelming majority of the 41 branches emanating from London are attributable to a handful of firms, namely Henry Jones, the Le Drays, the Mallans and the various members of the Mosely family. These branches are of a somewhat different nature to the provincially based ones; they are not the result of simple expansion of an individual into a neighbouring town to maximise his opportunities but of the use of the practice of dentistry as a vehicle for commercial enterprise.

According to trade directories, the earliest such ventures out of London were the Kent branches of Henry Jones. It would seem that he had begun dental practice in the late 1820s at 49, Old Broad Street[77] but by 1829 had entered into partnership with Alex at 26, New Bridge Street, Blackfriars.[78] Visits by Jones to Canterbury and Ramsgate are recorded in the local press but do not seem to have been on a regular basis. However, he gives a Dover address in an 1831 directory[79] and by 1834 his newspaper advertisements suggest permanent branches in Canterbury, Ramsgate and Dover, with attendance in Kent for the whole week.[80] In 1838 he established a new London practice in his own name and in 1848 a further practice of Jones and Bell. In all, at different dates in the period 1831-55, Jones had branches in five Kent towns[81] as well as maintaining his interests in London.

Le Dray's first directory entry appears to be in Liverpool in 1834. A contemporary advertisement states Monsieur Le Dray to be under the patronage of the courts of France and England[82] but some of his readers knew differently. Purland states, 'Le Dray is John Jordan, the quack doctor of Houndsditch. He also figures as 'Perry and Co' and 'Le Dray and Davis'...'.[83] By 1836 Le Dray had acquired a London address[84] and in subsequent advertisements in Liverpool states that he is from the capital.[85] The firm traded under various

titles in London until 1849. At different dates between 1834 and
1850 Le Dray had branches in Liverpool (1834-41?), Manchester (1837
and 1846), Newcastle (1838), Bristol (1845-46) and Bradford (1850).
As dentists, the firm of Le Dray were held in contempt by James
Robinson and cited by him as the epitome of all that was worst about
contemporary dental practice.[86]

If the Le Dray firm was pilloried by Robinson in *Forceps*, his
treatment of them was mild in comparison with the campaign he waged
against another London concern with multiple interests, the Mallans,
who, as we have already seen, were well known for giving newcomers to
the trade a brief initiation before sending them out to practise
under the firm's name.[87] Robinson's opinion of the Mallans is
encapsulated in his reply to an enquiry addressed to *Forceps*:[88]

> The change of names is an old 'dodge' of the parties alluded to.
> Our correspondent may rest assured there will be no change of
> practices; whether they advertise under the names of Messrs.
> Mallan, Messrs. Edwards, or any other *alias*, their object is the
> same -imposition and extortion.

From the beginning of their time as dentists, the Mallans
travelled outside London on visits,[89] advertising their 'Mineral
Succedaneum for filling decayed teeth' but not until 1834 did they
acquire a provincial directory entry, in Liverpool. There are
entries in Bristol between 1840 and 1843. However, the Mallans'
branches were not all they seemed, as was pointed out by Robinson in
his account of Abraham Mosely who ran their Bristol practice. It may
be that their Liverpool branch was operated in the same manner and
that they financed other provincial practices in the names of their
former trainees when their own reputation wore thin.

The last of the handful of London firms to open branches in the
provinces were the Mosely family, who between them appear to have
operated nearly thirty branches in the provinces in the 1840s and
1850s. Charles, Ephraim, Lewin and Simeon were brothers but it is
uncertain whether they were related to the Abraham who worked for the
Mallans in Bristol. Their London history is an extremely complex
one, with the brothers combining and recombining in different
practices throughout the period. It appears that their business
concerns may have been run as a large family firm, carried on by the
second generation. Whilst maintaining London addresses throughout the

period before 1855, they were all involved in provincial ventures:[90] Charles had six branches between 1848 and 1855,[91] Ephraim ten from 1842,[92] Lewin seven from 1843[93] and Simeon six from 1845.[94] Their commercial interests became even more extensive after 1855 as branches were opened in their own and their sons' names in Alnwick, Barnsley, Birmingham, Bradford, Derby, Hastings, Hexham, Leamington, Leeds, Leicester, Sheffield, York and elsewhere.

With such far-flung interests, even before 1855, it is clear that the brothers themselves cannot have operated all the branches personally as well as their London practices. In some cases it is clear that sons were involved[95] but managers and agents may also have been used, either in the provinces or in London itself.[96]

It might be thought that such widespread commercial involvement in dentistry would bring great wealth, but, although Ephraim appears to have been very successful in monetary terms, leaving nearly £12,000 at his death,[97] Charles and Lewin left under £2,000 each,[98,99] and Simeon's personal estate mounted to only £591.[100] This last surviving brother was described in his obituary as a father to the poor, a cultured Englishman of the old school, of gentle nature and keen human sympathies. A pillar of the Hull Hebrew Congregation,[101] (he was secretary of the Synagogue), he would be deservedly regretted by a large circle of friends of all religions throughout the north of England.[102] The leading rôle he appears to have played in Hull and his philanthropic acts may go some way to explaining the relatively small size of his estate.

The very presence of London based branches in the provinces suggests an expansion of the market there for dental treatment (particularly in the 1840s and 1850s) and the possibility of increased competition in the capital itself. The establishment of a branch is an indication both of an opportunity seized and of the impracticality of expansion at the home base. Perhaps the London reputation of the Le Drays and the Mallans in particular made it advisable for them to expand into pastures new.

Although few in number, the members of these last two firms had a disproportionate influence on the reputation of the dental profession as a whole. Many of the complaints against 'empirics' were levelled specifically at them and they became by-words for quackery.[103] By their involvement in the swift initiation of would-be dentists, they spread their malevolent tentacles into the provinces.

NOTES AND REFERENCES

1   See **A note on sources** (p.1 *et seq.*) for a discussion of the unsatisfactory nature of 1841 and 1851 census material.

2   *Br.J.dent.Sci.*, 1(1856-57), 185.

3   A. Hill, *The history of the reform movement in the dental profession in Great Britain* (1877), 87.

4   If the provincial total of practices is put at about 500 in 1856 and that for London at about 350 (from trade directories), this leaves a potential total for assistants of 50, using Rymer's estimates.

5   J. Gray, *Dental practice* (1837), 15.

6   *ibid.,* 9. London trade directories show an increase from 69 dentists in 1821 to 290 in 1851. (Sources: Robson, *London commercial directory* (1821) and Kelly, *P.O. London directory* (1851)).

7   An address to a conference of dentists in Edinburgh, 6 October 1877, reported in *Br.J.dent.Sci*, 20(1877), 603.

8   Statements about manpower status are based on a complete survey of all provincial trade directories published before 1856. See introduction for a description of the principles on which this was conducted.

9   Calculated from London trade directories.

10   Defined as a greater number of dentists than in any other previous year.

11   This early period might well be thought to be that most affected by a lack of directory evidence. Whilst some directories must undoubtedly have disappeared, there are nevertheless a number of towns with surviving directories from the 18th century which specifically show the absence of a resident dentist. Brighton, Cardiff, Carlisle, Leeds, Newcastle upon Tyne, Sheffield, Shrewsbury, Southampton and York all have directories which have yielded such negative results. Seven of the towns with dentists in the late 18th century (Bath, Birmingham, Bristol, Chester, Hull, Liverpool and Manchester) show negative results before positive ones, which would suggest that resident dentistry was a new phenomenon even in the large places where it might be expected to appear first.

12   Brighton, Burton on Trent, Newcastle upon Tyne, Preston, Reading, Romsey, Sheffield, Southampton, Stonehouse.

13   Barnsley, Berwick, Burslem, Bury St. Edmunds, Carlisle, Derby, Ipswich, Leamington Spa, Lincoln, North Shields, Plymouth, Portsea, Sleatord, Shrewsbury, Weymouth, York.

14   Bolton, Braintree, Cambridge, Canterbury, Chatham, Cheltenham, Chichester, Devonport, Dover, Gateshead, Guernsey, Hastings, Henley, Hereford, Isle of Man, Isle of Wight, Oxford, Portsmouth, Rochdale, Salisbury, St. Helier, Sunderland, Taunton, Tunbridge Wells, Uxbridge, Woolwich, Yarmouth.

15   Banbury, Barnstaple, Birkenhead, Blackburn, Bradford, Brecon, Bridgewater, Camborne, Colchester, Coventry, Croydon, Darlington, Devizes, Dodbrook, Eastbourne, East Grinstead, Gloucester, Gravesend, Greenwich, Guildford, Hanley, Huddersfield, Kendal, Kingsbridge, King's Lynn, Kingston, Lancaster, Landport, Lewisham, Louth, Ludlow, Macclesfield, Maidstone, Margate, New Alresford, Northampton, Penzance, Poole, Richmond (Surrey), Ripon, Ross, Runcorn, Spilsby, Stockton on Tees, Stockport, Stowmarket, Stratford on Avon, Swansea, Tavistock,

Teignmouth, Torquay, Truro, Warwick, Whitchurch, Wigan, Wolverhampton, Worthing, Yeovil.

16   Abergavenny, Alderney, Aylesbury, Bedford, Boroughbridge, Brampton, Bromley, Bury, Cardiff, Chelmsford, Chepstow, Chertsey, Doncaster, Dorchester, Dorking, Durham, Enfield, Evesham, Pakenham, Falmouth, Penny Stratford, Folkestone, Foulsham, Frome, Hanwell, Heaton Norris, Hertford, High Wycombe, Huntingdon, Lewes, Liskeard, Loughborough, Lyme Regis, Malvern, Melcombe Regis, Monmouth, Newark, Newbury, Reigate, Retford, Rochester, Saffron Walden, Scarborough, Shepton Mallet, Southsea, Stafford, Stoke on Trent, Tetsworth, Tipton, Wakefield, Whitehaven, Winchester, Wisbeach, Woburn.

17   Beverley, Buckingham, Chesterfield, Dawlish, Dunstable, Exmouth, Hartlepool, Mansfield, Newcastle under Lyme, Newport (Mon.), Penrith, Shelton, Shipley, Sleaford, South Shields, Wimborne.

18   11,000 was the median population size for a town with its first dentist in the 1820s. By 1850-55, this had fallen to 6,000. The overall median was 9,000.

19   P.S. Brown, 'Notes on some advertising dentists in the 18th century', *Notes and Queries for Somerset and Dorset*, 30(1977), 278-282.

20   A.D.M. Phillips and J.R. Walton, 'The distribution of personal wealth in English towns in the mid-nineteenth century', *Trans.Inst.Brit.Geogr.*, 64(1975), 35-48.

21   They point out that many small towns are omitted from the study.

22   'Suaviter et Fortiter', 'Quackery and country practice', *Br.J.dent.Sci.*, 2(1858), 49. The author may be S. Phillips, the only dentist listed as living in Tavistock in Kelly's *P.O. Directory of Devonshire* (1856).

23   e.g. many of the dentists visiting the Isle of Man were from Liverpool, Edinburgh and Glasgow.

24   Anne Tupholme.

25   Howard Plattin.

26   G.A. Cranfield, *The development of the provincial press, 1700-1760* (Oxford, 1962), 23.

27   *ibid.*, 27.

28   C. Robinson, 'Dental manpower ratios: factors influencing dentists' choice of practice location' (unpublished M.Sc.(Community Dentistry) dissertation, University of Manchester (1978), 51).

29   'Nemo', 'Professional reminiscences', *Quart.J.dent.Sci.*, 1(1857), 209.

30   Those dentists with their own practices and whose names appear in trade directories. Even when the figures are corrected to take into account a possible 20% underestimation of the directory evidence, the ratios remain substantially of the same order (1: 165,000 to 1: 22,000).

31   From Registrar General, *Report of the 1861 census* (1861), table 15: 'Population of England and Wales (exclusive of Army, Navy and Merchant Service abroad) estimated to the middle of each of the years 1801 to 1861'. It should be pointed out here that the number of dentists did not simply increase in line with the rapid growth of population over this same period. Dentistry was set on a course of expansion, unlike some other paramedical specialties, such as cupping, which was simultaneously in decline and had almost disappeared by 1850.

32   From British Dental Association, *Dental manpower requirements to 2020* (1982).

33   e.g. Pilleau in the first decade; Jullion 'at the sign of the deficient and rectified heads' in the 1750s; Scardovi in the 1780s (T. Purland, *Dental memoranda [Purland scrapbook]*, MS 63518 Wellcome Institute, 63, 72, 79).

34   Foreign-sounding names still appear in London trade directories in the early part of the 19th century: Bourquin, Landzelle, Ravizzotti and Finzi.

35   e.g. Grimaldi, 'many years in Paris' (*ABG*, 18 June 1759); Moor, 'native of Berlin' (*ibid.*, 28 July 1777); C. Anthony Therenez, 'pupil to the late ... Mr. Mouton, Dentist to ... Louis XV' (*ibid.*, 7 May 1785); Mr. and Mrs. Sedmon, 'of Berlin' (*LMJ*, 14 and 21 Dec 1776).

36   e.g. H. Samuel of Hamburg (*Leicester Journal [LJ]*, 5 Mar 1813) and the Mallans touring the provinces from the 1820s.

37   Here he lived in some style, counting the Duke of Gloucester among his invited guests to a supper in 1809 (Sir George Jackson, *The Bath archives-diaries and letters*, ed. Lady Jackson (1873), 32-33. Quoted by P.S. Brown, 'Notes on some advertising dentists').

38   Some of his early directory entries name him as 'Pierre Michel'.

39   B. Williams, *The making of Manchester Jewry* (1976), 124.

40   Samuel died in Chester in 1865, Louis in Göttingen in 1863.

41   Williams 1976, 197. Dreschfeld, very involved in local political and religious affairs, was a founder member of Manchester Dental Hospital.

42   *Leeds Mercury (LM)*, 4 Jan 1840. He disappears from the provinces after 1855 but died in London in 1869.

43   *Forceps*, 1(1844-45), 230.

44   W. Cooper, *Post Office directory of Southampton* (1847).

45   *Liv M*, 3 Feb 1831.

46   R. Ward, *North of England directory* (1853).

47   W. White, *Directory and gazetteer of Leeds & the clothing districts of Yorkshire* (1853).

48   e.g. Bew in Chester (*CC*, 22 Mar 1805); Leigh in Banbury (*Jackson's Oxford Journal*, 14 Jan 1826, *MCC* 504); King and Lyon in Kent (*Kentish Gazette*, 15 July 1834, *Kent Herald*, 27 June 1839, *MCC* 734); Normansell in Northampton (*Northampton Herald*, 29 Feb 1840, *MCC* 744).

49   *Morning Herald*, 3 June 1824, *MCC* 450.

50   *J.Br.Dent.Assoc.*, 2(1881), 309.

51   *Liv M*, 15 Aug 1828.

52   Ward 1853.

53   W. Leppard, *Brighton and Hove directory* (1845).

54   G. Rowe, *Illustrated Cheltenham Guide* (1845).

55   e.g. William Hunt -Plymouth/Yeovil (*Br.dent.J.*, 26(1905), 638); James Orrock -Leicester/Nottingham (*Br.dent.J.*, 34(1913), 550); Thomas Sheffield -Carlisle/Exeter (*J.Br.Dent.Assoc.*, 5(1884), 697); Thomas Gill Palmer -Southampton/Peterborough (*Br.J.dent.Sci.*, 18(1875), 685).

56   That Liverpool, Manchester and Birmingham felt the effects of this mobility to a greater extent than other cities may be seen as reflecting the expansive phase through which they were passing. It is noticeable that Bristol shows only 4 cases of moves made by established dentists in nearly 100 years (2 losses and 2 gains).

57   Known moves to and from London, moves within the provinces and the inclusion of a nominal representative of each of the families thought to have practised in both London and the provinces.

---

58   *Forceps*, 1(1844-45), 123.
59   74 provincially based, 41 London based.
60   J. Williams, *Directory of the principal market towns in Hertfordshire* (1850).
61   Craven, *Commercial directory of the county of Huntingdon and the town of Cambridge* (1855).
62   Directory advertisements have been disregarded for this purpose as their survival is a matter of pure chance. They were frequently removed by libraries before a directory was permanently bound.
63   e.g. the Clarke family's branch in Mansfield and G.A. Manne's in Beverley.
64   e.g. W.K. Bridgman's branch in King's Lynn and James Prew's in Bristol.
65   Ward 1853.
66   *Cheltenham Free Press and Gloucestershire Herald*, 16 May 1835. (Tibbs was visiting the town from London at this date). The occasional advertisement is found for managers: e.g. *Br.J.dent.Sci.*, 1(1856-57), 197, where A.J.R. of Hereford seeks such a post.
67   *Liv M*, 23 Mar 1832. Williams states that Frederick Eskell of Manchester sent out members of the firm to satellite towns in the 1840s (Williams 1976, 142).
68   Charlton and Archdeacon, *Directory of Leeds* (1849).
69   J. Smith, *Topography of Maidstone and its environs* (1839).
70   I. Slater, *Directory...of Yorkshire and Lincolnshire* (1839).
71   M. Billing, *Directory and Gazetteer of Devonshire* (1857).
72   *Worcester Herald*, 10 Oct 1840.
73   I. Slater, *Directory...of...Lincolnshire...*(1850).
74   Moncrieff, *Visitors' new guide* (1822).
75   The gross 1839 income (£924) from operating the Bristol branch for two days a week might be compared with the resources of Thomas Carlyle's household in 1834, namely £300 (quoted by J. Burnett, *A history of the cost of living* (1969), 235).
76   Thomas Eden, John William Mitchell, T. and W. Read, J.V. Cherriman. Thomas Henry Harding appears for one year (1851) in a directory of Richmond, Surrey.
77   *Courier*, 16 Sept 1828 (*MCC* 1057).
78   W. Robson, *Classification of trades and street guide* (1829).
79   I.T. Hinton, *The watering places of Great Britain ...* (1831).
80   e.g. *Kentish Observer*, 19 June 1834; *Kentish Gazette*, 17 June 1834.
81   Canterbury, Ramsgate, Dover, Maidstone and Tunbridge Wells.
82   *Liv M*, 13 June 1834.
83   *Purland scrapbook*, 104. Purland also identifies De Berri as being part of 'Le Dray' (120).
84   60, Newman Street (J. Pigot, *London ... directory* (1836)).
85   e.g. *Liv M*, 4 Aug 1837.
86   e.g. *Forceps*, 1(1844-45), 135.
87   *Age*, 25 Aug 1837 (*MCC* 720): 'established 1826'. Mallan claimed to have been a pupil of Monsieur Valade and to have treated English visitors to Paris (*Courier*, 24 Mar 1828 (*MCC* 1074)).
88   *Forceps*, 1(1844-45), 195.
89   e.g. *Warwick and Warwickshire General Advertiser and Leamington Gazette*, 1 Oct 1831 (visits to Warwick, Leamington and Birmingham); *Liv M*, 23 Nov 1832 (visits to Liverpool and Manchester); *Bath Journal*, 2 Feb

1829.
90   It would appear that the mechanical work was sometimes sent back to London (F. White, *General directory of Hull* (1846) (*MCC* 775)).
91   Blackburn, Carlisle, Kendal, Preston, Penrith and Liverpool (with Lewin).
92   Hull (with Simeon), Newcastle (with Simeon or with his own son), Stockton on Tees (sometimes with his son), South Shields, Durham, Darlington, Hartlepool, Sunderland (with his son), Bath, Dunstable. He also had a branch in Paris.
93   Exeter, Newbury, Reading, Torquay, Banbury, Cardiff and Liverpool (with Charles).
94   King's Lynn, Hull (with Ephraim), Newcastle (with Ephraim), Wolverhampton (with Drake), Newcastle under Lyme (with Drake) and Scarborough.
95   Ephraim had three sons in dentistry: Benjamin Ephraim Mosely, Alexander Mosely Morley [sic], Alfred Isaiah Mosely. The last, who carried on the practice in Newcastle, died in the cause of duty while travelling by railway from Calais to the Paris branch in 1879 (*Calendar of Probate*, 1880).
96   All the Moselys did not remain based in the capital for the whole of their careers; whilst Lewin's permanent address at death was in London, Charles was living in Preston when he died, Simeon in Hull and Ephraim in Paris.
97   *Calendar of Probate*, 1874.
98   *ibid.*, 1861.
99   *ibid.*, 1875.
100   *ibid.*, 1889.
101   Williams 1976, 243.
102   *Jewish Chronicle*, 16 Nov 1888.
103   Purland's comment on a 1769 advertisement for Hamilton's tincture: 'beats Ledray or Mallan' (*Purland's Scrapbook*, 76).

CHAPTER 4: TREATMENT

Before about 1840, most English dentists acquired their techniques in a somewhat haphazard and pragmatic manner, either in imitation of claims made in other dentists' advertising pamphlets or from their preceptor during apprenticeship. There appear to have been no contemporary translations of major works by foreign writers[1] and the few books of worth in English on the anatomy, physiology and treatment of the teeth[2] comment only very generally on restorative and prosthetic techniques. Bell[3] has more to say on the filling of teeth, but like Robertson[4] he does not discuss artificial replacements. The early dentist had to wait until 1839 before the need for a textbook of dentistry in English was fulfilled by Chapin Harris's *The Dental Art* .[5] This was followed in 1846 by Robinson's *Surgical, Mechanical and Medical Treatment of the Teeth* [6] which gave step-by-step instructions in dental techniques.

However, this dearth of reliable literature did not deter dentists from attempting to provide remedies for much the same problems as confront their modern counterparts: they offered to extract, restore, regularise and replace teeth and to treat periodontal diseases. The limits imposed upon them were the absence of anaesthetics, unsophisticated materials, hand instruments and a lack of knowledge of the aetiology and pathology of dental disease.[7] There was still radical disagreement as to the cause of caries; the proponents of toothworms and inflammation of the pulp as the initiating cause still had their followers, despite the arguments of Robertson in 1835 who convincingly demonstrated that caries began externally, in the enamel. There was gross confusion over the disease processes observable in periodontal conditions. Not until considerably later was there an agreed consensus on the pathology of dental disease.

Unsolved problems promote diverse attempts at their solution. Dentists jealously kept their trade secrets to themselves and there must have been a wide variation in the treatments offered to the patient, for each of which some theory could be called upon for support. Whether the average provincial dentist, with his frequently inadequate training and limited access to dental literature, was able to execute the available techniques proficiently, or even safely, depended very much on the level of his skill, experience and willingness to exercise his powers of observation rather than to perpetuate ill-founded procedures. An American visitor in 1859 summed up his observations on English dentists thus:[8] 'They appear greatly wedded to old practices, and altogether inclined to follow leaders, to do this or that in consequence of some personal precedent much apart from all question of merit'.

Filing

The practice of filing the teeth exemplifies the diversity of practice arising from differences of understanding of the nature of decay. Fox and Bell recommend filing to prevent caries, being of the opinion that it was lateral pressure from other teeth which initiated decay. Gray deprecated this, pointing out that close contact points were natural and that filing only produced additional places for the stagnation of food debris. Bell, since he believed that caries began on the surface of the dentine and spread outwards to the enamel, considered that the minimum of enamel need be removed with the file; Robertson, on the other hand, who rightly observed that caries began in the enamel, considered that in dealing with small cavities on the sides of teeth, inaccessible to contemporary excavators and filling instruments, it was essential to remove enough tooth substance to render the surrounding area level with the bottom of the carious cavity, thus ensuring that 'no lodgement can take place in that situation for the future'.[9] He emphasised that filing is most appropriate in the early stages of decay, when the procedure will only involve the enamel.

The over-zealous or misguided use of the file as practised by many dentists of the day may well have led to hypersensitivity where dentine was exposed or to further decay when only the caries was removed, providing an ideal niche for the lodging of food debris.

Filling

The decay was scraped away with hand instruments and the cavity plugged with one of a variety of filling materials. Robertson was very scathing of those who did not consider it necessary to remove all the caries in the belief that it was only necessary to exclude the air to prevent recurrence of the decay. He pointed out that caries will continue to spread underneath the filling material. Gray, on the other hand, was of the opinion that dentists were overprescribing in this field, bemoaning[10]

> the iniquitous system of filing and picking holes in the sound teeth...for no other apparent purpose than that of affording themselves the opportunity of plugging up these holes of their own making. In the hollows of the grinding surfaces of the side or molar teeth, some dark specks are seen, or supposed to be seen; the patient is gravely told that these specks will degenerate into holes, to prevent which they must be dug out, by way of eradicating the disease, and the cavities thus formed stopped with gold. So a hole is to be made in the tooth to prevent the tooth from making a hole in itself......certain dentists perceive in these specks *fees for stopping.*

On the one hand it would appear that caries was not always sufficiently removed whilst on the other cavities were being opened up by dentists who may not have been capable of filling them adequately to prevent caries recurring.

Gold foil was the material of choice as a filling material, although early dentists also used silver, platinum and lead for this purpose. Because of the expense of gold, a number of cheaper substitutes and amalgams were being tried out in the early nineteenth century, to the disapprobation of such commentators as Levison who revealed their contents in a letter to the *Lancet* in 1831.[11] 'Mineral cement' he described as being composed of bismuth, tin and lead; 'terro-metallic cement' was three parts calcium sulphate and one of rust of iron; 'mineral succedaneum' was made up of silver filings mixed with mercury. Levison considered that all these filling materials were unstable chemically and soon crumbled in the mouth. Bismuth, tin, lead and mercury are all highly toxic in the appropriate concentrations. Fillings composed of these materials, if the results were as impermanent as Levison maintained, can have brought the patient no ultimate benefit and probably positive harm. Contemporary advertisements, however, show the various 'cements' in wide use in the early nineteenth century.

A well-executed gold filling, inserted in the manner recommended by Levison and Robertson, with all the decay removed and the metal tightly plugged into the carefully dried cavity, might well last as many years as would a modern one; however, contemporary comment makes it clear that many dentists lacked either the skill or the knowledge to carry out such a technique.

Crowns

Harris described the technique of fitting a new crown to an existing root as one that has 'on account of its simplicity, been more extensively practised than any other method of inserting artificial teeth',[12] and yet it is one which, from the present-day point of view, must have presented the early dentist with a host of opportunities for failure.   It was a procedure which had evolved from ill-fated attempts in the eighteenth century to transplant complete teeth[13] and was performed where the crown of a tooth was beyond restoration but where the root remained sound.   The remains of the decayed crown were removed with files and excising forceps and the nerve destroyed with a pointed instrument or a hot wire.   These last were inserted only as far up the root canal as was necessary for the accommodation of the post which was to bear the new crown.   (Robinson suggests that the patient should be allowed to rinse out the mouth at this stage with warm water containing a few drops of laudanum).   After further enlargement of the canal, the new crown, natural or porcelain, was then prepared so that it fitted on to the root perfectly.   The post, or 'pivot', was then inserted in the root and the prosthesis pressed firmly home.

Many stages during this procedure were fraught with potential failure.   Modern orthodoxy considers that any nerve tissue remaining behind in the root canal if not already necrotic soon becomes so and is a potential focus for infection leading to apical abscesses, bone loss and apical cysts.   No attempt was made to fill the root canal and seal it completely at the apex, now considered to be essential to the success of the procedure.   The risk of cross-infection throughout must have been high, given that there was no sterilisation of instruments and modern antibiotics were unknown.

Early dentists were themselves aware that this operation could result in infection.   Harris recommends that 'sufficient time should elapse for the subsidence of any irritation that this operation may have occasioned, previously to the placing of the tooth.   A neglect of this precaution not infrequently gives rise to inflammation of the periosteum of the root, and alveolar process'.[14]   He suggests making a groove in the pivot to afford drainage for infection.

Considerable skill was needed to obtain a perfect fit between root surface and crown, since no mention is made of the use of any cement between the two parts which might have accommodated slight inaccuracies and made for an air-tight seal.   An irregularity at the

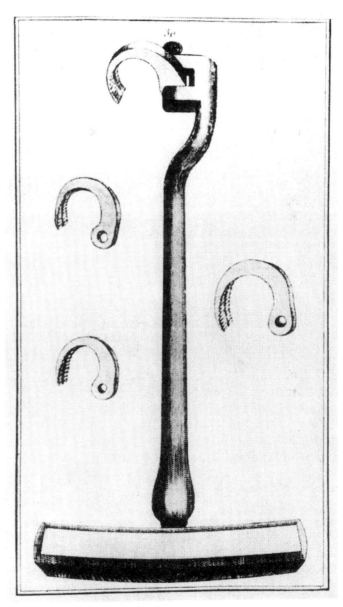

illus. 1: Key, with interchangeable claws
(L. Laforgue, *L'art du dentiste*, Paris, 1802)

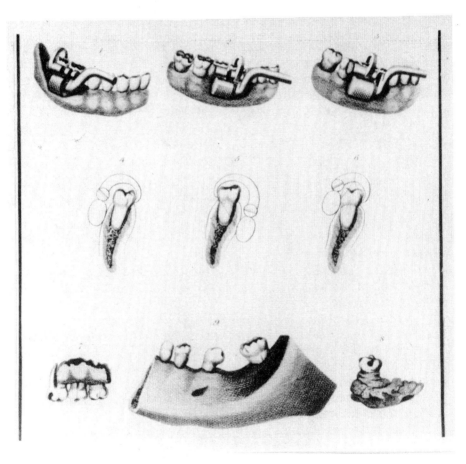

illus. 2: The use of the dental key
(J. Fox, *The history and treatment of the diseases of the teeth*,
London, 1806)

junction of the two would promote stagnation of food debris and hence caries and periodontal disease. When the technique was extended to include a bridge,[15] then the problem of stagnation could be compounded without careful design.

Harris and Robinson favoured gold for use as the pivot but hickory was frequently used for this purpose, its properties of expansion in a moist environment being relied upon for retention in the root. Such a practice was also known to split the root.

At the hands of a skilled and knowledgeable operator, such a crown prosthesis may well, with good fortune, have lasted for years. Apical cysts may have developed but since they are generally painless, the patient may have enjoyed many years' service from such a restoration. Undoubtedly, there must have been cases of apical abscesses resulting from the treatment, some as a direct result of ignorance on the part of the dentist.

Extraction

> The extraction of a tooth, if conducted by a skilful hand, is a safe and easy operation; but, if attempted by the unskilful, may occasion the most frightful and dangerous consequences.[16]

When it was to be performed without the benefit of anaesthesia, there was, perhaps, even greater need for the dentist to be a quick and efficient operator.

Horrific tales are to be found in dental literature of fractured jaws and of whole groups of teeth unintentionally extracted at the hands of the inept. Some of the lack of success can be laid at the door of the instrument most frequently used in England at the time, the key (*illus. 1 and 2*). It looked rather like an old-fashioned corkscrew, except that where the screw should be there was provision for the attachment of a claw at right angles to the shaft. With this claw hooked round the offending tooth and the shaft resting against the gum, the handle of key instrument was then turned through 180° and the tooth removed sideways.

That there were so many individual modifications made to the design of the key indicates that it was not in itself the ideal extracting instrument. Its mode of action made it more damaging to the tissues than the modern forceps, the greatest hazard being the fracture of the alveolar process against which the fulcrum was levered. If a claw of the incorrect size was applied, there was a high risk of the tooth fracturing. It also had the disadvantage of operating in one direction only; the tooth could not be rotated in the socket to separate the adherent fibres prior to extraction, as with forceps. Although this last instrument was gaining ground as the implement of choice by 1850, the key remained the most commonly used. By its very design it seems likely to have made extraction a more traumatic operation than it is in the present day, especially as it was often wielded by those with only the most cursory knowledge of anatomy and mechanics.

Orthodontic treatment

Offers to 'regulate' the dentition of both adults and children were widespread. Particularly in the eighteenth century, much is made of the possibility of a 'double row' of teeth in children and the necessity of consulting a dentist regularly, especially when the permanent teeth are erupting. The orthodontic techniques of the late eighteenth and early nineteenth centuries were, in essence, no different from present-day procedures. They aimed to correct overcrowding, anterior cross-bite and class 3 malocclusion (where the lower teeth project in front of the upper) and, in addition to judicious extraction, employed prototypes of the modern appliances to do so. Arches were widened by expansion plates of gold or ivory and bite planes used to separate the jaws, affording space into which realigned teeth could move.

If carried out by a knowledgeable dentist, there was every likelihood of success. Bell, however, was of the opinion that this expertise was often lacking. This was particularly evident where deciduous teeth were extracted too early, actually promoting the crowding which the procedure was designed to prevent. And we have already seen the disastrous results of a combination of half-knowledge of the principles of regulation and almost total ignorance of the anatomy of the mouth in the case of the eight year old girl deprived of four erupting permanent incisors (p.34). Overzealous intervention also manifested itself in the excessive use of the file to relieve a minor degree of overcrowding, often with the potentially harmful effects we saw earlier. So routine was this practice in the 1830s that Gray stated that children at boarding schools were having their teeth filed without the prior knowledge of their parents, 'their first information on the subject being derived from the item in the bill of school charges'.[17]

Artificial teeth

The main claim made for artificial teeth in the late eighteenth and early nineteenth centuries was that they would not be distinguished from natural ones. If the individual human crowns attached to existing roots (described earlier) are included in 'artificial teeth', then this assertion could probably be made with some justification by a skilled dentist, even though the replacement crowns were of necessity non-vital and so lacking in translucence. The same might perhaps be said for those partial appliances consisting only of teeth, with no attempt to replace the gum. Less convincing must have been the full dentures with teeth mounted on an ivory or gold plate. Ivory soon changed its appearance in the mouth and where the teeth were also carved from ivory, a most unnatural appearance must soon have been produced. Any colour applied to the gum area had a very short life and the early enamelled gum prostheses were not entirely convincing. The production of porcelain teeth obviated some of these deficiencies but it was some time before they became aesthetically acceptable replacements for natural teeth.

Features of the design of dentures of the period made them less likely to be successful as appliances than their modern counterparts. The poor impression materials available to the early dentist (beeswax for most of the period, used without an impression tray until the 1820s) must have made most dentures a poor fit and hence led to traumatic ulceration of the oral mucosa in load-bearing areas.

Before the realisation that a complete upper denture was best retained by extending the prosthesis over the palate, such appliances were normally held in position by spiral springs joining the denture and a swivel device fixed on to the lower teeth or denture. This frequently resulted in traumatisation of the cheek. Partial dentures were attached to adjacent teeth by silk ligatures or gold or ivory clasps, both capable of stripping the gum and the second of exerting deleterious lateral pressure on the teeth to which they were fixed, leading to potential further tooth loss. Gray was particularly scathing about the havoc wrought with clasps and ligatures by the ignorant or unscrupulous dentist of the 1830s.[18]

It is clear from advertisements that dentures were often fitted over retained roots or stumps; potential patients were assured that it was not necessary to undergo the ordeal of extraction before artificial teeth could be fitted. As in the case of crowns, there was no attempt to fill the root first, as modern orthodoxy would require. Apart from the possible reservoir of infection contained in the roots, the main deficiency of this technique lay again in the limitations of the materials available to the early dentist. A precise fit to the irregular surface of the mouth would have been unlikely with a beeswax impression and a base carved freehand from ivory; a denture produced using these materials could be expected to be painful to the wearer, especially if he attempted to wear it to eat with.

Periodontal disease

The accumulation of salivary calculus on the teeth was seen as a condition in itself. Writers accurately described the results of its accretion to the teeth (loss of gum and resorption of bone) but, with no knowledge of the existence of plaque and its bacterial content, wrongly assumed that the process was a purely mechanical one, with the growing bulk of calculus separating the gum from the tooth. Plaque was on occasions described, but only because it was considered to be the first stages of calculus.

The standard treatment recommended was scaling until all calculus had been removed, the use of an astringent[19] and regular, thorough brushing to prevent its re-establishment. The use of strong acids to dissolve the calculus was universally condemned by writers, although there is ample advertising evidence of their being used for this purpose, particularly in the eighteenth century, even after 1768 when Berdmore had demonstrated their disastrous effects on the enamel.

Offers to fasten the loose teeth consequent on periodontal disease featured prominently in early advertisements. However, since the means employed was to attach them by ligatures and wires to adjacent teeth, the problems must have been compounded.

Most early dentists promised to cure 'scurvy of the gums'.[20] This can be identified as embracing the modern concepts chronic periodontitis and acute ulcerative gingivitis. Although Bell saw 'scurvy' as constitutional in origin, it was generally thought to arise from such local irritation as a dead or loose tooth, calculus or irregular teeth. It was not appreciated that these were the likely sites for the collection of plaque. The remedy advocated was the removal of such irritants; in the case of calculus, this could only have been beneficial, but many sound teeth must have been lost in the course of the treatment without the realisation that it was the plaque which needed to be removed, not the sites of its collection.

Scarification and the application of leeches were also practised to reduce swelling of the gums, probably to little effect. Harris was an advocate of gingivectomy where the gums were grossly enlarged, a technique still used for this condition. However, surgical procedures carried out with no knowledge of the germ theory of disease must have carried a high risk of cross-infection and recurrence.

Treatment offered in a Bath practice in 1843

Throughout the period up to 1850, most dentists advertised their services at some time in their careers, with varying degrees of flamboyance. Any assumption that these offers of treatment were mere exaggeration and that in reality 'dentists' were self-advertising toothdrawers, is dispelled by an examination of the account books of James Prew (in practice in Bath and Bristol from the 1820s until 1846).[21] Although somewhat haphazardly organised, these accounts afford useful insight into the practice of dentistry in the provinces at the period:

type of treatment	number of cases[22]
prosthetic	82
extraction	72
plumbing (filling)	20
pivot crown	11
cleaning	15
filing	4
'operations'	113

table 1: Treatment carried out by Prew in 1843

About half the prosthetic cases (40) in 1843 involved the provision of small partial dentures (usually of only one or two teeth) or the replacement of broken teeth on old dentures. A further 20 larger prostheses were made (described as 'pieces'), ranging in price from £3 – £14 (average about £5). During the year Prew made, rather surprisingly, only eight complete sets, usually at a fee of £20. The remainder of the prosthetic cases involved repairs to springs or remaking old dentures, by fitting new ivory blocks[23] or new teeth to an old plate.

Prew appears to have been using mineral (porcelain) teeth for most of his prostheses at this date, natural teeth being specifically mentioned in only eight cases. Receipted bills survive for his purchases of mineral teeth from Claudius Ash[24] and Thomas Smale[25] in 1843 and from Thomas Lemale in 1844.[26]

Because the teeth treated are not identified, it is difficult to see whether Prew's prosthetic intervention caused further loss of teeth. Whilst cases can be identified of the fitting of pivot teeth or partial dentures being succeeded by the extraction of teeth or the insertion of a 'piece', it cannot be said with certainty whether the same teeth were involved in both instances.

It might be thought that extracting teeth would form a major part of Prew's dental practice in 1843. In fact, he had, on average, only 1.4 cases per week. Even fewer were the number of fillings he appears to have inserted, only 20 patients in the entire year. He was, however, no stranger to filling teeth. On 31 October 1845 Prew notes with evident pleasure, 'saw a tooth I plumbed 20 years.' A bill from Lemale for January 1843[27] shows him purchasing both gold leaf and '4 oz fine grain silver', both of which might be used as filling materials. Pivot crowns also seem to have formed an insignificant part of his practice, as did cleaning and filing the teeth.

However, by far the most frequent entry in Prew's book is 'operations'. This seems likely to represent mixed treatments; unfortunately, since his fees for the same procedure vary, perhaps with the complexity of the task in hand, it is not possible to decide which treatments were performed on those patients who received 'operations'. The average fee for this category was £2 (the median £1.15.6.) which makes it unlikely that any major work was being undertaken. The fact that there were 40 different charges made for 'operations' lends weight to the suggestion that these represent individual combinations of items of treatment. Scaling and treatment of the gums seem likely candidates for inclusion in the category, since both could be expected to be in demand. Occasionally the entry 'operations' is followed by one recording the sale of 'lotion', 'brush' or 'dentifrice', suggesting that in these cases, at least, scaling had been performed, followed by advice on oral hygiene.

Some of the extractions Prew performed in 1843 were on children, probably to regulate the teeth to relieve crowding, but there were no cases of orthodontic appliances in that year. These were a rarity in Prew's practice, with only the occasional case being recorded, as when in 1840 Miss Pooley had two teeth extracted on 27 July and the following day her teeth were filed and 'regulated with a plate'.[28] Miss Graham was another of the select band of orthodontic patients: on 28 September 1842 she had two teeth extracted and her front teeth 'regulated on the silver plate'.[29]

Fees charged by provincial dentists

	A	B	C a	C b	C c	C d	D	E	F single	F set
18th century										
Paul Jullion[30]	2.6.	10.6.	5.0.	7.6.	---	---	2.6.	2-5gn	10.6-3gn	10-30gn
Grimaldi[31]	---	10.6.	5.0.	10.6.	---	---	---	---	10.6.	---
James Blair[32]	---	5.0.	---	5.0.	2.6.	---	---	1gn	10.6-1gn	20gn
Crawcour[33]	2.6.	---	---	2.6.	---	---	---	---	1gn	---
1830s										
J.H. Wilcock[34]	---	5.0.	---	2.6.	2.6.	3.0.	---	---	---	---
De Berri[35]	---	---	---	---	---	2.6.	---	---	5.0.	£4-20gn
Le Dray[36]	---	---	---	---	---	---	---	---	10.0.	5-20gn
1840s										
James Prew[37]	2.6.-2gn	10.6.-£2	---	2.6.-£2	---	---	2.6.-£1	£1-2	10.6.-£1.10.0.	£20
James Evatt[38]	---	2.0.	---	2.6.	---	---	---	---	5-10.0.	£5-15gn
J.C. Browne[39]	1.0.	2.6.	---	2.6.	---	1.0.	---	---	10-15.0.	£5-20
Isaiah Jones[40]	---	---	---	5.0.	---	---	---	---	10.0.	£5+
F. Richeraud[41]	---	5.0.-1gn	---	2.6.	---	---	---	---	7.6.-1gn	5-20gn
1850s										
Charles Smartt[42]	---	---	---	2.6.	---	---	---	---	5.0.	£5-10
R.H. Wall[43]	---	3.6.-5.0.	---	5.0.	---	2.6.	---	---	3.6.-18.6	---
H. Lyon[44]	---	5.0.	---	2.6.-3.6.	---	---	---	---	10.6.-1gn	---

key: A extraction D filing
B cleaning/scaling E crown
C a lead b gold c silver d cement F artificial teeth

table 2: Specimen fees (in pre-decimal currency) charged in the 18th century, the 1830s, 1840s and 1850s

Although there was variation, depending on the difficulty of the case, the materials used and the value placed by the individual dentist on his services, fees remained substantially the same over a long period.   It will be seen from *table 5* that some dentists were reticent to advertise their fees for disagreeable operations such as extractions, but this is no indication in itself that they did not perform them.

The greatest variation in fees is to be seen in those charged for artificial teeth.   The maximum price of about £20 remained the standard charge for a set of teeth on a gold plate.   The lower charges reflect the use of various types of ivory.   Robinson pointed out (in 1846) that 'the *cheap* teeth commonly advertised at £5 or £10 a set' were made of hippopotamus ivory, for which the inferior walrus ivory was often substituted.[45]   The single artificial teeth referred to included those made of porcelain by the 1830s.   Most cost the dentist 1s.6d. each in the 1840s.

The variety of fees for fillings is again a reflection of the materials used.   Dentists of the eighteenth century were more specific than their successors;   many of the charges quoted for fillings in the 1840s and 1850s were probably for 'mineral paste' restorations, so decried by Levison but very popular with the advertising dentist.

NOTES AND REFERENCES

1   e.g. P. Fauchard, *Le chirurgien dentiste* (1728).
2   e.g. J. Hunter, *The natural history of the human teeth* (1771) and *A practical treatise on the diseases of the teeth* (1778); J. Fox, *The history and treatment of the diseases of the teeth* (1806).
3   T. Bell, *The anatomy, physiology and diseases of the teeth* (1829).
4   W. Robertson, *Practical treatise on the human teeth* (1835), 4th ed. 1846.
5   C.A. Harris, *The dental art, a practical treatise on dental surgery* (1839).   Although produced in the United States, this had a wide circulation in England.
6   J. Robinson, *The surgical, mechanical, and medical treatment of the teeth* (1846).
7   The following brief outline is based on the writings of Bell, Harris, Robertson and Robinson (works likely to be available to the provincial dentist) together with the advertisements of ordinary dentists in the provincial press. A full exposition of dentistry at this period is to be found in e.g. W. Hoffmann-Axthelm, *History of dentistry* (1981).
8   *Am.Jnl.Dent.Sci.*, 9(1859), 353.

9   Robertson 1846, 119.
10   J. Gray, *Dental practice* (1837), 16.
11   J.L. Levison, 'Exposure of quackeries in dental surgery', *Lancet* (1831), 764.
12   Harris 1839, 318.
13   This was a short-lived vogue encouraged by John Hunter's suggestion of its possibility. Despite almost inevitable failure of the operation, 18th century dentists offer transplanting as one of the available treatments.
14   Harris 1839, 319.
15   Two crowns supporting a small number of replacement teeth between them to bridge a gap.
16   Harris 1839, 177.
17   Gray 1837, 22-23.
18   *ibid.*, 12. Clasps are still in use but a further 150 years of research into their use has not entirely eliminated their potential harmful effects.
19   The favourite, based on tincture of myrrh, may have had little effect on the progress of the disease but the brushing involved in its application was beneficial.
20   Recognised at the time as being unrelated to the deficiency disease.
21   *Account books (1830-46) of James Prew*, MS 5208-5214, Wellcome Library. The year 1843 has been chosen for analysis as one where it is clear that all the account holders have been listed.
22   Some of these cases may be the same patients since no names are generally given in the cash books.
23   Fitted in place of individual teeth in the molar region.
24   Prew, MS 5214/3.
25   *ibid.*, MS 5214/5.
26   *ibid.*, MS 5214/7.
27   *ibid.*, MS 5214/2.
28   *ibid.*, MS 5211, 8.
29   *ibid.*, MS 5121, 8.
30   Quoted in T. Purland, 'Dental Memoranda', *Quart.J.dent.Sci.*, 1(1857), 492.
31   *ABG*, 28 June 1773.
32   *LJ*, 8 December 1787.
33   *LMJ*, 4 February 1775.
34   Mathews, *Bristol directory* (1838).
35   *Midland Counties Herald, Birmingham and General Advertiser*, 21 June 1838.
36   *Liv M*, 11 August 1837.
37   Account books, MS 5208-5214, Wellcome Library.
38   Charlton and Archdeacon, *Directory of Leeds* (1849).
39   *ibid.*
40   Forbes and Knibb, *Directory of Southampton* (1849).
41   *Fleetwood Chronicle*, October 1845.
42   Large, *Gravesend...directory* (1851).
43   McAulay, *Berkshire Almanac* (1853).
44   Craven, *Commercial directory of the county of Huntingdon and the town of Cambridge* (1855).
45   Robinson 1846, 177-178.

CHAPTER 5: SPURS AND CONSTRAINTS

Whilst the writers of the 1830s and 1840s were aware that the numbers of dentists had increased by their day, most did not express any view on why this had come about as opposed to how it had occurred. Gray does offer some clues, but these scarcely seem adequate as a total explanation of the phenomenon. We need to look further to try to determine why this growth occurred when it did and which were the enabling and limiting factors in the spread of dentistry in provincial England.

5.1 Predisposing factors

A change in demand for treatment

This must surely be the basic factor involved. Gray himself talks of 'the increasing demand for artificial teeth'[1] which opens up a rich field for the enterprise and encouragement of ingenious mechanics. Elsewhere he remarks that[2]

> in the last century, when a person lost a tooth, even in the front of the mouth ... the space remained vacant; ... when such an accident now occurs, and the person seeking a remedy for his deficiency has the misfortune to fall into the hands of one of the unprincipled quacks with which the metropolis abounds, he is supplied with a tooth ... which the empiric fastens to the adjoining teeth, perfectly aware that such fastening will destroy them. When this is accomplished, the patient is next supplied with a piece of three teeth, which is soon followed by the like result; and, if the sufferer has the patience to go on, he is supplied with pieces more extensive in proportion to the havoc made in his teeth by the fastenings of those which are artificial.[3]...It seems a hard case that teeth should suffer in proportion to the care bestowed on them.

There may well be an element of prelapsarian nostalgia here, but if his clinical observations are true (and it seems likely that this is the case, bearing in mind the design of contemporary partial dentures held in place by ligatures), then Gray is pointing to a situation where the iatrogenic disease caused by some gives more

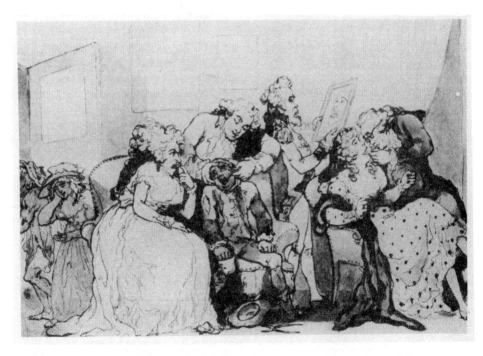

illus. 3: 'Transplanting of teeth' depicted by Rowlandson, 1787
(7766 in the *British Museum Catalogue of political and personal satires*)

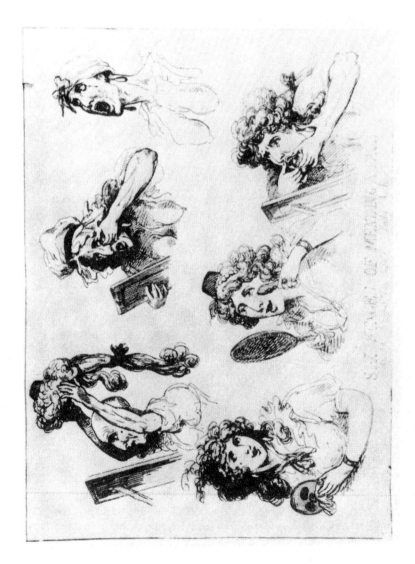

illus. 4: 'Six stages of mending a face', Rowlandson, 1792
(8174 in the *British Museum Catalogue of political and personal satires*)

opportunities to others and potentially increases the number of dentists. This is borne out by the not uncommon offer of advertising dentists to re-do the inadequate work of others: 'badly-applied Artificial Teeth remodelled', declares Eskell of Leeds;[4] 'artificial teeth out of repair Re-Modelled and made to fit to the greatest nicety', echoes Mr. Orme of London.[5]

But although poor treatment might well lead to an increase in the volume of dental work performed and thus contribute to an increase in the number of dentists needed to carry it out, this would seem to offer only a partial explanation of the ever growing numbers of provincial dentists. If disastrous treatment were the only stimulus to the doubling of the number of practices every ten years after 1810, one would surely expect to arrive at a point where dental practice began to decline, as the public at large became aware of its empty promises. This was patently not the case. It would seem that factors other than self-generating treatment were at work in promoting a change in demand.

One of Gray's most pertinent comments is that[6]

> many young persons are in the habit of attending the dentist from a mere feeling of vanity, when no real necessity exists for his services;...provided that he be a person who is supposed to be *fashionable*, his fitness for his profession is never questioned.

This link between seeking dental treatment and fashion is one which emerges from other evidence. Whereas the extraction of teeth had always been a popular target for illustrators, in the late eighteenth and early nineteenth centuries there appear a number of caricatures by artists such as Rowlandson using the subject of dental operations to satirise current fashionable society,[7] suggesting these activities were considered the current fad and something new (*illus. 3 and 4*). Extraction had always been an inevitable part of life, but restoration of lost tooth substance was to most a novelty.

Contemporary with these caricatures are a wealth of advertisements offering dental products[8] and treatments designed to beautify the mouth. Every late eighteenth and early nineteenth century newspaper seems to have its advertisement for such products, be it Hemet's Dentifrice[9] or Butler's Restorative Tooth Powder, which brings redness to the gums, sweetens the breath and renders teeth pearly white.[10] Advertisements for dentists offering artificial teeth, fillings, crowning and the removal of tartar became more

common in the provincial press. They are usually addressed to the
Ladies and Gentlemen of the town or to 'the Nobility, Gentry and a
Kind Public'.   Mr.   Moor   from   Bath   brings   to   Birmingham
'Recommendations from several Persons of Distinction ... to some of
the most eminent Families'.[11]

The emphasis is placed mainly on the cosmetic and social
benefits of seeking dental treatment.   Signor Grimaldi, with his
fashionable Paris and London connections, assures his readers that
'Persons, every other way agreeable, shall not go one Day longer with
a foul and disfigured Mouth, and interrupted Speech, proceeding from
the Loss of their Teeth, if they will apply to him'.[12]

The writers of dental tracts develop the same themes.   Edward
Breham favours the blunt approach: 'many ladies owe the acquisition
of a husband to the attraction of a beautiful set of Teeth. Without
them   the   most   regular   features   are   uninteresting,   if   not
repulsive'.[13]   He is typical of his fellow writers in referring to
his eminent patients, recounting that he has those 'who although they
annually visit the metropolis, are so well pleased with his practice,
that they delay any operation, until their return to the country'.[14]
Even the eminently respectable William Robertson of Birmingham, whose
book was of a more serious intent than most, refers to Lord Lyttleton
as a patient.[15]   Dentists enjoying royal patronage[16] were equally not
averse from advertising the fact.[17]

One comes away from the writers and advertisers of this early
period with the distinct impression that the reader is being invited
to make an association between repair of tooth loss and genteel
living, between care of the mouth and the emulation of his social
superiors.   This would seem to re-inforce the evidence of the
Rowlandson caricatures that, in the early years at least, fashion
played a not inconsiderable part in stimulating the growing demand
for the 'decency' of dental treatment, over and above the occasional
necessity of an extraction.

This change in attitude can be seen as an expression of the
consumer   revolution   of   the   eighteenth   century   identified   by
McKendrick, when, 'spurred   on   by   social   emulation   and   class
competition, men and women surrendered eagerly to the pursuit of
novelty'[18] and when the desire to spend was accompanied by an
increased ability to do so.[19]   Dental treatment can be seen as one
more of the consumer services on offer whose marketing McKendrick
chronicles.

When dentists visit towns in the late eighteenth and early nineteenth centuries, they often operate from the premises of a hairdresser,[20] toyman,[21] jeweller[22] or even a china shop,[23] thus finding their natural home among the consumer products of the day. Some of the early dentists combined one or other of these fashionable occupations with dentistry.

Many common factors can be discerned in the spread of dentistry and McKendrick's description of the commercialisation of fashion: the importance of France as a trend-setter at an early stage, London seen as the 'radiant centre of the fashion world' and the encouragement to emulate what is presented as the life style of a social élite.[24] French goldsmiths offering artificial teeth begin to appear in the London press from the beginning of the eighteenth century, vying with native-born toothdrawers and 'operators for the teeth'. The French influence on the field was considerable in the early eighteenth century, due in no small part to the publication by Pierre Fauchard in 1728 of the first book devoted entirely to a full exposition of the techniques of dental surgery.[25]

By the middle of the century the French term 'dentist' was being used, much to the disgust of the *Edinburgh Chronicle* of 15 September 1759: 'Dentist, figures it now in our newspapers and may do well enough for a French puffer, but we fancy Rutter [a prominent London dentist] is content with being called a tooth-drawer'. (Rutter's obituary in 1761 resolutely describes him as 'a famous operator for the teeth').[26] Certainly the renowned Thomas Berdmore would have agreed with the *Edinburgh Chronicle* 's view. When he died in 1785, aged 45, he left directions that his memorial tablet should declare that he 'acquired an ample fortune by tooth-drawing'. His executors presumably felt they knew better, for the actual tablet in Nottingham read, 'acquired a liberal And ample Fortune By the Profession of *Dentist*'.[27] The term 'dentist' seems to have gained ground during Berdmore's career. Advertisements in the Birmingham press from 1757[28] show 'operator' as the common term in the eleven advertisements before 1771, although Foy and Isdael describe themselves as 'surgeon dentist' in 1759. Grimaldi (1759), Whitlock (1768) and Lewis (1771) show the transition by declaring themselves 'dentist and operator', thus highlighting the new element (restoration) represented in the term 'dentist'. After 1771, the descriptions 'dentist' or 'surgeon dentist' are used.

Insufficient work has yet been done on dental advertisements in the provincial press of the early eighteenth century to be able to say with certainty whether dentistry was diffused from London to the rest of the country or arose in the provincial centres simultaneously, but certainly few opportunities were lost in advertisements to claim a London connection. This advertisement by a Norwich staymaker of 1788 could, with the substitution of 'practices' for 'shops', serve as an announcement for a dentist: 'their Orders [will be] executed in a Height of Taste not inferior to the *first Shops in London* '.[29]

There are other aspects of eighteenth century social history which can be seen as playing a part in the change in demand for dental treatment and thus in the growth of the numbers of dentists. Plumb points out that 'by the 1740s, a new attitude to children was spreading steadily among the middle and upper classes'.[30]   With the greater expectancy of seeing their children survive into adulthood, parents began to view their offspring as 'a less risky vehicle for capital investment'.[31]   Plumb finds a great upsurge in the number of private schools, especially after 1770, children's literature booming and the young becoming a new consumer market.   This is strikingly reflected in the number of advertisements by dentists urging parents to seek professional advice about their children's teeth.   'As Attention to Children at the casting of their Teeth is indispensably requisite for their future regular growth,' declares Mr. Restieaux, 'he will give Advice on that Head, and attend on the shortest Notice either in Town or Country'.[32]   James Blair announces to the Ladies and Gentlemen of Manchester that[33]

> too great an attention cannot be paid to the Teeth of Children, between the age of Six and Fourteen The utmost care is absolutely Necessary at the time of changing the Teeth, for it too frequently happens that the old Teeth, by continuing too long, force the young ones into a wrong Direction, and that sometimes to such a degree, as to cause the Appearance of a double Row. This is truly unbecoming, and the timely Assistance of a Dentist should be called to remove or prevent it; for if it is suffered to remain any length of Time, it will not be in the Power of the ablest Artist to cure the Deformity; and the Person who is so unfortunate as not to have proper Assistance at this critical Period, will be ever subject to all the Inconvenience which proceeds from a bad set of Teeth. It is almost unnecessary to add, that where due Attention has been paid to the Teeth at an early Age, and particularly at the Time of shedding them, a very small Degree of Attention to cleaning, etc., is afterwards sufficient to preserve their Soundness and Beauty even to Old Age.

In Denbigh[24]

> he particularly recommends to parents, as they value the comforts
> of their children, in a good set of teeth, to examine the state of
> their teeth ... and should they perceive any irregularities, to
> make immediate application, as they are during that age [six to
> fourteen], for the most part, easily regulated.

George Bott jun. offers a further operation: 'Infants' Gums
judiciously opened at the first Dentition'.[35] Mr. Moor is equally
convinced of the indispensability of his services and undertakes to
advise parents and the governesses of boarding schools.[36] Dentists
offer their services to such establishments, quarterly or yearly, 'on
most reasonable terms'.[37] These include the enterprising Mrs.
Hunter, who used her sex as an added recommendation to the mistresses
of ladies' schools.[38] So common a practice had this become by the
1830s that, as we have seen, Gray states that children in boarding
schools are having their teeth filed without their parents knowing
anything about it.[39]

This pressure on parents continued into the nineteenth century,
frequently with explicit emphasis on the moral responsibility they
should exercise towards their offspring. Purland declares: 'a duty
parents too often neglect, is the attention to children *at the period
of shedding the teeth*; ... it rests solely with the parent, whether a
child has a good, or ill-regulated, or decayed set'.[40] John
Nicholles, himself a visitor of boarding schools 'upon advantageous
terms to the proprietor'[41] dedicates a whole book to 'Mothers of the
Rising Generation'.[42]

The addition of duty to the catalogue of reasons for seeking
dental treatment is one which obtrudes more as the nineteenth century
progresses. Purland speaks of 'the impropriety of neglecting the
teeth'.[43] Without teeth, he says, 'we become an annoyance to our
friends and a burthen to ourselves'.[44] Thomas Bell considers that
people 'have no right to shock the senses of others' with their
offensive breath.[45] Henry Jordan, with a mid-Victorian sense of
purpose, tells his readers, 'nature has formed nothing in vain —we
are not furnished with a single tooth more than we need ... to lose
only one ... unnecessarily, is wrong, and to sacrifice our teeth
carelessly is to be guilty of a species of suicide'.[46]

Interacting with these factors designed to stimulate demand for
dental treatment, was the intermittent suggestion that dental disease

was at the root of a myriad of systemic ills. Edward Breham details the horrors of toothache and questions 'might it not eventually plunge them [the sufferers] into dejection and want, or hurry them, though reluctant, in search of parochial relief?'[47] He appeals to parents to consult the bills of mortality, where they will see that one third of all children die before the age of two; two thirds of these deaths, he claims, are brought about 'by convulsions and consumption, originating in dentition'.[48] Purland is of the opinion that the absence of teeth leads to bad breath, feeble stomach and a debilitated constitution.[49] John Nicholles reminds his readers that in his first edition he had said that 'a multitude of diseases, apparently originating in the remoter parts of the body, might yet be traced to the teeth; and this doctrine was thought by many to belong to that spirit of exclusiveness and exaggeration'; yet, he reiterates, 'from neglect and loss of the teeth, must arise imperfect mastication, and from that cause indigestion and its inseparable affections'.[50] 'Caries of the teeth will sometimes give rise to ... tic douloureux, to disorders of the ear, of the stomach, and other organs; it has even been known to set up excruciating pain in the limbs analogous to rheumatism'.[51] He cites abscesses and even a case of epilepsy cured by the removal of decayed teeth and stumps.[52] 'The influence of bad teeth on the state of general health must be very great, and some have even considered it as a cause of pulmonary consumption'.[53] Henry Jordan is more concise but every bit as damning: dental disease leads to 'the impoverished state of the blood, and the derangement of the whole system'.[54] Indeed, many writers of the nineteenth century can cite a case which foxed an eminent doctor but which they were able to cure completely by judicious treatment of the teeth.

This line of approach, which gives hope to those suffering from chronic complaints and sows apprehension in the minds of those with poor teeth, surfaces from time to time and is still not completely dead in some quarters, particularly in the realm of popular medical myth. In the nineteenth century it is a doctrine used by dentists who wished to stress their allegiance to medicine and conversely by surgeons who wanted to reserve the treatment of the mouth for themselves. It reached its apogee at the beginning of this century when the theory of focal sepsis led doctors to recommend the wholesale extraction of teeth as a remedy for intractable ills. For the anxious early nineteenth century reader, it was an added incentive to seek the attention of a dentist.

If more encouragement were needed to demand treatment, it was to be discovered in the well-founded theories of such writers as William Robertson, who stressed that by the time caries was obvious and pain experienced, the damage had already been done. He urged upon his readers the imperative of seeking treatment early and of regular checks to detect caries and gum disease in their first stages.

A change in demand for dental treatment occurred, then, in the eighteenth century, springing initially out of the contemporary fascination with novelty and fuelled by the socially emulative attitudes of the day. The few dentists then in practice were not slow to encourage this new interest, becoming masters of manipulation of the field. By nurturing this concern for the restoration of the ravages of dental disease, playing on a changing attitude towards the care of children and making out fresh arguments for dental treatment as a necessity of life, they were able, to use the words of McKendrick,[55]

> to take full advantage of that *existing* demand, to release the potentiality of *latent* demand, and by creating new wants and provoking new needs, to create *new* demand which would not have become economically operational without the requisite entrepreneurial skills to conjure it into existence.

The demand generated by such techniques was such as to lead to an increase in the numbers of dentists over the period covered by this study. Demand, existing and created, was not the only factor in the growth of the profession but certainly must have been at the root of the phenomenon.

The need for dental treatment

The increased level of demand for dental treatment from the eighteenth century onwards may be seen as something new, but one can deduce[56] that the need for it had been there for a long time. It is very evident from eighteenth century advertisements that there was a high incidence of dental disease in the sector of society to which dentists addressed themselves. Their offers of artificial teeth ('from one to a complete set'), fillings, transplantations, crowns, the extraction of 'stumps not perceivable within the gums'[57] and the removal of calculus as a means to encouraging the gums to become reattached, all point to severe dental disease as a commonplace among the readers of the eighteenth century newspapers. As if to reinforce this, Sinclair, in his examination of 96 old men in Greenwich Hospital who were products of the eighteenth century, described 21 as having 'not a tooth left', 9 with 'very bad teeth', 48 with 'bad teeth', 11 with 'middling teeth', 2 with 'middling good teeth' and only 5 with 'good teeth'.[58]

Early nineteenth century writers suggest that the situation did not improve with time. Gray devotes a whole section of his treatise to 'The Defective State of the Teeth of the present day, compared with that of the last Century':[59]

> In the higher ranks of society, it is scarcely possible to find a person of the age of twenty-four, who has not lost some teeth, and so many of the remainder are stopped with gold, that their mouths have some resemblance to the window of a jeweller's shop. I am often waited on by elderly ladies with their daughters; the mother has often excellent teeth, but the daughter is as often half toothless. The mother eagerly inquires the cause of the teeth being so generally defective now-a-days, compared with what they were forty or fifty years ago.

His conclusion that this was all iatrogenic in origin does not detract from his observations.

The eminent Joseph Fox contradicts the view of John Hunter published in the 1770s that caries does not occur after the age of fifty; he has met with several persons who had no decay until the age of sixty but who thereafter had to undergo extractions 'on account of the extreme pain, which the influence arising from caries had occasioned'.[60] He may possibly be observing cervical caries, more prevalent in the older age groups, but there may also be contained in his statements the suggestion of an increase in the caries incidence even in less prone subjects after the turn of the century.

A number of writers make unfavourable comparisons between the teeth of those in 'civilised' societies and those who live elsewhere. Robertson states,[61]

> I have had ample opportunities of comparing the teeth of the inhabitants of warm climates, who continue to live in a state of nature, with those of the human races whose habits and modes of living may be said to be artificial; and I have found the teeth of the former much more perfect in the formation of the enamel than those of the latter.

He advances this as one of the reasons for greater decay among those in 'artificial' societies. De Loude has not such comparisons to make, but in describing the state of teeth in his own day (1840), he bemoans[62]

> the fearful increase of unhealthy and decayed teeth ... It is really alarming to see the thousands and tens of thousands of young people, scarcely arrived at the age of puberty, with most of their teeth decayed or lost.

Modern epidemiological studies would confirm this state of affairs. In a series of studies of the teeth of ancient British populations, Moore and Corbett have discerned a change in the pattern and incidence of carious attack. Their first three papers examine the Anglo-Saxon period,[63] the Iron Age[64] and the seventeenth century.[65] They found the incidence of caries rising from a low overall prevalence until by the seventeenth century it became much closer to modern levels. The site of carious attack had changed from the cemento-enamel junction to a higher occurrence on the interstitial surfaces of the teeth. Cavities in occlusal fissures had also increased in numbers. They concluded that by the seventeenth century the modern pattern of caries attack was well established.

Their nineteenth century study[66] was based on the examination of 255 skulls from a pre-1850 graveyeard in Ashton-under-Lyne (average year of death 1841) and 305 skulls from the adjoining post-1850 cemetery (average year of death 1876). Because of problems of identification of the remains in all the studies, skulls were divided into age groups on the criteria of tooth eruption and attrition.[67] 'Both the nineteenth century populations in age groups 1, 2 and 3, showed significantly higher caries rates for all teeth than did the Anglo-Saxon, mediaeval and seventeenth century populations, demonstrating the trend for a progressive increase throughout the centuries'.[68] However, the most marked increase in caries rate was seen in the cemetery skulls, buried after 1850; the total caries prevalence peaked at 47% compared with 32% for the pre-1850 graveyard. The pattern of caries was close to that observed in the modern (1976) British population. It would seem from this work that dental disease was significantly more prevalent among those alive in the late eighteenth and early nineteenth centuries than it had been among their ancestors, even if it had not yet reached the levels found towards the end of the century. Moore and Corbett attribute this rise in caries prevalence to change in diet over the centuries –and particularly to the increased consumption of sugar– as do other writers. Hardwick chronicles the history of the use of refined sugar.[69] He links its arrival in southern Europe to the conquest of the Arabs, recounting that by the early fifteenth century Venetian ships were carrying 100,000 lbs. per year to England. By the end of the sixteenth century sugar was an important export of the South American colonies and its consumption in Europe continued to rise. (He suggests that before this date what dental references there are in the medical literature make little mention of decayed or hollow teeth). Burnett puts the *per capita* consumption of sugar in Britain (excluding Ireland) at 4 lb. in 1740, 13 lb. in 1788[70] and 30.6 lb. in 1801.[71] Although the amount fell during the first decades of the nineteenth century in response to the higher price, when the tariff was reduced in 1845 consumption again soared, reaching 110 lb. per head in 1957.

So inseparable are dental disease and the indiscriminate consumption of sugar, that there can be no doubt that an increase in the ingestion of the second must lead to a higher rate of incidence of the first, especially in a period such as the eighteenth and early nineteenth centuries when the relationship between the two might be hinted at but certainly was not proved. With surplus income available to more people, luxuries such as tea, coffee and chocolate, generally accompanied by sugar, became the necessities of more social groups, bringing with them the doubtful blessing of dental disease. Finer flour promoted the production of better cakes, biscuits and fruit pies, further vehicles for sugar. (The increase in the number of cookery books aimed at the affluent, such as Mrs. Glasse's *The Compleat Confectioner* of 1770, might perhaps have a part to play here). Burnett sees spending on food in the early nineteenth century as a matter 'of high social importance and class demarcation'.[72] The introduction of afternoon tea from 1840 can have done little for the teeth of a social élite.

The modern day explanation of the rise in the incidence of caries during the period in question, validates the tentative suggestions of contemporary writers such as Robertson. In his comparison of the teeth of those in simpler societies with those in his own, he says that in the latter 'the greater part of the mischief is occasioned by the softer and more adhesive portions of our nutriment' whereas in simpler societies 'the food itself possesses less of those adhesive qualities which it acquires from our own more varied and refined modes of preparing it'.[73] Robertson's comments, though misunderstanding the rôle of sucrose, formed the basis of later scientific investigations which were to reveal the causative relationship between sugar and caries. However, while a contemporary such as Chapin Harris, whose textbook on dental surgery continued to be reprinted throughout the century, could support the fantasy of the noble savage with his statement that 'barbarous people are usually possessed of better teeth than those of civilised nations, because their systems are not enervated by luxurious living',[74] there was a long way to go before the cause of caries was understood and this knowledge could begin to have any effect on the ever rising incidence of dental disease.

5.2 Enabling factors

The supply of manpower

No amount of demand or need could have led to the promotion of dentistry without there being a supply of men ready to take up the challenge and opportunities afforded by the coincidence of these two factors. The period in which dentistry first began to expand was one which saw great enterprise and an explosion of consumer spending. The trades which provided the first generation of the new dentists were well established throughout the country. Nineteenth century writers were correct in their assertions that many early dentists had originally been jewellers, ivory turners, hairdressers, perfumers, druggists and watchmakers. However, not all those who were engaged in these trades turned to dentistry when the opportunity arose. For those who did, an altered local demand for their services may well have been a factor in their diversification but individual case histories suggest that it was the opportunity to try something new, in the spirit of the age, which probably attracted them as much as anything. James Blair (of Leicester, Chester and Liverpool) was, at different times in his life, a hairdresser and perruke maker, dresser and occasional performer with a company of travelling actors, perfumer, toyman, keeper of a register office, jeweller and dentist.[75] George Bott of Nottingham (1748-1820) started out in life as a wool-comber and sorter. His later activities as a patent medicine vendor and manufacturer led him into bleeding and toothdrawing and finally into dentistry.[76] Both these men were very much products of the age, seizing opportunities to expand their businesses, especially in their younger years.

Not only was dentistry a novelty to be tried, but like chiropody and optics (also phenomena of the same period), it attracted those men who wanted to operate in a para-medical field without the expense in time and money needed for an orthodox medical education. The Apothecaries' Act of 1815 demanded an apprenticeship (lasting a minimum of five years) followed by attendance at lectures at an approved institution. Loudon has shown that the medical education of Henry Peart, who began provincial medical practice in the 1830s, probably cost his family over £1,000.[77] From the 1820s onwards, as Loudon points out,[78] there were constant complaints that the medical profession was overcrowded. By 1834 it was estimated that the ratio of general medical practitioners to population was about 1:1,000, with even fewer of the population likely to demand the surgeon-apothecary's services, many either being too poor or belonging to a social group which retained physicians as their family doctors. It may be that some potential medical students, who could not count on as much family support as could Peart in his early years of practice, were diverted into dentistry where a comfortable income was more assured.[79] Indeed, it did not take long for those in search of an occupation to realise that a lucrative living could be made from this new form of treatment. The typical fee for a full denture in the second half of the eighteenth century and the beginning of the nineteenth was about 20 gns.,[80] a whole year's income for a Berkshire agricultural labourer and his family[81] and enough to keep Parson Woodforde and his household of six in food for a good two and a half months.[82]

By 1839 Chapin Harris was complaining, 'on account of the facility with which a superficial knowledge of some of its [dentistry's] principles may be obtained, the supposed emolument arising from its practice, and the want of better employment, many have resorted to it as a means of support'.[83] James Robinson talks of 'those who are ... studious of gain, by whatever means obtained'.[84]

That the expectation of a handsome income was one of the reasons for trying dentistry, cannot be denied. It was presumably an important motive for mechanics breaking away on their own, having compared the fees commanded by the dentist with the amount they themselves received for their side of the work. This is not to say that there were not those who, like Gray, wanted to contribute 'to the lessening of human suffering, and the consequent increase of general happiness',[85] but the reasons for continuing in a career are not always the same as those for taking it up in the first place.

On a more elevated plane, dentistry must have appealed to the intellectual curiosity of some of its practitioners. The eighteenth and early nineteenth centuries saw a great upsurge of interest in the wonders of nature, whether revealed by the telescope or the microscope. John Hunter's works brought rigorous scientific observation to bear for the first time on the teeth and established them as worthy of serious study. He was on intimate terms with a number of London dentists, including the Spences, Martin Van Butchell and William Rae, who gave a course of lectures on the teeth at Hunter's Leicester Square house in 1785.[86] From Hunter's day onwards, most dental treatises had their token scientific chapter, some more original than others. An element of scientific kudos had entered into dentistry, even if it was over-exploited at times.

It is clear that throughout the period in question, dentistry was able to draw on a more than adequate pool of those with business enterprise, medical or scientific leanings and financial expectations, even when the market was so dispersed, outside the large towns, as to oblige dentists to travel around to find patients. As dental practice became established, so did family firms and the profession was able to draw on a new ready-made source of manpower, the sons and relations of dentists channelled into the business, probably with little or no say in the matter. As we have seen, the number of such family businesses in the provinces can be conservatively put at 110 and this aspect must have made a considerable contribution to increasing the numbers of dentists in practice. By the early decades of the nineteenth century it was not only dentists' sons who were entering the profession. The serious practice of dentistry had acquired enough respectability to attract such men as James Robinson and John Tomes, one the son of a sea captain[87] and the other of a gentleman 'rather deficient in business capacity'.[88] With dentistry once established as a normal part of life, what had been a steady flow of recruits at later dates developed into a positive flood.

Transport

Provincial dentistry could not have developed at the rate it did without the changes which took place in road transport in the eighteenth century. Most newspaper advertisements are placed by visiting dentists, especially in the eighteenth century. One has to conclude that, despite the growing market for dental treatment, potential clients were still spread rather thinly and needed to be sought out. As we have seen, even as late as 1858, a Tavistock dentist was pointing out that he could not hope to make a decent living by practising in that 'unfashionable town' alone, with a population of only just over 8,000.   Birmingham's visiting practitioners in the eighteenth century emanated from as far afield as London, Bath, Oxford and Nottingham, Liverpool's between 1788 and 1792 largely from London.

Just how extensively some early dentists were in the habit of travelling is seen from the case of James Blair.   He regularly embarked on at least two tours a year, each lasting several weeks and taking in a number of places. In 1798, for example, he made a tour of the Manchester area in April, one of Chester and North Wales in June and a final visit to the Cambridge district in November. Towards the end of his career, now based in Liverpool, he made two visits a year to Chester and a further two to Shrewsbury, and that at the age of sixty-five. In addition he established agencies for his toothpowder all over the Midlands and East Anglia. It is to be noted that, even well established in a large centre such as Liverpool where an ample supply of patients might be expected, he still took to the road.   His successor in the practice, Thomas Whitfield Lloyd, continued the same pattern of visits until the 1840s.

In another part of the country, William Lukyn of Oxford was making extensive tours of the area to the north-west of the city. A printed handbill of his has survived which gives details of his visits for a whole year in the 1830s.[89] In March, June, September and December he would set out on his tours, each taking place in the first and third weeks of the month. The first week seems to be the time for collecting orders and the third week for delivering appliances, after a week in Oxford making them up. His reconstructed timetable for June (*table 1*) exemplifies his method of operation. It will be seen that Lukyn moved on each day, his hour of arrival in the next town being governed, presumably by the coach timetable. In all, he visited   twenty different   places   between Oxford and

date	town visited	inn	time of arrival
Mon 2 & 16 June	Charlbury	Crown	11
Tues 3 & 17 June	Shipstone	George	11
Wed 4 & 18 June	Bromyard	Falcon	1
Th 5 & 19 June	Leominster	Red Lion	9
Fri 6 & 20 June	Tewkesbury	Swan	11
Sat 7 & 21 June	Burford	Bull	1

table 1: William Lukyn's visits in June

Leominster, there being some overlap between the places on his September and December circuits. Altogether, he devoted twelve weeks a year to the work generated by these tours and there is no saying that he did not have similar circuits for which the evidence has not survived.

None of this kind of travelling would have been practicable before the eighteenth century. Defoe certainly travelled around the country, but one feels that there were certain roads he would not have gone along repeatedly with any enthusiasm. 'Coach travel, rapidly increasing in popularity during the seventeenth century, was slow, uncomfortable and often dangerous, particularly at any distance from London'.[90]

The tours of Blair, Lukyn and innumerable others were only really feasible when the road improvements of the eighteenth century made it possible to get from point A to point B with relative certainty and in increasingly short times. Albert challenges the Webbs' view that turnpike development was scattered and unconnected and shows that there was, on the contrary, a coherent pattern to the changes.[91] He considers that by 1750 many of the arterial routes out of London were completely turnpiked and that the major interprovincial arterial routes were virtually completed by the mid-1770s.[92] He quotes John Byng as saying in 1781[93]

> I wish with all my heart that half the turnpike roads of the Kingdom were plough'd up which have imported London manners, and depopulated the country -- I meet milkmaids on the road, with the dress and looks of strand misses.

Here we have contemporary evidence for improved roads as an important agent in the spread of fashionable ideas.

By 1800 a network of coach routes had been built up every bit as complex as the present passenger rail system. Porter gives as his example of the growth in the number of coach services the fact that in 1740 there had been only one coach a day from Birmingham to London, whereas by 1763 there were thirty.[94]   Improvements in the design of coaches themselves contributed to speedier travel. Burnett states that the mid-century average distance covered of 50-60 miles a day doubled by the end of the century.[95]

When Blair was wanting to travel around in the late 1790s, Leicester could boast a daily coach to London at 11 am, with another at either 2 pm or 8 pm, Monday to Fridays. There was a daily coach to Manchester at 8 am with an additional 10 pm service three days a week.   In addition to these were the daily mail and post chaises to London.   The route of the London to Manchester coach is given in full: London, St. Albans, Hockliffe, Stoney Stratford, Northampton, Harborough, Leicester, Loughborough, Derby, Ashburn, Leek, Macclesfield, Stockport, Manchester.[96]   If Blair caught the London to Leeds coach when it stopped in Leicester, then he also had access to Nottingham, Mansfield, Chesterfield, Sheffield, Barnsley, Wakefield and Leeds itself, together with all the interconnecting coaches along the way.[97]   Not that journeys were completely without excitement. George Bott jun., who had set up dental practice in Birmingham, had to place an advertisement in the *Aris's Birmingham Gazette* on 31 August 1799 informing his clients in his home town that he had been thrown out of a carriage near Derby, breaking his leg. He was now laid up for an expected two weeks at the New Inn there, but he would be sure to inform his patients of his return.

With the development of the roads came the growth in the number of inns to act as staging posts along the route. These are the very places where dentists often offered their services when visiting a town. They were also the resort of many of the clients the dentist had come to seek, since this improved transport brought together in one place precisely the people who comprised the potential market for dental treatment, as they came into the town for the races, the assizes, a social gathering at the Assembly Rooms, a big fair or the visit of a travelling theatre company, all ready to indulge themselves in a bout of consumer spending. Thus the improvement of the roads worked to the advantage of both parties. More people were able to converge on the town for festive occasions and the dentists, who could not find enough clients if they stayed put in a small town, took advantage of the same improvements to extend their business.

Some of the early dentists were already used to this travelling way of life, even if they perhaps saw it as an unfortunate necessity. R.A. Cohen's unpublished research has pointed out that a number of pre-1855 dentists came from theatrical families or were involved with the acting profession at some time in their lives.[98] He cites as examples Arman Talma (a member of the family of the French tragedian), Charles Bew of Brighton (actor manager and dentist to the Prince Regent) and Signor Grimaldi, who came to England as dentist to Queen Charlotte in 1760. Once here, he resigned his position, became a dancing master and was appointed ballet master at Drury Lane and Sadler's Wells Theatres. Although the evidence is somewhat confused, he would appear to have been the father of Grimaldi the clown and the son of 'Iron Legs' Grimaldi who appeared on the London stage in the 1750s and 1760s.[99] To this list might be added James Blair, who in the late 1760s left his London job with a fashionable hairdresser and perfumer in Rupert Street to join Mr. Miller's Company of Comedians as dresser and occasional player of rôles. Charles Whitlock had a more extensive experience and more elevated connection with the theatrical profession. He played only small parts when his company of Comedians visited Newcastle in 1744, spending the rest of his visit offering his services as a dentist. He appears to have combined his two occupations during annual visits to the city, even becoming manager of the new Theatre Royal from 1788 to about 1797. After a ten year tour of America, he returned to Newcastle and appears in a trade directory of 1811 as a dentist. His wife was Elizabeth Kemble, the sister of Mrs. Siddons.[100]

Certainly, histrionic talents would be as great an asset to the dentist as they were to the itinerant toothdrawer, the subject of so many caricatures of the time, with his assistant to divert the crowd while the master operates. A neat picture of the qualities demanded of such assistants is contained in an advertisement which appeared in the *Newcastle Courant* in 1761:[101]

> Wanted immediately a brisk active man to serve a travelling doctor as an Andrew. He must be a person of drollery and ready wit, if he has followed that calling before he will be the more acceptable, or if he plays an instrument. Like wise wanted a second-hand trumpet, cheap.

If the improved road communications of the eighteenth century were an important enabling factor in the development of dentistry, this must have been even more true of the advent of the train from the 1830s onwards. By the 1840s and 1850s the rail network should have removed much of the remaining difficulty of travelling around in pursuit of patients. The increase in the number of branch practices in these decades may owe something to the greater ease of travel, both for dentist and patient.

Newspaper advertising

Just as important an enabling factor in the promotion of provincial dentistry was the spectacular growth of that other organ of communication, the newspaper.

When the Printing Act expired at the end of the seventeenth century, the London press proliferated, with as many versions of the news as there were newspapers. The provincial press came into existence in part to provide a digest of these varying reports for provincial readers who were just as avid for news but unlikely to be able to afford subscriptions to all the London papers.[102]

The first newspaper to be published outside London is considered to be the *Norwich Post* (1701), closely followed by the *Bristol Postboy* in 1702.[103] The growth in this new field of publication was such that after 1719 the number of papers in any one year never fell below twenty and after 1737 never below thirty. By 1760, 130 different newspapers had been started in 55 towns, although by no means all of them survived for long.[104] As regards the geographical distribution of provincial newspapers before 1760, whilst acknowledging that the size of a town, its strategic position in relation to London (the source of news) and its tradition as a county capital, might all contribute to the promotion of a newspapers, Cranfield points out that some small towns acquired newspapers at an early date (e.g. Maidstone in 1725) whilst some of the more obvious candidates had to wait until quite late for a successful paper to be established (e.g. Liverpool until 1756). He suggests that the profits from newspaper production were meagre in the first half of the eighteenth century[105] and that the presence of a newspaper during this period is less a reflection of the importance of a town than of the decision of an individual printer to take the risk of production.

It can be estimated that the earliest newspapers each produced only 100-200 copies a week but that this figure had risen to 1000-

2000 by 1760, when the total annual output of the provincial press probably reached 2 million copies.[106] Burnett considers that the sales of newspapers in the country as a whole doubled between 1753 and 1792.[107] Bearing in mind Addison's view that each newspaper bought probably had twenty readers,[108] it is clear that newspapers reached increasingly large numbers of people during the period when dentistry was itself developing.

The circulation of provincial newspapers was not restricted to the town in which they were printed, aiming as they did, initially, to serve several counties. Cranfield suggests that success or failure depended largely on the efficiency of the distribution system adopted.[109] Newsmen were employed to deliver supplies to agents anything up to 40 miles away from the town of printing, collecting advertisements and selling the patent products promoted by the paper en route. The system was 'so effective that it reached even those readers in the most remote and isolated hamlets and farmhouses'.[110] By 1743 the *York Courant* had 43 agents scattered between Scarborough and Manchester.[111]

In the middle of the century competition from the increasing number of new papers curtailed expansion somewhat, but the list of agents for the *Leeds Mercury* in 1800 shows that spheres of influence were still extensive at the end of the century. This newspaper was distributed in Huddersfield, Bradford, Rochdale, Elland, Wakefield, Pontefract, Rotherham, Barnsley, Dewsbury, Kendal, Lancaster, Doncaster, Knaresborough, Ripon, Tadcaster, Settle, Colne, Keighley, Otley, Burnley, Skipton, Pateley, Grassington, Threshfield and Bingley.[112] Production continued to increase. The readership of the *Leeds Mercury* in 1839 has been estimated as 150,000, certainly not all in Leeds. Manchester newspapers circulated throughout the cotton area and Sheffield papers in the whole of South Yorkshire.[113]

Taking all this evidence into consideration, it can confidently be said that, although many small towns could not boast their own newspapers in the eighteenth and early nineteenth centuries, there can have been few which did not fall within the circulation area of a larger one which did.

Advertisements were few and far between in the early years of provincial newspaper production, but by the 1750s a paper such as the *York Courant* regularly gave up more than three quarters of its space to them.[114] From the middle of the century, papers were carrying anything from 10 to 40 independent[115] advertisements per issue, the

most common figure being about 20.[116]   A striking feature of the new
trade notices were those placed by skilled men arriving in a
provincial town from London.   Cranfield finds quack doctors and
surgeons feature prominently among their number, as do those
connected in some way with the world of fashion, all making the most
of their London connection.[117]   Just as motorways of two hundred
years later opened up new commercial avenues, so the improved roads
of the second half of the eighteenth century appear to have prompted
a wave of business intitiative from tradesmen prepared to try new
markets and enabled to do so effectively by the burgeoning provincial
newspapers.   Dentists are to be found among their number.

Throughout the period up to 1855, dentists relied on newspaper
advertisements to a large extent to publicise their services,
unencumbered as they were by a code of professional ethics.   The tone
of their announcements might vary from the restrained to the
outrageous, but there can have been few who did not use them at some
time in their careers.

The most obvious use dentists had of advertisements was to alert
their potential clients of a visit, actual or imminent.   An efficient
advertiser might give advance warning, like Mr. Wooffendale of
Sheffield, who announces in the *York Courant* on 25 December 1772 that
he 'will be at York the thirteenth of January next'.   Many, however,
seem to have placed their first notice to co-incide with their
arrival ('Mr. Jeffs, Dentist, is just arrived from Ireland'),[118] but
it may be that they had previously arranged for the printer to
distribute handbills in advance.   (Mrs. De St. Raymond on her visit
to York in 1775, refers readers to her handbill for detailed
fees).[119]

The dentist who has his tour planned out is committed ahead,
states the length of the visit ('From his indispensible engagements
at Leicester, he cannot protract his stay beyond three weeks'),[120]
whereas those whose visit is perhaps a little more speculative can
sometimes be prevailed upon to extend their stay by popular demand:
Benjamin Hornor, on a visit to Leeds in 1800 decided to remain
another two or three weeks.[121]   In both cases, the date of departure
serves as a spur to encourage patients to waste no time in seeking
treatment.

A stay of some time in a town might include subsidiary visits
to smaller places: James Blair, having arrived in Chester at the

SIGNIOR GRIMALDI, Dentift and Ope-rator for the Teeth and Gums, has practiced with furprifing Succefs many Years in Paris and London, not only for the Prefervation, but likewife for every Reparation of every Deficency in the Mouth ; Perfons, every other way agreeable, fhall not go one Day longer with a foul and diffigured Mouth, and interrupted Speech, proceeding from the Lofs of either of their Teeth, if they will apply to him, and thave their Deficiencies fupplied with artificial Teeth, that will leave every Ufe without being painful or difcernible.——N. B. On Fridays the Poor may apply to him Gratis: He lodges at the Pell Office, in New Street, Birmingham.

from *Aris's Birmingham Gazette,* 18 June 1759

P. MICHEL, *Surgeon-Dentist,*
No. 11, YORK-STREET, BATH,

RETURNS thanks to the Nobility, Gentry and Public in general, for the liberal patronage he has already received, and begs to inform them, that he makes ARTIFICIAL TEETH, in Gold Sockets, with a brilliant Enamel, equal to the firft natural teeth.

He likewife makes, and fixes in peculiar manner, from one to a whole fet of Natural Teeth, Compofition, fo neatly that they cannot be difcovered by the nicest obferver from real Teeth.

P. M. performs every operation of Cutting, Stopping, Cleaning, and Faftening the Teeth, in the moft perfect manner; and trufts that his peculiar facility of extracting Teeth will enfure a continuance of general fupport, which he will be moft emulous of deferving.

N. B. He fells, as ufual, his incomparable TOOTH POWDER and LOTION, which is held in the greateft efteem of many by the Nobility and Gentry, for Cleanfing, Beautifying, and effectually Faftening the Teeth, and giving a healthy hue to the Gums. [3060]

from *Bath Chronicle ,* 22 February 1810

DENTAL SURGERY.

MR. ALEX'S

VISITS TO LEICESTER FOR THE YEAR 1842,

Are One Week in each Month, as under :—

FROM		FROM	
Monday, Jan. 17, until the 22nd		Monday, July 11, until the 23rd	
—— Feb. 14,	—— 19th	—— Aug. 15,	—— 20th
—— Mar. 14,	—— 19th	—— Sept. 19,	—— 24th
—— April 18,	—— 23rd	—— Oct. 17,	—— 22nd
—— May 16,	—— 21st	—— Nov. 14,	—— 19th
—— June 13,	—— 18th	—— Dec. 12,	—— 17th

HOURS OF ATTENDANCE, from *Ten* until *Four*, at **Miss CLARKE'S, Gallowtree Gate.**

Communications addressed to Messrs. ALEX and JONES, 26, *Bridge Street, Blackfriars, London*, will at all times meet with attention.

from Cook's *Leicestershire Almanack*, 1842

MR. LEIGH,

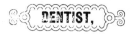

90, PORTLAND CRESCENT,

LEEDS,

In respectfully and gratefully acknowledging the liberal patronage he has experienced during nearly SIX Years residence in Leeds, begs to assure his Patients and the Public that he lays no claim to

Wonderful and Astounding

DISCOVERIES

in DENTAL SCIENCE, nor would he pay them so poor a compliment as to ask them to believe Impossibilities; but combining all modern SURGICAL Improvements in the treatment of the Teeth and Gums, and all Mechanical Improvements in the manufacture and adaptation of Artificial Substitutes, he pledges himself that his patients shall, on all occasions, meet with kind, liberal, and *strictly honorable* treatment; the best guarantee to which is a permitted reference to any number from a list of upwards of Three Hundred patients of high character and respectability, principally resident in Leeds.

from White's *Directory of Leeds and the clothing districts of Yorkshire ,* 1853

beginning of May 1799, announces a two-day visit to Denbigh on 10 and 11 June, returning to Chester for the remainder of his visit and not leaving until nearer the end of the month.[122] The facility to advertise such a short stay in advance must have been almost indispensible if there was to be enough work waiting to make the journey worthwhile.

The newspaper advertisement also allowed the dentist to publicise more widely just what wonders he could perform, from artificial teeth which could not be distinguished from real ones (a universal claim) to the ability of Mrs. De St. Raymond to transplant 'teeth from the front of the jaws of poor lads into the heads of any Lady or Gentleman'[123] 'without putting both patients to any anguish'.[124] When dental treatment was a novelty, only publicity could reach enough potential clients. As discussed earlier, hopes and fears were encouraged and new demands created. Parents learned from many a dentist of the dreadful havoc which could result from neglecting to seek professional advice when their children began to lose their first set of teeth. Fortunately, men like Mr. Leigh were at hand to advertise: 'the care of Children's Teeth, from its great importance in regulating their form and beauty, he has made an ornament of particular study'.[125]

Other advertising techniques make their presence felt. Dentists arrived, like Mr. Restieaux, with recommendations 'not only from the most eminent Physicians and Surgeons at Norwich, (where he has resided nine years), but also from Nottingham, and every other Place in which he has practised'.[126] They might be from exotic parts, like Hemet Hart from Mannheim[127] or merely from London, like Mr. E. King of Canterbury.[128]

They offered inducements, often in the form of free treatment for the poor at certain hours, even if, as in the case of Robertson of Birmingham, there were strings attached: he 'will attend gratuitously on the mornings of Tues and Thurs, from 9 till 10, on any of the poorer class who bring recommendatory notes from respectable persons'.[129] Crawcour gives 'best advice gratis'[130] and 'will forfeit ten times the sum of money if his operation and his advertisement shall not prove alike'.[131] Grimaldi 'will give immediate Ease, and make an effectual Cure or receive nothing for his Trouble. He requires no Payment for one Year or two after the Cure is perfected if required'.[132] Users of Amboyna toothpowder are promised £1,000 if they experience toothache or decay after using the product as directed.[133]

While on a visit to a town, a dentist would establish agencies for his own products, whose advertisement would keep his name in the public eye until his next visit. This was a common technique practised by any number of dentists, including Mr. Crawcour, whose twelve day visit to Leicester in 1799[134] was followed up with three advertisements later during the year for his products. In fact, advertisements for products outnumber those for dentists themselves, although not all the products were marketed by dentists.

Through the medium of the provincial newspaper advertisement, the dentist was able to project an image of the educated, literate, well-connected conveyor of valuable pseudo-scientific information and provider of relief and repair for one of the chief ills to beset mankind. Whilst soliciting custom in the most deferential of terms, some dentists also managed to give the impression that they were so much in demand that they were actually doing the public a favour by yielding to pleas to visit a town. Particularly in the eighteenth century, the aim appears to be to establish a stance of respectability. Nothing has yet been found in the provincial press to rival the extraordinary publicity campaign of Patence who over a twenty year period from 1770 kept his name in the public eye with regular verses and anecdotes in the London press.[135] 'Testimonials' appeared:

> To Mr. PATENCE
> SURGEON AND DENTIST
> No. 103, Strand, near Southampton Street
> Sir,
> Good Heavens! What are you made of! (cried I after a month's experience of your artificial teeth!)- the public indeed owes you much, and amongst the rest your humble servant,
> A NOBLEMAN

Nor had Patence any hesitation in attacking the opposition:

> He [De Chémant] offered his Teeth and Services gratis to Mr. Ruspini, Pall Mall; but Mr. Ruspini had character to lose, and had more honour than to propose such ridiculous stuff to mankind.

Sadly, the provincial press is altogether more sober; perhaps eccentricity was a commercial risk which it was not advisable to take in smaller communities where passing trade was not so easy to come by.

Dentists were not always on the move, of course; they had equal need of newspapers to advertise their services at their permanent base, especially when setting up a practice. Even the most respectable dentist, who might never advertise again in the press of his home town, like Robertson of Birmingham, can be expected to place notices in the newspaper when he commences practice.[186] When competition is fierce, as in Liverpool in the 1820s and 1830s, new dentists scarcely miss an issue for months on end in an effort to keep their names in the public eye.[187] The Mallan family make sure they maximise their investment in a Liverpool branch by placing advertisements in the *Liverpool Mercury* virtually every week of operation in the 1830s.[138]

As the nineteenth century progressed, vast amounts came to be spent on advertising by dentists such as the Mallans. Mortimer claims, 'it has been calculated that each advertiser spends from 10 1. to 20 1. *weekly* in them'.[189] Certainly, things had got so out of hand by the mid-century that abstinence from quackish advertising was one of the prerequisites for joining the two professional organisations, the College of Dentists and the Odontological Society.

Without a complete survey of the provincial press, it is impossible to say how many dentists made use of newspapers. Partial searches have discovered that at least 22 of the 45 eighteenth century dentists in trade directories were in the habit of advertising and this figure seems very likely to prove higher if more extensive searches were made. Of the fifty-one pre-1840 dentists in Liverpool trade directories, advertisements have been found for thirty-seven (72.4%). One thing is certain: in the 1760s, only a handful of advertisements for dentists are to be encountered in a whole year's production of a provincial newspaper; by 1860, that number had increased to about five per issue. The newspaper had proved itself indispensible in creating and nurturing demand and thereby swelling the numbers of dentists.

Technical advances
The main advance during the period before 1855 was in the field of prosthetics.[140] The traditional choice of material for the construction of dentures in the eighteenth century was ivory, that from the hippopotamus being the most expensive. It had the merits of being initially white, very hard and yet carvable and of producing results of passing verisimilitude. Great skill and ingenuity went

into the production of full and partial dentures, either carved in one piece or with separately fashioned teeth attached to an ivory plate with gold pins. However, such prostheses had their drawbacks, from the very nature of the material. They had a short life, being as subject to degradation in the mouth as the teeth they replaced and producing a particularly offensive odour in the process.

Various attempts were made to circumvent these detractions. Natural teeth were tried. By the early nineteenth century these could be bought in bulk in matched sets from suppliers. In theory, they came from healthy bodies taken off the battlefield and hence became known as 'Waterloo teeth'. However, as De Loude pointed out, 'battles are not fought every day nor is the supply 100,000th part sufficient'.[141]   In practice the teeth emanated from the dissecting rooms, graveyards and mortuaries. In a letter from London (dated 6 March 1782) to her brother in Paris, Anne Gertrude Talma writes (in translation):[142]

> Father asks you to do everything you can to get him some teeth, and if you can get into the mortuary, to take advantage of the opportunity. If that is not possible, you must try and get to know the brother friar who is in charge of the place and ask him to let you have some. You will have to pay for the large incisors and the small laterals. Father used to pay his predecessor 12 [livres] a hundred for the canines.

The foreign origin of many of the natural teeth used in denture manufacture in England is again suggested by the following advertisement placed by Robert Wooffendale in the London press on 10 February 1792:[143]

> WANTED - Several Human Front Teeth. To avoid unnecessary applications, those only are wanted that are sent from the Continent.

Gold was introduced as a denture base by Bourdet in 1757 and continued to be used for the most expensive prostheses well into the nineteenth century and beyond.[144]   However, the real step towards the prosthesis immune to decay was taken by Nicholas Dubois de Chémant when he patented his method of using porcelain for dentures in 1791.[145]   Whilst these one-piece dentures had the potential additional advantage of realistic colouring of teeth and gums, they can scarcely have been practicable to wear because of their weight and doubtful fit. Problems were experienced in the firing, shrinkage and cracking of glazes being major difficulties. They attracted a certain amount of ridicule, as is evidenced by Rowlandson's cartoon of 1811 entitled 'A French Dentist shewing a specimen of his artificial teeth and false palates'.[146]

Whilst not the complete answer to the problems experienced by wearers of ivory dentures, De Chémant's work formed the basis for the major technical innovation of the early nineteenth century, the individual porcelain tooth, first introduced by Da Fonzi in 1808, which in one form or another was not superceded until the advent of plastics. It took some time to perfect the technique of production of these 'mineral teeth'. Nicholles, writing in 1834, could still complain that they were 'glazed with lead or arsenic' and 'soon lose their colour'.[147] He describes another type of porcelain tooth (the 'terro-metallic') as having a poor colour, being liable to fracture, of great weight and instrumental in grinding away any opposing natural teeth. However, by 1839, Chapin Harris considers porcelain teeth are much improved over the last five to six years and are generally accepted.[148]

By 1840 they were being produced in huge numbers. De Loude states that half a million were being exported annually from Paris alone.[149] Ivory teeth on gold plates are quite out of date, he considers, although human teeth are still being used.[150] In 1845 Mortimer is of the opinion that mineral teeth should have superceded natural ones and recommends those made by Claudius Ash of London.[151] For the first time the universal promise of artificial teeth 'not to be distinguished from real ones' came near to being fulfilled, at least as far as appearance of the teeth themselves was concerned.

The press and directory advertisements (particularly from the 1830s onwards) make much of this new invention[152]

> guaranteed to restore to the wearer every advantage equal to nature.... The peculiar composition of the Metallic Teeth renders them particularly desirable, as they can be made to match Teeth of any shade, and never decompose, change colour, or become offensive in the mouth.

Mr. Evatt of Leeds is still offering a full range of materials in 1849[153] but his 'best' teeth, if quality can be equated with price, are the mineral ones at £12 on an ivory plate or 15 gns. on gold. His competitor in the town, Thomas Dixon, offers 'every description of English and Foreign new improved MINERAL TEETH, of the latest designs in shape, shade, and colour, with a perfect knowledge of the present progressive Improvements in DENTAL MECHANISM'.[154]

There are no figures available to show the actual numbers of porcelain teeth used in the first half of the nineteenthth century in provincial England.   However, it is clear from such writers as Robinson that the home supply was insufficient to satisfy the demand created and by 1846 large quantities were being imported from Brussels.[155]   Whilst no strict correlation can be postulated between the increased use of incorrodible teeth and the numbers of dentists, it seems more than co-incidental that the development of this new product should be contemporary with startling increases in dental manpower from the 1830s onwards.   It can be argued that this first major advance on the techniques of more than a century played a not inconsiderable part in the growing demand for dental treatment and thus in the numbers of its practitioners.

5.3 Limiting factors

Whilst there were circumstances operating to promote the spread of dentistry, there were at the same time checks on its expansion. The most obvious of these was the high cost of dental treatment.

The need for treatment may well have been there, but the number who could afford the fee of anything up to 20 gns. for a full set of artificial teeth must have been exceedingly limited.   Not only this but the wearing of dentures incurred recurrent costs.   Jordan was of the opinion that whilst some people might keep a set for between 8 and 15 years, others needed to have them replaced in only 3-4 years. A well-made set might be expected to last 5-6 years.[156]   Ephraim Mosely considered that any natural teeth used in dentures needed annual replacement.[157]   And how many not already committed to the preservation of their teeth would pay up to 10s.6d. to have a tooth filled by a dentist when they could have it extracted for 6d. or 1s. by the chemist?

Dentists themselves were only too well aware of the problem. J.H. Wilcock of Bristol states the situation most clearly: 'The high charges that are usually made for everything connected with Dental Surgery, has hitherto placed it far beyond the reach of many to obtain that relief, ease, and comfort, which this truly useful branch of surgical science affords to the afflicted'.[158]   To counteract this financial barrier, 'in order that all classes may obtain proper attention in the Dental department',[159] and also of course to attract custom, dentists frequently stress in their advertisements that their fees are strictly moderate, 'unprecedentedly low',[160] or that treatment is performed 'at the lowest remunerating charges'.[161] On occasion they are prepared to reduce their fees to draw in patients, or, as Montague Alex puts it, 'to render the Dental Art more extensively useful'.[162] Thomas Dixon of Leeds claims that his new improved mineral teeth enable him to greatly reduce his charges in 1849;[163] J.H. Parsons attributes his own philanthropy in 1840 to the fact that he has removed to cheaper premises, making his treatment less expensive before ten in the morning and after five in the afternoon.[164]

Consultations and advice were given free by many dentists. In addition, the poor might be treated without charge at certain hours of the day. Although it should be pointed out that this gave assistants the opportunity to learn the skill of extraction without harm to fee-paying patients, nevertheless, behind the practice lay the same charitable sentiment which led to the founding of the dental dispensaries and hospitals for the poor from the middle of the nineteenth century.[165]

All the evidence points to the dentist's clientèle being drawn from an affluent sector of society. The surviving account books of the Lloyd practice of Rodney St, Liverpool, reinforce this view.[166] (Although the records refer to the 1860s, there seems no good reason for believing that they are inappropriate to the first half of the century). Of the 154 account holders with James Blair Lloyd of Liverpool, 105 can be identified with some certainty. The largest single group are the 35 merchants, followed by 20 of independent means, 12 tradesmen, 12 brokers, 4 bankers, 4 clerics, 2 each of attorneys, agents, bookkeepers, servants (presumably sent by their employers), and one each of surgeons, veterinary surgeons, shipping masters, farmers, architects and artists. Lloyd also had among his patients the staff and pupils of three convents and a school.

However, membership of the middle classes cannot be equated directly with a desire to seek dental treatment. In her work on the remains from Ashton-under-Lyne graveyard, Corbett concluded: 'from the evidence of gravestones and coffins, it must be presumed that those remains examined were from the middle classes of an urban industrial population'[167] and yet 'there was little evidence of conservative work having been carried out and the few fillings seen were of poor quality'.[168] Of 255 bodies buried before 1850, only four had fillings and three of these belonged to one wealthy family. A few gold dentures were recovered from vaults. Although one might expect the number of gold dentures buried with bodies to be low, the amount of restorative work is surprising when one sees that this aspect of dentistry formed up to 60% of the items of treatment carried out by Lloyd in 1865.

Money might be an important check on seeking treatment, but then, as now, the ultimate determinant was that of social attitude.

NOTES AND REFERENCES

1   Gray, *Dental practice* (1837), 7.
2   *ibid.*, 11-12.
3   *ibid.*, 14.
4   W. White, *Directory and gazetteer of Leeds and the clothing district of Yorkshire* (1853).
5   Tallis, *A comprehensive gazetteer of Gravesend...* (1839).
6   Gray 1837, 15.
7   e.g. 'Transplanting of teeth', 1787 (7766 in *British Museum Catalogue of political and personal satires*) and 'Six stages of mending a face', 1792 (8174, *ibid.*).
8   P.S. Brown's sample of medicines advertised in Bath newspapers (1744- the end of the century) revealed dental preparations as the third most commonly advertised specialised product (10.33% of the total number of 7988 advertisements and 13.03% of the specialised advertisements). Of the 302 medicines to emerge from the survey, the largest single category was dental products (17.22%) (P.S. Brown, 'Medicines advertised in the 18th century Bath newspapers', *Med.Hist.*, 20(1976), 152-168).
9   Patented 22 January 1773 (no.1031 in B. Woodcroft, *Abridgement of specifications relating to medicine, surgery and dentistry, 1620-1866*, 2nd ed. (1872)).
10   *CC*, 25 Jan 1805.
11   *ABG*, 28 July 1777.
12   *ibid.*, 18 June 1759.
13   E. Breham, *Treatise on the structure, formation, and various diseases of the teeth and gums*, 3rd ed. (1821), iii.
14   *ibid.*, xii.
15   W. Robertson, *Practical treatise on the teeth*, 4th ed. (1846).
16   Royal appointments had been made at least as early as 1727 (J. Dobson, 'The Royal dentists', *Annals of the Royal College of Surgeons of England*, 46(1970), 277-291).
17   e.g. Heath, surgeon dentist to the Duke of Clarence (*Times*, 18 Dec 1798) and Charles Bew, dentist to the Prince Regent (*Wright's Brighton Perambulator* (1818)).
18   N. McKendrick, J. Brewer and J.H. Plumb, *The birth of a consumer society* (1982), 11.

19   *ibid.*, 23.
20   e.g. Mr. and Mrs. Sedmon's at Hextall's (*LJ*, 3 Feb 1787).
21   e.g. Restieaux at Blair's (*LMJ*, 27 Aug 1785).
22   e.g. Ruspini at Lloyd's, Shrewsbury (*ABG*, 8 Aug 1763).
23   e.g. Crawcour at Mrs. Ayres' (*Williamson's Liverpool Advertiser*, 18 Feb 1788).
24   McKendrick 1982, ch.2.
25   P. Fauchard, *Le chirurgien dentiste* (1728).
26   *Gentleman's Magazine*, 7 Nov 1761.
27   L. Lindsay, 'The London dentist of the 18th century', *Proc.R.Soc.Med.*, 20(1927), 355-366.
28   E. Robinson, unpublished *Compilation of lectures, advertisements etc. ... taken from Aris's Birmingham Gazette in the 18th century* (1972).
29   McKendrick 1982, 49.
30   J.H. Plumb, 'The new world of children in 18th century England', in McKendrick 1982, ch.7.
31   Plumb, *ibid.*, 287.
32   *LMJ*, 27 Aug 1785.
33   *MM*, 27 May 1794.
34   *CC*, 7 June 1799.
35   *ABG*, 8 May 1797.
36   *ABG*, 3 May 1784.
37   Alex in *Cheltenham Chronicle*, 3 Oct 1833 (*MCC* 419).
38   1791 (*MCC* 122).
39   Gray 1837, 9.
40   T. Purland, *Practical directions for preserving the teeth; advice to parents* (1831), 2.
41   1822 (*MCC* 413).
42   J. Nicholles, *The teeth, in relation to beauty, voice and health*, 2nd ed. (1834).
43   Purland 1831, iv.
44   *ibid.*, 1.
45   T. Bell, *The anatomy, physiology and diseases of the teeth and gums* (1835),201.
46   H. Jordan, *Practical observations on the teeth* (1851), 14.
47   Breham 1821, xiv.
48   *ibid.*, 53.
49   Purland 1831, 1.
50   Nicholles 1834, 37.
51   *ibid.*, 39.
52   *ibid.*, 46.
53   *ibid.*, 48.
54   Jordan 1851, 16.
55   McKendrick 1982, 71.
56   Systematic surveys of dental health do not exist until the end of the 19th century.
57   *ABG*, 12 Feb 1759.
58   Sinclair, 'An essay on longevity', *Naval Chronicle*, 9(1803), p.388; quoted by M.E. Corbett, 'An investigation into the pattern of dental caries in a 19th century British urban population' (unpublished DDS thesis, University of Birmingham, 1975).
59   Gray 1837, 14.

60   J. Fox, *The natural history and diseases of the human teeth*, 2nd ed. (1814), 24.
61   Robertson 1846, 69.
62   L.C. De Loude, *Surgical, operative and mechanical dentistry* (1840), 70.
63   W.J. Moore and M.E. Corbett, 'The distribution of dental caries in ancient British populations: I, Anglo-Saxon period', *Caries Res.*, 5(1971), 151-168.
64   W.J. Moore and M.E. Corbett, 'The distribution of dental caries in ancient British populations: II, Iron Age, Romano-British and mediaeval periods', *Caries Res.*, 7(1973), 139-153.
65   W.J. Moore and M.E. Corbett, 'The distribution of dental caries in ancient British populations: III, 17th century', *Caries Res.*, 9(1975), 163-175.
66   M.E. Corbett and W.J. Moore, 'The distribution of dental caries in ancient British populations: IV, 19th century', *Caries Res.*, 10(1976), 401-414.
67   Group 0 was designated for stages between eruption of the 2nd and 3rd molar whilst gp. 3 contained permanent dentition with occlusal fissures obliterated by attrition;   gps. 1 and 2 showed intermediate degrees of attrition.
68   Corbett 1975, 136.
69   J.L. Hardwick, 'The incidence and distribution of caries throughout the ages in relation to the Englishman's diet', *Br.dent.J.*, 108(1960), 9-17.
70   J. Burnett, *Plenty and Want* (1968), 24.
71   J. Burnett, *A history of the cost of living* (1969), 180.
72   Burnett 1968, 77.
73   Robertson 1846, 70.
74   C.A. Harris, *The dental art, a practical treatise on dental surgery* (1839), 143.
75   C. Hillam, 'James Blair (1747-1817), provincial dentist', *Med.Hist.*, 22(1978), 44-70.
76   D.G. and C. Hillam, 'The Bott family of dentists', *Dent.Hist.*, 11(1985), 1-10.
77   I.S.L. Loudon, 'A doctor's cash book: the economy of general practice in the 1830s', *Med.Hist.*, 27(1983), 254.
78   *ibid.*, 257.
79   Some, like C. Spence Bate, originally started out as medical students but did not complete their training and turned to dentistry (*Lancet* (1846), 1, 231).   Tomes himself could be counted among their number.
80   e.g. in *LJ* 8 Dec 1787, *MM* 17 Apr 1798; account books of James Prew of Bath covering 1842 (MS 5213, 22).
81   Burnett 1969, 165.
82   *ibid.*, 161.
83   Harris 1839, 22.
84   J. Robinson, *The surgical, mechanical and medical treatment of the teeth* (1846), 4.
85   Gray 1837, 77.
86   J.M. Campbell, *Dentistry then and now* (1981) 105.
87   *Dent.Rev.*, 4(1862), 189.
88   Sir Z. Cope, *Sir John Tomes, pioneer of British dentistry* (1961),

4.
89   *MCC* 673.
90   W. Albert, *The turnpike road system in England, 1663-1840* (1972), 8.
91   *ibid.*, ch.3.
92   It will be remembered that this is the period when visiting dentists begin to appear in the provinces.
93   In the *Torrington diaries*, ed. C.B. Andrews (1935) vol.1, 6, quoted in Albert 1973, 11.
94   R. Porter, *English society in the 18th century* (1982), 209.
95   Burnett 1969, 157.
96   *LJ*, 20 Jan 1797 and 7 June 1798.
97   J. Binns and G. Brown, *A directory for ... Leeds* (1800).
98   Personal communication.
99   'Boz' (Charles Dickens), *Memoirs of Joseph Grimaldi* (1838).
100   J. Boyes, 'Medicine and dentistry in Newcastle upon Tyne in the 18th century', *Proc.R.Soc.Med.*, 50(1957), 229-235.
101   Quoted by Boyes, *ibid.*
102   For a full exposition of the origins of the provincial press see G.A. Cranfield, *The development of the provincial press, 1700-1760* (1962), ch.1.
103   *ibid.*, 16.
104   *ibid.*, v and 27.
105   *ibid.*, 245 *et seq.*
106   *ibid.*, 169 and 176.
107   Burnett 1969, 156.
108   *Spectator*, 12 Mar 1711. Quoted by Cranfield 1962, 177.
109   Cranfield 1962, 190.
110   *ibid.*, 204.
111   *ibid.*, 202.
112   *LM*, 15 Feb 1800.
113   D. Read, *Opinion in three English cities* (1961).
114   Cranfield 1962, 208.
115   i.e. ones not placed by the printer.
116   Cranfield 1962, 210.
117   *ibid*, 212.
118   *LJ*, 18 Nov 1786.
119   *YC*, 10 Feb 1775.
120   *Cambridge Chronicle*, 2 Dec 1797.
121   *LM*, 10 May 1800.
122   *CC*, 7 June 1799.
123   *YC*, 10 Mar 1775.
124   *YC*, 10 Feb 1775.
125   *Jackson's Oxford Journal*, 14 Jan 1826 (*MCC* 504).
126   *LJ*, 27 Aug 1785.
127   *YC*, 31 July 1778.
128   *Kentish Gazette*, 15 July 1834.
129   *ABG*, 23 Sept 1822.
130   *LJ*, 4 Feb 1775.
131   *LJ*, 18 Feb 1775.
132   *ABG*, 28 June 1773.
133   *CC*, 3 May 1805.
134   *LMJ*, 26 June 1779.

135   B.R.Townend, 'Mr. Patence, quack', *Dent.Mag.*, 59(1942), 169-181.
136   *ABG*, 21 Jan *et seq.* 1822.
137   e.g. Samuel Berend in *Liv M*, 1822.
138   The branch was not operated absolutely full-time for the whole decade; advertisements suggest the firm was in the town for 3 months in 1835, 1837, 1839; 4 months in 1836; 5 months in 1831; 10 months in 1832 and the whole year in 1833, 1834 and 1838. They also had interests in Manchester at the same time.
139   W.H. Mortimer, *Observations on the growth and irregularity of children's teeth* (1845), 4, notes.
140   For a full account of the development of dental prostheses see, for example, ch.11 in W. Hoffmann-Axthelm, *History of dentistry* (1981).
141   De Loude 1840, 163.
142   Quoted in R.A. Cohen, 'The Talma family', *Br.dent.J.*, 126(1969), 326.
143   Contained in a compilation of advertisements in the archive of the British Dental Association (publications/printed matter 399); dated but no source given.
144   One of the most interesting examples extant are the artificial teeth of the Duke of Wellington, the subject of a paper by C.B. Henry, 'The Iron Duke's dentures', *Br.dent.J.*, 125(1968), 354-356.
145   When in England De Chémant obtained supplies of materials from Josiah Wedgwood (see R.A. Cohen, 'Messrs. Wedgwood and porcelain dentures, correspondence 1800-1815', *Br.dent.J.*, 139(1975), 27-31 and 69-71).
146   11798 in *British Museum Catalogue of political and personal satires.*
147   Nicholles 1834, 128.
148   Harris 1839, 19.
149   De Loude 1840, 163.
150   *ibid.*, 162.
151   Mortimer 1845, 119. The dental manufacturing firm of Claudius Ash (founded 1837) is still in existence as Dentsply.
152   *Kentish Gazette*, 9 Oct 1829.
153   A complete set of teeth, £5; a complete set wih natural teeth, £10.
154   Charlton and Archdeacon, *Directory of Leeds* (1849).
155   Robinson 1846, 178-179.
156   Jordan 1851, 102.
157   B. Mosely, *Teeth, their natural history* (1862), 45.
158   Mathews, *Bristol directory* (1835).
159   *Fleetwood Chronicle*, Oct 1845.
160   H. Davies, *Cheltenham Annuaire* (1840).
161   Forbes and Knibb, *Directory of Southampton* (1851).
162   G. Rowe, *Illustrated Cheltenham Guide* (1845).
163   Charlton and Archdeacon 1849.
164   *Liv M*, 6 Nov 1840.
165   See E.M. Spencer, 'Notes on the history of dental dispensaries', *Med.Hist.*, 26(1982), 47-66.
166   Held by the Museum of the School of Dentistry, University of Liverpool.
167   Corbett 1975, 31.
168   *ibid.*, 115.

APPENDIX 1

DIRECTORIES EXAMINED

1. Those listed in J.E. Norton, *Guide to the national and provincial directories of England and Wales, excluding London, published before 1856* (London,1950)
   (Identified by Norton number)

2. Those not listed in Norton, in alphabetical order of publisher.
   (Locations are public libraries unless otherwise stated)

1. Listed in Norton

1-4, 6-8, 13, 15, 18-21, 23-24, 29-36, 43, 47, 53, 56-57, 59, 61-62, 64, 67, 70-71, 74, 76-79, 81-86, 89, 91, 93, 95-97, 99

100-102, 105-110, 112-118, 120-139, 141-146, 148, 150-160, 163-199

200-207, 210-212, 214-219, 221-222, 224, 227, 229, 233-235, 238-299

300-315, 318-321, 323-338, 340-349, 352-354, 356-384, 386, 388, 390, 392-393, 395-399

400-407, 409-414, 416-419, 422-424, 427, 430-445, 447-451, 453-466, 468-481, 484, 487-499

500-510, 512-515, 517-518, 521, 523-525, 528, 530-536, 538-548, 550-563, 565-568, 570-572, 574-582, 584-598

600-618, 620-631, 633-640, 642, 644, 646-674, 677-678, 680-684, 686-696, 699

700-703, 705, 708-709, 711, 713, 716-717, 719, 721, 723-731, 733-739, 741-742, 744-757, 759-760, 762, 768, 775, 777-781, 783-786, 788-790, 794-799

800-804, 806-832, 834-838, 840-863, 867-878

2. Directories not listed in Norton

date of publication	publisher	Short title	Location
1839	-----	Wolverhampton directory	Wolverhampton
1852	-----	Wigan directory	Wigan
1854	-----	Directory of Hampstead	Guildhall
1855	-----	Directory of Scarborough	Scarborough
1852	Archdeacon	Greenwich & Woolwich directory	British Library
1823	Baines	Directory of Hull	Hull
1853	Barbet	Almanack for the Channel Islands	Guille-Allès Library Guernsey
1831	Bartlett	Blandford directory	British Library
1853	Bass	Deptford guide	British Library
1827	Batten	Key and companion to Clapham	Guildhall
1828, 41	Batten	Clapham with its common	Guildhall
1844	Batten	List of inhabitants of the parish of Clapham	British Library
1840, 41, 42, 45, 48	Beck	Leamington guide	Leamington
1845	Burgess	Directory of Northampton	Northampton
1851	Collinson & Burton	West Riding worsted directory	British Library
1849	Cook	Annual guide to Leicester	Leicester
1847, 53	Cooke	Westminster local directory	Guildhall
1829	Cowslade	Berkshire Commercial directory	Reading
1834	Cowslade	Directory and gazetteer for...Berkshire	Reading
1773, 76	Cruttwell	New Bath guide	Bath
80, 82, 84, 93, 94, 96	Cruttwell	New Bath guide	Guildhall
1850	Dobson	Guide and directory to Cleethorpes	Lincoln
1810, 14, 22, 25	Easton	Salisbury guide	Salisbury
1834	Fairfax	New guide and directory to Leamington Spa	Leamington
1839	Fletcher	Directory of Southampton	Southampton
1841	Fordham	Kentish advertiser and Chatham directory	British Library
1853, 54, 55	Hall	Gravesend & Northfleet directory	Gravesend
1847	Hickman	Directory of Northampton	Northampton
1828	Hollinsworth	Portsmouth guide	Guildhall
1841, 44, 46, 47	Johnston	Addenda to Moore's Almanack, Milton and Gravesend directory	Gravesend
1853	Lascelles	Directory and gazetteer of the county of Oxford	Bodleian
1849, 50, 51	Large	Gravesend, Milton & Northfleet directory	Gravesend
1845	Law	Directory of Birkenhead	Birkenhead
1832	Le Cras	Englishman's Almanack [Jersey]	Société Jersiaise
1843	Lewis	Berkshire Almanac, directory...	Reading
1846	Longbottom	Directory of King's Lynn	Guildhall
1843	Lucas	Paddington directory	Guildhall
1855	Mannex	History, topography & directory of mid-Lancashire	St. Helens
1852	Mason	Greenwich & Blackheath directory	British Library
1853	Mason	Brentford directory	Guildhall
1822, 24, 29	Moncrieff	Visitors' new guide [Leamington]	Leamington
1840, 47	Moody	Winchester directory	British Library
1843, 48, 49, 52, 54, 55	Naftel	British Press Royal Jersey Almanac	Société Jersiaise
1851, 53	Oakey	Comm. trade directory of Preston	Preston

date of publication	publisher	Short title	Location
1851, 54	Osborne	Birkenhead directory	Birkenhead
1835	Parsons	Tourists' companion from Leeds through Selby to Hull	Guildhall
1830	Pigot	Comm. directory of Birmingham & Sheffield	Sheffield
1837	Pigot	Directory of Worcestershire	Worcester
1839	Reeve	Guide to Royal Leamington Spa	Leamington
1836	Richardson	Directory of Newcastle and Gateshead	Guildhall
1811	Risdon	Chorographical description of Devon	Guildhall
1801	Robbins	Bath directory	British Library
1802	Roper	Trades and professions in Wolverhampton	Guildhall
1801, 04, 08-12,14-20, 22, 25-40, 43, 45-48, 52, 55	Rusher	Reading guide and Berkshire directory [annual]	Reading
1802-03, 05-07, 13, 21, 24, 41, 44.			Guildhall
1817, 18, 23, 25	Sharpe	New guide of Leamington and Warwick	Leamington
1822	Smith	Leamington guide	Leamington
1844, 47	Snare	Berkshire advertiser	Reading
1839	Tallis	Gazetteer of Gravesend	Gravesend
1791, 96, 1822	Trewman	Exeter pocket journal	Exeter
1855	Trounce	Islington directory	Guildhall
1847	Turner	Directory for Islington, Holloway and Pentonville	Guildhall
1844	Vint & Carr	Directory of Sunderland	Durham University
1848	Whetstone	Directory of Richmond [Surrey]	Guildhall
1833	White	Directory and topography of Leeds, Bradford, Halifax and the clothing districts of the West Riding	Sheffield
1855	White	Directory of S. Staffordshire	Salt
1818	Wright	Brighton perambulator	Guildhall
1837	Whittle	History of the borough of Preston	Institute of Historical Research
1841	Whittle	Commercial directory of Preston	Preston

APPENDIX 2

REGISTER OF PROVINCIAL DENTISTS WHOSE NAMES APPEAR IN PRE-1855 TRADE DIRECTORIES, WITH BIOGRAPHICAL NOTES ON SOME OF THE DENTISTS

2.1 Register of names p.154
- Components of entries: names, date, trade description(s), address, town, directory code, location code for directory
- Abbreviations: acc [accoucheur], apoth [apothecary], barbsur ⌊barber-surgeon⌋, bleed ⌊bleeder⌋, chem ⌊chemist⌋, cup [cupper], dent [dentist], drug [druggist], man ⌊manufacturer⌋, mech ⌊mechanical⌋, med electr ⌊medical electrician⌋, MCDE [Member of the College of Dentists], MRCS [Member of the Royal College of Surgeons], perf ⌊perfumer⌋, sur [surgeon⌋, surdent ⌊surgeon dentist⌋
- * Indicates a second occupation
- These are edited directory entries and should not be seen as a record of a dentist's entire career. Further investigation would probably reduce the number of individual dentists by confirming, for example, that A. Andrews is the same person as Alfred Andrews. There are forty-four dentists to whom this applies

2.2 Directory codes p.251
- Abbreviations: Nat [National], Comm ⌊Commercial⌋, P.O. ⌊Post Office⌋
- Since this list forms part of a larger survey, there are gaps in the sequence of codes
- for D241 read D734, for D145 read D788

2.3 Location codes p.269
- public libraries unless otherwise stated

2.4 Biographical notes on some pre-1855 provincial dentists p.272

2.1 Register of names

Name	Year	Type	Address	City	Code1	Code2
ABBOTT JOHN	1822	SURDENT	ST AUBYN ST	PLYMOUTH	D877	L022
	1823	SUR DENT	ST AUBYN ST	PLYMOUTH DOCK *	DB51	L025
	1823	DENT	5 ST AUBYN ST	PLYMOUTH DOCK	D142	L011
ADAMS EDWARD CHARLES	1839	DENT	BOCKING END BOCKING	BRAINTREE	D584	L020
ALABONE A	1855	DENT	113 HIGH ST	NEWPORT I OF W	DA84	L011
ALABONE ALFRED	1852	DENT	113 HIGH ST	NEWPORT I OF W	D346	L017
ALBERT EDWARD	1848	DENT	91 PICCADILLY	MANCHESTER	D475	L020
	1848	DENT	91 PICCADILLY	MANCHESTER	D332	L016
	1852	DENT	55 GEORGE ST	MANCHESTER	D216	L009
ALDRIDGE J L	1855	DENT	CROSS ST	RYDE I OF W	DA84	L011
ALDRIDGE JOHN	1844	DENT	116 HIGH ST	PORTSMOUTH	D144	L068
ALEX	1842	DENT	GALLOWTREEGATE	LEICESTER	D662	L024
ALEX & JONES	1850	DENT	9 SHIP ST	BRIGHTON	D603	L047
	1851	DENT	9 SHIP ST	BRIGHTON	DA77	L011
	1852	DENT	9 SHIP ST	BRIGHTON	D604	L047
	1854	DENT	9 SHIP ST	BRIGHTON	D605	L047
	1855	DENT	9 SHIP ST	BRIGHTON	D594	L046
ALEX & LEVASON	1840	SURDENT	98 HIGH ST	CHELTENHAM	D833	L069
	1842	SURDENT	18 PROMENADE VILLAS	CHELTENHAM	D835	L069
	1842	DENT	18 PROMENADE VILLAS	CHELTENHAM	DB46	L049
	1842	DENT	21 RODNEY TCE	CHELTENHAM	DB46	L049
	1843	SURDENT	18 PROMENADE VILLAS	CHELTENHAM	D836	L069
	1844	SURDENT	18 PROMENADE VILLAS	CHELTENHAM	D837	L069
ALEX (& LEVASON & LEVASON)	1839	SUR DENT	90 HIGH ST	CHELTENHAM *	D654	L068
	1841	SURDENT	98 HIGH ST	CHELTENHAM	D834	L069
ALEX ISAIAH	1830	DENT	414 HIGH ST	CHELTENHAM	D119	L020
ALEX J	1835	DENT	HIGH ST	OXFORD	D639	L050
ALEX M	1839	SURDENT	90 HIGH ST	CHELTENHAM	D957	L068
	1839	SURDENT	98 HIGH ST	CHELTENHAM	D832	L069
	1845	SURDENT	21 RODNEY TCE	CHELTENHAM	D838	L069
	1846	SURDENT	21 RODNEY TCE	CHELTENHAM	D839	L069
	1847	SURDENT	21 RODNEY TCE	CHELTENHAM	D840	L069
	1848	SURDENT	21 RODNEY TCE	CHELTENHAM	D841	L069
	1849	SURDENT	21 RODNEY TCE	CHELTENHAM	D842	L069
	1849	DENT	21 RODNEY ST	CHELTENHAM	DB81	L082
	1850	SURDENT	21 RODNEY TCE	CHELTENHAM	D843	L069
	1851	SURDENT	21 RODNEY TCE	CHELTENHAM	D844	L069
	1852	SURDENT	21 RODNEY TCE	CHELTENHAM	D845	L069
	1853	SURDENT	21 RODNEY TCE	CHELTENHAM	D846	L069
	1853	SURDENT	21 RODNEY TCE	CHELTENHAM	D847	L069
ALEX MONTAGUE	1843	DENT	18 PROMENADE BACK OF	CHELTENHAM	D955	L068
	1844	SURDENT	18 PROMENADE VILLAS	CHELTENHAM	D959	L069
	1845	SURDENT	21 RODNEY TCE	CHELTENHAM	D958	L068
	1847	DENT	21 RODNEY TCE	CHELTENHAM	D890	L068
	1848	DENT	21 RODNEY TCE	CHELTENHAM	D954	L069
	1850	DENT	21 RODNEY TCE	CHELTENHAM	DA74	L011
	1851	DENT	21 RODNEY TCE	CHELTENHAM	D953	L069
	1852	DENT	21 RODNEY TCE	CHELTENHAM	D78B	L020
	1852	DENT	21 RODNEY TCE	CHELTENHAM	D952	L069
	1853	SURDENT	21 RODNEY TCE	CHELTENHAM	D956	L068
ALLAWAY WILLIAM	1834	DENT	18 ST THOMAS BDGS	LIVERPOOL	D236	L009
	1835	DENT	17 SIR THOMAS BDGS	LIVERPOOL	D406	L016
	1837	DENT	18 SIR THOMAS BDGS	LIVERPOOL	D566	L020
	1837	DENT	17 SIR THOMAS BDGS	LIVERPOOL	D407	L016
	1839	DENT	35 SIR THOMAS BDGS	LIVERPOOL	D408	L016
	1841	DENT	33 ST ANNE ST	LIVERPOOL	D409	L016
	1841	DENT	35 SIR THOMAS BDGS	LIVERPOOL	D409	L016

ALLAWAY WILLIAM	1843 DENT	35 SIR THOMAS BDGS	LIVERPOOL	D410 L106
	1843 DENT	35 SIR THOMAS BDGS	LIVERPOOL	D434 L019
	1845 DENT	7 SLATER ST	LIVERPOOL	D411 L016
	1845 DENT	35 SIR THOMAS BDGS	LIVERPOOL	D411 L016
	1846 DENT	7 SLATER ST	LIVERPOOL	D879 L072
	1846 DENT	SIR THOMAS BDGS	LIVERPOOL	D303 L014
	1847 DENT	7 SLATER ST	LIVERPOOL	D412 L016
	1848 DENT	7 SLATER ST	LIVERPOOL	D332 L016
	1849 DENT	7 SLATER ST	LIVERPOOL	D413 L016
	1851 DENT	3 SLATER ST	LIVERPOOL	D414 L016
	1851 DENT	3 SLATER ST	LIVERPOOL	D438 L020
	1852 DENT	3 SLATER ST	LIVERPOOL	D216 L009
ALLCOUD M	1853 DENT	COMMERCIAL ARCADE	GUERNSEY	DC68 L088
ALLDRIDGE J	1848 DENT	116 HIGH ST	PORTSMOUTH	D357 L017
	1852 DENT	116 HIGH ST	PORTSMOUTH	DB72 L025
ALLDRIDGE J L	1855 DENT	143 HIGH ST	PORTSMOUTH	DA84 L011
ALLDRIDGE JOHN LUMLEY	1852 DENT	143 HIGH ST	PORTSMOUTH	D346 L017
ALLDRIDGE JOHN LUMLY	1852 DENT	143 HIGH ST	PORTSMOUTH	D788 L020
ALLEN W H	1850 DENT	KING ST	MAIDSTONE	D592 L045
ALLEN WILLIAM HART	1845 DENT	15 KING ST	MAIDSTONE	DA66 L011
	1847 DENT	KING ST	MAIDSTONE	D586 L044
ALLEN WILLIAM,	1821 BLEEDER TOOTHDRAWER	PHILIP STREET	BIRMINGHAM *	D051 L002
ALLEOUD E	1852 DENT	35 COMMERCIAL ARCADE	GUERNSEY	DB72 L025
ALLISON G	1851 DENT	CHERTSEY ST	GUILDFORD	DA77 L011
ALMOND WILLIAM	1842 SURDENT	1 TEMPLAR ST	LEEDS	D060 L015
	1845 SURDENT	1 TEMPLAR ST	LEEDS	D275 L015
	1846 SURDENT	1 TEMPLAR ST	LEEDS	D713 L061
	1846 DENT	1 TEMPLAR ST	LEEDS	D879 L072
	1847 SURDENT	1 TEMPLAR ST	LEEDS	D276 L015
	1848 DENT	1 TEMPLAR ST	LEEDS	D332 L016
	1849 DENT	6 TEMPLAR ST	LEEDS	D277 L015
	1851 DENT	5 TEMPLAR ST	LEEDS	D283 L015
	1852 DENT	5 TEMPLAR ST	LEEDS	D216 L009
	1853 SURDENT	5 TEMPLAR ST	LEEDS	D261 L010
	1855 DENT	5 TEMPLAR ST	LEEDS	D222 L009
ALSOP EDWARD	1781 BARBSUR DENT PERF	BACK KING ST	MANCHESTER *	D449 L020
ANDERTON JOHN	1842 DENT	HIGH ST	WHITCHURCH	D123 L043
ANDREWS A	1852 SURDENT	ST CLEMENTS	OXFORD	D645 L050
	1854 DENT	69 ST GILES ST	OXFORD	DA71 L011
ANDREWS ALFRED	1853 SURDENT	CORN MARKET ST	OXFORD	DB80 L082
	1854 SURDENT	CORN MARKET ST	OXFORD	D628 L049
ANTHONY C	1822 SURDENT	9 PORTLAND PL	CLIFTON	D005 L020
ANTHONY CHARLES	1821 SURDENT	9 PORTLAND PL CLIFTON	BRISTOL	D920 L075
	1822 SURDENT	9 PORTLAND PL CLIFTON	BRISTOL	D921 L075
	1823 SURDENT	9 PORTLAND PL CLIFTON	BRISTOL	D922 L075
	1824 SURDENT	1 MALL CLIFTON	BRISTOL	D923 L075
	1825 SURDENT	1 MALL CLIFTON	BRISTOL	D924 L075
	1826 SURDENT	1 MALL CLIFTON	BRISTOL	D925 L075
	1827 SURDENT	1 MALL CLIFTON	BRISTOL	D926 L075
	1828 SURDENT	1 MALL CLIFTON	BRISTOL	D927 L075
ARANSON MR	1839 SURDENT	27 HURST STREET	BIRMINGHAM	D083 L002
ARANSON PASCO	1807 SUR DENT	43 UPPER PITT ST	LIVERPOOL *	D394 L016
	1811 SUR DENT	UPPER PARLIAMENT ST	LIVERPOOL *	D284 L011
	1814 SUR DENT	5 DUNCAN ST	LIVERPOOL *	D398 L016
	1814 SURDENT	5 DUNCAN ST	LIVERPOOL	D330 L016
	1816 DENT	DUNCAN ST	LIVERPOOL	D049 L016
ARANSON PASCOE	1824 SURDENT	2 PRINCESS ST	MANCHESTER	D401 L019

ARANSON PASCOE	1828 SURDENT	21 PRINCESS ST	MANCHESTER	D025 L020
	1829 SURDENT	21 PRINCESS ST	MANCHESTER	D465 L020
	1829 SURDENT	21 PRINCESS ST	MANCHESTER	D565 L020
	1830 SURDENT	21 PRINCESS ST	MANCHESTER	D466 L020
	1841 DENT	27 HURST STREET	BIRMINGHAM	D058 L002
	1842 DENT	27 HURST STREET	BIRMINGHAM	D075 L002
ARANSON PASCOW	1816 SUR DENT	25 DUNCAN ST	LIVERPOOL *	D431 L016
ARSON	1832 DENT	BOND ST	ST HELIER	DC57 L088
ASPINALL JOSEPH	1848 DENT	DEANSGATE RES WOOD ST	BOLTON	D486 L011
ASPINWALL JOSEPH	1845 SUR DENT	DEANSGATE	BOLTON *	D786 L020
	1848 DENT	163 DEANSGATE	BOLTON	D332 L016
	1851 DENT	DEANSGATE	BOLTON	D438 L020
ATKINSON (& FATH J)	1845 SURDENT	20 EAST PDE	LEEDS	D275 L015
	1846 DENT	20 EAST PDE	LEEDS	D879 L072
	1846 SURDENT	20 EAST PDE	LEEDS	D713 L061
	1847 SURDENT	20 EAST PDE	LEEDS	D276 L015
	1848 DENT	20 EAST PDE	LEEDS	D332 L016
	1849 DENT	14 EAST PDE	LEEDS	D277 L015
	1851 DENT	14 EAST PDE	LEEDS	D283 L015
	1852 DENT	20 EAST PDE	LEEDS	D216 L009
	1855 DENT	14 EAST PDE	LEEDS	D222 L009
ATKINSON (& FATHER J)	1853 SURDENT	14 EAST PDE	LEEDS	D261 L010
ATKINSON J	1817 SUR DENT MRCS	MEADOW LANE	LEEDS	D038 L015
ATKINSON JOHN	1822 SURDENT	EAST PDE	LEEDS	D255 L010
	1822 SURDENT	EAST PDE	LEEDS	D005 L020
	1826 SUR	9 PARK SQ	LEEDS	D040 L015
	1826 SURDENT	18 EAST PDE	LEEDS	D040 L015
	1828 DENT	20 EAST PDE	LEEDS	D025 L020
	1833 SURDENT	EAST PDE	LEEDS	D778 L066
	1834 DENT	20 EAST PDE	LEEDS	D042 L015
	1834 DENT	20 EAST PDE	LEEDS	D236 L009
	1837 SURDENT	20 EAST PDE	LEEDS	D257 L010
	1837 DENT	20 EAST PDE	LEEDS	D566 L020
	1839 SURDENT	EAST PDE	LEEDS	D082 L015
	1840 SURDENT	20 EAST PDE	LEEDS	D734 L063
	1841 DENT	20 EAST PDE	LEEDS	D331 L016
	1841 SURDENT	20 EAST PDE	LEEDS	D241 L009
	1842 SURDENT	20 EAST PDE	LEEDS	D060 L015
ATKINSON JOHN & J H	1846 DENT	41 PICCADILLY	MANCHESTER	D879 L072
ATKINSON JOHN & JOHN HASTINGS	1845 DENT	41 PICCADILLY	MANCHESTER	D474 L020
ATKINSON JOHN & SON	1845 SURDENT	20 EAST PDE	LEEDS	D275 L015
	1846 DENT	20 EAST PDE	LEEDS	D879 L072
	1846 SURDENT	20 EAST PDE	LEEDS	D713 L061
	1847 SURDENT	20 EAST PDE	LEEDS	D276 L015
	1848 DENT	20 EAST PDE	LEEDS	D332 L016
	1849 DENT	14 EAST PDE	LEEDS	D277 L015
	1851 DENT	14 EAST PDE	LEEDS	D283 L015
	1852 DENT	20 EAST PDE	LEEDS	D216 L009
	1853 SURDENT	14 EAST PDE	LEEDS	D261 L010
	1855 DENT	14 EAST PDE	LEEDS	D222 L009
ATKINSON JOHN HASTINGS	1848 DENT	41 PICCADILLY	MANCHESTER	D332 L016
	1848 DENT	41 PICCADILLY	MANCHESTER	D475 L020
ATKINSON JOHN HASTINGS (& J)	1845 DENT	41 PICCADILLY	MANCHESTER	D474 L020
	1846 DENT	41 PICCADILLY	MANCHESTER	D879 L072
ATLEE D	1850 DENT	31 RICHMOND PL	BRIGHTON	D603 L047
	1852 DENT	31 RICHMOND PL	BRIGHTON	D604 L047
ATLEE D & CO	1848 DENT	31 RICHMOND PL	BRIGHTON	D602 L047

AYTON J	1848 DENT	NORTHGATE ST	DEVIZES	D357 L011
	1855 DENT MD	NORTHGATE ST	DEVIZES	DA84 L011
AYTON JACOB	1848 SURDENT MD	NORTHGATE ST	DEVIZES	D125 L075
	1852 SURDENT	NORTHGATE ST	DEVIZES	D788 L020
BAILEY W H	1833 SURDENT	7 CHAPEL ROW QUEENS SQ	BATH	D120 L007
BAKER M	1829 DENT	PECK LANE	BIRMINGHAM	D055 L002
	1830 DENT	PECK LANE	BIRMINGHAM	D056 L002
BAKER STEPHEN	1822 SURDENT CUPPER	30 NEW KING ST	BATH *	D005 L020
BALL F	1850 DENT	36 CARLIOL ST	NEWCASTLE	D214 L009
	1851 SURDENT	15 CARLIOL ST	NEWCASTLE	D215 L009
	1853 DENT	15 CARLIOL ST	NEWCASTLE	D243 L009
BALL FRED	1847 SURDENT	36 CARLIOL ST	NEWCASTLE	D242 L009
BALL FREDERICK	1848 DENT	36 CARLIOL ST	NEWCASTLE	D332 L016
	1852 DENT	36 CARLIOL ST	NEWCASTLE	D216 L009
BALLANTYNE GEORGE	1851 DENT	4 CHRISTIAN ST	LIVERPOOL	D438 L020
	1852 DENT	4 CHRISTIAN ST	LIVERPOOL	D216 L009
BALLARD GEORGE	1852 DENT	BATH ST	FROME	D788 L020
BALLS W	1844 DENT	CARLIOL SQ	NEWCASTLE	D213 L009
BAMTON FRANCIS	1852 DENT	WORCESTER VILLA ST SAVIOURS	BATH	D128 L007
BANNISTER	1843 DENT	BURRARD ST	ST HELIER	DC58 L088
BANNISTER W F	1845 DENT	BURRARD ST	ST HELIER	DA82 L011
	1847 SURDENT	BURRARD ST	ST HELIER	DB53 L025
	1848 SURDENT	PROVIDENCE ST	ST HELIER	DC59 L088
BANNISTER WILLIAM F	1839 DENT CUPPER	3 WATERLOO ST	JERSEY *	D654 L011
BARCLAY J	1855 DENT	19 MARKET PL	DERBY	D511 L023
BARCLAY JAMES	1854 DENT	MARKET PL	DERBY	D660 L057
BARNARD	1839 DENT	11 TERRACE	ST HELIER	DB43 L078
	1843 DENT	11 TERRACE	ST HELIER	DC58 L088
	1845 DENT	VAL PLAISANT	ST HELIER	DA82 L011
	1847 SURDENT	VAL PLAISANT	ST HELIER	DB53 L025
BARNARD A	1848 SURDENT	STOPFORD TCE	ST HELIER	DC59 L088
	1849 SURDENT	STOPFORD TCE	ST HELIER	DC60 L088
BARNARD J F	1836 DENT	184 HIGH ST	SOUTHAMPTON	D336 L017
	1846 SURDENT	8 CORNWALLIS CRESC	BRISTOL	D941 L075
BARNARD JOHN FREDERICK	1847 DENT	1 GUILDFORD LAWN	DOVER	D586 L044
BARNES	1829 APOTH CHEM DENT ETC	37 SOUTHGATE ST	BATH *	D118 L007
BARNES J W	1826 SURDENT	40 SOUTHGATE ST	BATH	D117 L007
	1849 SURDENT	40 SOUTHGATE ST	BATH	D126 L007
BARNETT MOSES	1840 DENT	22 GARTSIDE ST	MANCHESTER	D471 L020
	1841 DENT	22 GARTSIDE ST	MANCHESTER	D472 L020
BARRETT JOHN SMITH	1850 DENT	29 ROCK ST	BURY	D728 L020
BARRITT THOMAS	1818 DENT	7 NEW COCK YD	PRESTON	D524 L020
	1824 DENT	7 NEW COCK YD	PRESTON	D463 L020
BARRON W	1823 SURDENT CUP	12 UNION STREET	BIRMINGHAM *	D052 L002
	1825 SURDENT CUP	12 UNION STREET	BIRMINGHAM *	D053 L002
BARRON WILLIAM	1828 DENT	12 CHERRY ST	BHAM	D025 L006
	1829 DENT	12 CHERRY STREET	BIRMINGHAM	D055 L002
	1833 SURDENT	12 CHERRY STREET	BIRMINGHAM	D079 L002
BARRON WILLIAM.	1830 DENT	12 CHERRY STREET	BIRMINGHAM	D056 L002
BARRON WILLIAM.HENRY	1835 DENT	12 CHERRY STREET	BIRMINGHAM	D057 L002
BARROW THOMAS	1798 DENT		WINDSOR	D279 L011
BARTLETT H M	1853 DENT	FOULSHAM	DEREHAM	D655 L051
BARTLETT HENRY VALENTINE	1848 DENT	113 NORFOLK ST	SHEFFIELD	D332 L016
BARTLETT JOHN	1793 SURDENT	DENMARK ST	BRISTOL	D893 L075
BASS HENRY	1851 SURDENT	BATH TCE	BOROUGHBRIDGE	DB54 L025
BATE CHARLES	1844 DENT	6 OCTAGON	PLYMOUTH	D492 L022
	1844 DENT	6 OCTAGON	PLYMOUTH	D144 L008

BATE CHARLES	1850 DENT	7 OCTAGON	PLYMOUTH	D147 L008
	1850 DENT	DYNEVOR ST	SWANSEA	DC50 L085
	1852 DENT	7 OCTAGON	PLYMOUTH	D493 L022
	1852 DENT	6 OCTAGON	PLYMOUTH	D145 L008
	1852 DENT	6 OCTAGON	PLYMOUTH	D788 L020
BATE CHARLES SPENCE	1844 DENT	WIND ST	SWANSEA	D144 L078
	1848 DENT	3 DYNEVOR PL	SWANSEA	DC49 L085
	1853 DENT	DYNEVOR PL	SWANSEA	D951 L075
BATE G	1847 DENT	7 OCTAGON	PLYMOUTH	D152 L008
BATE JAMES JOSEPH ROGERS	1851 DENT	CASTLE HILL	LANCASTER	D438 L019
	1855 DENT	87 MARKET ST	LANCASTER	D222 L011
BATES CHARLES	1840 DENT	OCTAGON	PLYMOUTH	D143 L008
BAYLEY	1824 DENT	4 EAST ST	BRIGHTON	D599 L047
BAYLEY H	1822 DENT	4 EAST ST	BRIGHTON	D598 L047
BAYLY WILLIAM HENRY	1822 DENT	CASTLE SQ	BRIGHTON	DA68 L011
	1823 DENT	4 GREAT EAST ST	BRIGHTON	D142 L011
BAYNTUM F	1854 DENT	7 VINEYARDS	BATH	D129 L007
BAYNTUM F	1840 DENT	PARAGON BDGS	BATH	D143 L020
BAYNTUM FRANCIS	1837 SURDENT	6 PARAGON BDGS	BATH	D121 L007
	1841 SURDENT	6 PARAGON BDGS	BATH	D122 L007
	1842 SURDENT	6 PARAGON BDGS	BATH	D123 L007
	1846 SURDENT	1 BARTLETT ST & 26 NEW KING ST	BATH	D124 L007
	1848 SURDENT	26 MILSOM ST	BATH	D125 L007
	1850 SURDENT	7 WORCESTER PL	BATH	D127 L007
BAYNTUM FREDERICK	1852 SURDENT	BARTLETT ST	BATH	D788 L020
BEACAL EDWIN	1855 DENT	10 NORFOLK ROW	SHEFFIELD	D222 L009
BEACALL EDWARD	1854 DENT	BATH BDGS 203 GLOSSOP RD	SHEFFIELD	D757 L066
BEACALL EDWIN	1852 SURDENT	10 NORFOLK ROW	SHEFFIELD	D260 L010
	1852 DENT	10 SURREY ST	SHEFFIELD	D216 L009
BEAL MRS MARY ANN	1854 DENT	9 CARVER ST	SHEFFIELD	D757 L066
BEAL RICHARD	1849 SURDENT	15 CARVER ST	SHEFFIELD	D756 L066
	1855 DENT	9 CARVER ST	SHEFFIELD	D222 L009
BEALE RICHARD	1852 SURDENT	15 CARVER ST	SHEFFIELD	D260 L010
	1852 DENT	15 CARVER ST	SHEFFIELD	D216 L009
BEAUMONT ALFONSO RODOLPH	1849 DENT MD	40 SILVER ST	LINCOLN	D681 L056
	1849 DENT OCULIST	39 SILVER ST	LINCOLN *	D333 L016
	1850 DENT OCULIST	39 SILVER ST	LINCOLN *	D013 L020
BEDFORD	1843 DENT	47 KING ST	ST HELIER	DC58 L088
BEDFORD E R	1845 DENT	KING ST	ST HELIER	DA82 L011
	1847 SURDENT	DON ST	ST HELIER	D853 L025
	1848 SURDENT	DON ST	ST HELIER	DC59 L088
BELL (& JONES)	1849 DENT	BRIDGE ST	CANTERBURY	D587 L011
	1850 DENT	WEEK ST	MAIDSTONE	D592 L045
	1850 SURDENT	CHAPEL PL	TUNBRIDGE WELLS	DA52 L011
	1851 DENT	WEEK ST	MAIDSTONE	DA77 L011
	1851 DENT	BRIDGE ST	CANTERBURY	DA77 L011
	1854 DENT	WEEK ST	MAIDSTONE	D882 L082
	1855 DENT	12 LOWER BRIDGE ST	CANTERBURY	D594 L046
BELL JAMES	1822 SURDENT	PEMBROKE ST	PLYMOUTH	D877 L022
BELL JOSEPH	1840 SURDENT	36 PEMBROKE ST	DEVONPORT	D143 L020
BELLABY G W	1855 DENT	17 DERBY RD	NOTTINGHAM	D511 L023
BELLABY G WOOD	1854 DENT	17 TOLLHOUSE HILL	NOTTINGHAM	D510 L023
BELLAMY J C	1852 DENT CUPPER	14 GEORGE ST	PLYMOUTH *	D493 L022
BELLAMY JOHN C	1850 DENT	14 GEORGE GATE	PLYMOUTH	D147 L008
BELLAMY JOHN CREMER	1852 DENT	14 GEORGE ST	PLYMOUTH	D145 L008
	1852 DENT	14 GEORGE ST	PLYMOUTH	D788 L020
BELLHOUSE HARRY	1841 DENT	2 BOND ST	MANCHESTER	D331 L016

BELLIS W	1844 DENT	CALLOW PL	DOUGLAS I OF M	DB52 L025
BELLIS WILLIAM ANDREW	1843 DENT	MT PLEASANT	DOUGLAS I OF M	DC55 L087
BENNETT JAMES	1830 DENT	19 UNION ST	PLYMOUTH	D119 L008
	1830 SURDENT	UNION ST	PLYMOUTH	D491 L022
BENSUSAN J	1855 DENT	LAWN LODGE	PECKHAM	D594 L046
BERDMORE THOMAS	1783 SURDENT	RACQUET CT FLEET ST	LONDON	D272 L011
BEREND LEWIS	1837 DENT	41 GEORGE ST	MANCHESTER	D566 L020
	1838 DENT	41 GEORGE ST	MANCHESTER	D470 L020
BEREND LOUIS	1829 DENT	70 BOSTOCK ST	LIVERPOOL	D404 L016
	1832 DENT	70 BOSTOCK ST	LIVERPOOL	D445 L016
	1834 DENT	75 MT PLEASANT	LIVERPOOL	D405 L016
	1835 DENT	75 MT PLEASANT	LIVERPOOL	D406 L016
	1840 DENT	41 GEORGE ST	MANCHESTER	D471 L020
	1841 DENT	41 GEORGE ST	MANCHESTER	D472 L020
	1841 DENT	41 GEORGE ST	MANCHESTER	D331 L016
	1843 DENT	39 GEORGE ST	MANCHESTER	D473 L020
	1845 DENT	39 GEORGE ST	MANCHESTER	D474 L020
	1846 DENT	39 GEORGE ST	MANCHESTER	D879 L072
	1848 DENT	49 GEORGE ST	MANCHESTER	D332 L016
	1848 DENT	49 GEORGE ST	MANCHESTER	D475 L020
	1850 DENT	49 GEORGE ST	MANCHESTER	D476 L020
	1851 DENT	49 GEORGE ST	MANCHESTER	D567 L020
	1852 DENT	49 GEORGE ST	MANCHESTER	D216 L009
	1852 DENT	49 GEORGE ST	MANCHESTER	D477 L020
	1855 DENT	16 ST JOHN'S ST	MANCHESTER	D478 L020
BEREND S	1829 DENT	27 BOLD ST	LIVERPOOL	D404 L016
	1832 DENT	30 BOLD ST	LIVERPOOL	D445 L016
	1834 DENT	28 BOLD ST	LIVERPOOL	D405 L016
BEREND SAMUEL	1824 DENT	25 BOLD ST	LIVERPOOL	D401 L016
	1828 DENT	25 BOLD ST	LIVERPOOL	D025 L020
	1834 DENT	23 BOLD ST	LIVERPOOL	D236 L009
	1837 DENT	28 BOLD ST	LIVERPOOL	D566 L020
	1837 DENT	30 BOLD ST	LIVERPOOL	D407 L016
	1846 DENT	59 BOLD ST	LIVERPOOL	D303 L014
BEREND SAMUEL S	1835 DENT	28 BOLD ST	LIVERPOOL	D406 L016
	1839 DENT	59 BOLD ST 33 ST ANNE ST	LIVERPOOL	D408 L016
	1841 DENT	59 BOLD ST	LIVERPOOL	D409 L016
	1843 DENT	59 BOLD ST	LIVERPOOL	D410 L016
	1843 DENT	59 BOLD ST	LIVERPOOL	D434 L019
	1845 DENT	59 BOLD ST	LIVERPOOL	D411 L016
	1846 DENT	59 BOLD ST	LIVERPOOL	D879 L072
	1847 DENT	59 BOLD ST	LIVERPOOL	D412 L016
	1848 DENT	59 BOLD ST	LIVERPOOL	D332 L016
	1849 DENT	59 BOLD ST	LIVERPOOL	D413 L016
	1851 DENT	59 BOLD ST	LIVERPOOL	D438 L020
	1851 DENT	59 BOLD ST	LIVERPOOL	D414 L016
	1852 DENT	59 BOLD ST	LIVERPOOL	D216 L009
	1853 DENT	59 BOLD ST	LIVERPOOL	D415 L016
	1855 DENT	59 BOLD ST	LIVERPOOL	D416 L016
BERENDSON SAMUEL	1827 DENT	25 BOLD ST	LIVERPOOL	D402 L016
BERGER	1837 DENT	27 BERESFORD ST	ST HELIER	DB74 L080
	1843 DENT	WESLEY ST	ST HELIER	DC58 L088
BERGER A	1839 DENT	BERESFORD ST	ST HELIER	DB43 L078
BERGER M	1845 DENT	WESLEY ST	ST HELIER	DA82 L011
BERMINGHAM J	1848 DENT	2 TRINITY HOUSE LANE	HULL	D378 L018
BERMINGHAM JOHN	1848 DENT	2 TRINITY HOUSE LANE	HULL	D332 L016
	1851 SURDENT	2 TRINITY HOUSE LANE	HULL	D259 L010

BERMINGHAM JOHN	1851 DENT	2 TRINITY HOUSE LANE	HULL	D379 L018
	1852 DENT	2 TRINITY HOUSE LANE	HULL	D216 L009
BESWICK JOHN	1800 DENT MUSICIAN	21 SMITHY DOOR	MANCHESTER *	D453 L020
	1802 DENT MUSICIAN	21 SMITHY DOOR	MANCHESTER *	D454 L020
BEVERS E	1854 DENT	46 BROAD ST	OXFORD	DA71 L011
BEVERS EDMUND	1842 DENT	COWLEY ROW	OXFORD	D123 L007
	1846 SURDENT	LOWER COWLEY HO	OXFORD	D640 L050
	1851 DENT	46 BROAD ST	OXFORD	DA42 L011
	1852 SURDENT	46 BROAD ST	OXFORD	D645 L050
	1853 SURDENT	46 BROAD ST	OXFORD	DBB0 L082
	1854 SURDENT	46 BROAD ST	OXFORD	D628 L049
BEW	1818 DENT (PR REG ET AL) GREAT EAST ST		BRIGHTON	DB26 L011
BEW (& SINCLAIR)	1832 DENT	116 ST JAMES ST	BRIGHTON	D819 L011
	1833 DENT	116 ST JAMES ST	BRIGHTON	D583 L044
	1840 DENT	116 ST JAMES ST	BRIGHTON	D585 L044
BEW CHARLES	1822 DENT	69 EAST ST	BRIGHTON	DA68 L011
	1822 DENT	69 EAST ST	BRIGHTON	D598 L047
	1823 DENT	69 EAST CLIFF	BRIGHTON	D142 L011
	1824 DENT	69 EAST ST	BRIGHTON	D599 L047
	1826 DENT	69 GT EAST ST	BRIGHTON	D597 L011
	1831 DENT	12 PAVILION PDE	BRIGHTON	D582 L044
	1832 DENT	12 PAVILION PDE	BRIGHTON	DB19 L011
	1833 DENT	12 PAVILION PDE	BRIGHTON	D583 L044
BEW CHARLES DENT	1840 DENT	12 PAVILION PDE	BRIGHTON	D585 L044
BEWDLEY CHARLES	1830 DENT	61 FRIAR ST	READING	D119 L020
BEWLEY	1821 DENT		READING	DB19 L011
	1822 DENT		READING	DB86 L049
	1823 DENT		READING	DB20 L011
	1829 DENT		READING	DB87 L049
	1830 DENT		READING	DBB8 L049
	1831 DENT		READING	DB89 L049
	1832 DENT		READING	DB90 L049
	1833 DENT		READING	DB91 L049
	1834 DENT		READING	DBB3 L049
	1834 DENT		READING	DB92 L049
	1835 DENT		READING	DB93 L049
	1836 DENT		READING	DB94 L049
	1837 DENT		READING	DB95 L049
	1838 DENT		READING	DC03 L049
	1839 DENT		READING	DC04 L049
	1840 DENT		READING	DC05 L049
	1841 DENT		READING	DA87 L011
	1843 DENT		READING	DB96 L049
	1844 DENT		READING	DA88 L011
	1845 DENT		READING	DB97 L049
	1846 DENT		READING	DC06 L049
	1847 DENT		READING	DC07 L049
	1848 DENT		READING	DC08 L049
	1852 DENT		READING	DA89 L011
	1855 DENT		READING	DA90 L011
BEWLEY C	1847 DENT	21 CROWN ST	READING	D815 L011
BEWLEY CHARLES	1827 DENT	61 FRIAR ST	READING	D623 L049
	1837 DENT	153 FRIAR ST	READING	D624 L049
	1840 DENT	4 SOUTHAMPTON PL	READING	D143 L020
	1842 DENT	4 SOUTHAMPTON PL	READING	D625 L049
	1842 DENT	4 SOUTHAMPTON PL	READING	DB46 L049
	1844 DENT	LONDON ST	READING	D626 L049

BEWLEY CHARLES	1847 DENT	70 LONDON ST	READING	DB84 L049
	1852 DENT	4 QUEEN'S CRESC	READING	D788 L020
	1853 DENT	2 QUEEN'S CRESC	READING	D627 L049
BICKLEY FRANCIS	1855 DENT	12 PHOEBE ANN ST	LIVERPOOL	D416 L016
BINGHAM CHARLES	1839 DENT	53 GREAT CHARLES STREET	BIRMINGHAM	D083 L002
BIRD & MORES	1829 SURDENT	113 GREENGATE	SALFORD	D465 L020
BIRD JOHN	1837 SURDENT	34 HENRIETTA ST	BATH	D121 L007
BIRD M	1839 DENT	16 UPPER PRIORY	BHAM	D301 L002
BIRD W	1833 DENT	16 UPPER PRIORY	BIRMINGHAM	D079 L002
BISHOP T	1855 SURDENT	CHURCH ST	WOOLWICH	D594 L046
BLACKMORE & BLACKMORE	1852 SURDENT	129 BOUTPORT ST	BARNSTAPLE	D145 L008
BLACKMORE & SON	1852 DENT	129 BOUTPORT ST	BARNSTAPLE	D788 L020
BLACKMORE (& BLACKMORE)	1852 SURDENT	129 BOUTPORT ST	BARNSTAPLE	D145 L008
BLACKMORE (& E)	1850 DENT	129 BOUTPORT ST	BARNSTAPLE	D147 L008
BLACKMORE (& FARTHING)	1840 DENT	TANCRED ST	TAUNTON	D676 L055
BLACKMORE (& FATH)	1852 DENT	129 BOUTPORT ST	BARNSTAPLE	D788 L020
BLACKMORE EDWARD	1840 DENT	BOUTPORT ST	BARNSTAPLE	D143 L008
	1844 SURDENT	129 BOUTPORT	BARNSTAPLE	D144 L008
BLACKMORE EDWARD & BLACKMORE	1850 DENT	129 BOUTPORT ST	BARNSTAPLE	D147 L008
BLACKMORE JULIA ANNA	1848 DENT	FORE ST	TAUNTON	DA50 L011
BLACKMORE JULIA ANNA HARRIET	1852 DENT	24 FORE ST	TAUNTON	D788 L020
BLACKMORE RICHARD	1830 DENT	TANCRED COTTAGE	TAUNTON	D119 L020
	1840 DENT	TANCRED ST	TAUNTON	D143 L020
BLAIR & LLOYD	1818 DENT	41 BOLD ST	LIVERPOOL	D302 L002
	1818 DENT	42 BOLD ST	LIVERPOOL	D432 L016
	1819 DENT	41 BOLD ST	LIVERPOOL	D735 L064
	1821 DENT	51 BOLD ST	LIVERPOOL	D399 L016
	1823 DENT	51 BOLD ST	LIVERPOOL	D400 L016
BLAIR & TURNER	1824 DENT	51 BOLD ST	LIVERPOOL	D401 L016
BLAIR JAMES	1794 DENT	GALLOWTREEGATE	LEICESTER	D282 L011
	1794 DENT TOYMAN	GALLOWTREEGATE	LEICESTER *	D680 L024
	1807 SUR DENT	39 BOLD ST	LIVERPOOL *	D394 L016
	1810 DENT	39 BOLD ST	LIVERPOOL	D395 L016
	1811 DENT	41 BOLD ST	LIVERPOOL	D396 L016
	1813 DENT	41 BOLD ST	LIVERPOOL	D397 L016
	1814 SURDENT	41 BOLD ST	LIVERPOOL	D330 L016
	1814 DENT	41 BOLD ST	LIVERPOOL	D398 L016
	1816 DENT	41 BOLD ST	LIVERPOOL	D431 L016
	1816 DENT	41 BOLD ST	LIVERPOOL	D049 L016
BLAKENEY MRS MARY	1854 DENT	69 CHESTER ST	SHEFFIELD	D757 L066
BLUNDELL (& FISHER)	1845 DENT	9 SHIP ST	BRIGHTON	DA66 L011
	1845 DENT	9 SHIP ST	BRIGHTON	D606 L047
	1846 DENT	9 SHIP ST	BRIGHTON	D601 L047
BLUNDELL WALTER	1852 DENT	OLD STEINE	BRIGHTON	D604 L047
BOARDMAN	1822 DENT	FRANKFORT ST	PLYMOUTH	D877 L022
BOARDMAN MRS	1830 SURDENT	BEDFORD ST	PLYMOUTH	D491 L022
BOARDMAN WILLIAM	1823 DENT	265 FORE ST	EXETER	D142 L008
BOOTH ISAAC	1822 SUR DENT	MARKET ST	BURSLEM *	D005 L001
	1828 SUR DENT	NEWCASTLE ST	BURSLEM *	D025 L006
BORLASE WILLIAM GRENFELL	1850 DENT	BARBICAN TCE	BARNSTAPLE	D147 L008
	1852 SURDENT	BARBICAN TCE	BARNSTAPLE	D145 L008
	1852 DENT	BARBICAN TCE	BARNSTAPLE	D788 L020
BOTT GEORGE	1797 DENT	SQUARE	BIRMINGHAM	D081 L002
	1798 DENT		NOTTINGHAM	D279 L011
	1799 DENT	BRIDLESMITH GATE	NOTTINGHAM	D499 L023
	1800 SURDENT	NEWHALL ST	BHAM	D300 L002
	1800 SURDENT	32 NEWHALL ST	BHAM	D299 L002

Name	Year/Type	Address	City	Code
BOTT GEORGE	1800 SURDENT	32 NEWHALL STREET	BIRMINGHAM	D041 L002
	1803 SURDENT	8 THE PARADE	BIRMINGHAM	D043 L002
	1805 DENT	8 THE PARADE	BIRMINGHAM	D044 L002
	1811 DENT PATMEDDEALER	BRIDLESMITHGATE	NOTTINGHAM *	D284 L011
	1814 DENT	BRIDLESMITHGATE	NOTTINGHAM	D887 L023
	1819 DENT	BRIDLESMITHGATE	NOTTINGHAM	D735 L064
BOTT MRS	1839 DENT	8 PARADE	BIRMINGHAM	D083 L002
	1842 DENT	31 NEWHALL STREET	BIRMINGHAM	D075 L002
	1847 DENT	31 NEWHALL STREET	BIRMINGHAM	D061 L002
BOTT MRS.SOPHIA	1845 DENT	31 NEWHALL STREET	BIRMINGHAM	D077 L002
BOTT PARKER	1822 DENT	BRIDLESMITH GATE	NOTTINGHAM	D005 L020
	1825 DENT	BRIDLESMITH GATE	NOTTINGHAM	D500 L023
BOTT SOPHIA	1808 DENT	CANNON STREET	BIRMINGHAM	D045 L002
	1809 DENT	CANNON STREET	BIRMINGHAM	D046 L002
	1811 DENT	CANNON ST	BIRMINGHAM	D284 L011
	1812 DENT	CANNON STREET	BIRMINGHAM	D047 L002
	1815 DENT	CANNON STREET	BIRMINGHAM	D048 L002
	1816 DENT	27 CANNON ST	BIRMINGHAM	D049 L016
	1816 DENT	27 CANNON STREET	BIRMINGHAM	D049 L002
	1818 DENT	27 COLMORE ST	BHAM	D302 L002
	1818 DENT	CANNON STREET	BIRMINGHAM	D050 L002
	1821 DENT	PARADISE STREET	BIRMINGHAM	D051 L002
	1822 DENT	35 PARADISE ST	BIRMINGHAM	D005 L020
	1823 DENT	48 PARADISE STREET	BIRMINGHAM	D052 L002
	1825 DENT	48 PARADISE STREET	BIRMINGHAM	D053 L002
	1828 DENT	48 PARADISE STREET	BIRMINGHAM	D054 L002
	1828 DENT	8 PARADE	BIRMINGHAM	D025 L006
	1829 DENT	8 PARADE	BIRMINGHAM	D055 L002
	1830 DENT	8 PARADE SUMMER ROW	BIRMINGHAM	D056 L002
	1833 DENT	8 PARADE	BIRMINGHAM	D079 L002
	1835 DENT	8 PARADE	BIRMINGHAM	D057 L002
	1837 DENT	8 PARADE	BIRMINGHAM	D566 L020
	1839 DENT	8 PARADE	BHAM	D301 L002
BOULGER JOSEPH	1850 DENT	WILLOW LNE	NORWICH	D491 L011
BOULGER P J	1842 SURDENT	3 WILLOW LANE	NORWICH	D648 L051
	1853 DENT	WILLOW LANE	NORWICH	D655 L051
BOULGER PATRICK JOSEPH	1845 DENT	3 WILLOW LANE	NORWICH	D650 L051
	1850 DENT	WILLOW LANE	NORWICH	D652 L051
	1852 SURDENT	WILLOW LANE	NORWICH	D653 L051
	1854 DENT	WILLOW LANE	NORWICH	D651 L051
BOULNOIS DE (& FATH J J)	1826 SURDENT	2 COLLEGE GREEN	BRISTOL	D925 L075
BOULNOIS J	1809 SURDENT	39 GT KING ST	BRISTOL	D046 L011
	1811 SURDENT	63 QUEEN SQ	BRISTOL	D284 L011
BOULNOIS JAMES	1803 SURDENT	31 KING ST	BRISTOL	D903 L075
	1805 SURDENT	8 COLLEGE GREEN	BRISTOL	D904 L075
	1806 SURDENT	26 GT KING ST	BRISTOL	D905 L075
	1807 SURDENT	39 GT KING ST	BRISTOL	D906 L075
	1808 SURDENT	39 GT KING ST	BRISTOL	D907 L075
	1809 SURDENT	63 QUEEN SQ	BRISTOL	D908 L075
	1810 SURDENT	63 QUEEN SQ	BRISTOL	D909 L075
	1811 SURDENT	63 QUEEN SQ	BRISTOL	D910 L075
	1812 SURDENT	65 QUEEN SQ	BRISTOL	D911 L075
	1813 SURDENT	65 QUEEN SQ	BRISTOL	D912 L075
BOULNOIS JAMES JOSEPH	1814 SURDENT	63 QUEEN SQ	BRISTOL	D913 L075
	1815 SURDENT	63 QUEEN SQ	BRISTOL	D914 L075
	1816 SURDENT	63 QUEEN SQ	BRISTOL	D915 L075
	1816 DENT	63 QUEEN SQ	BRISTOL	D948 L075

BOULNOIS JAMES JOSEPH	1817	DENT	63 QUEEN SQ	BRISTOL	D949 L075
	1818	DENT	59 QUEEN SQ	BRISTOL	D950 L075
BOULNOIS JAMES JOSEPH DE	1817	SURDENT	59 QUEEN SQ	BRISTOL	D916 L075
	1818	SURDENT	59 QUEEN SQ	BRISTOL	D917 L075
	1819	SURDENT	59 QUEEN SQ	BRISTOL	D918 L075
	1820	SURDENT	59 QUEEN SQ	BRISTOL	D919 L075
	1821	SURDENT	59 QUEEN SQ	BRISTOL	D920 L075
	1822	SURDENT	59 QUEEN SQ	BRISTOL	D921 L075
	1823	SURDENT	59 QUEEN SQ	BRISTOL	D922 L075
	1824	SURDENT	2 COLLEGE GREEN	BRISTOL	D923 L075
	1825	SURDENT	2 COLLEGE GREEN	BRISTOL	D924 L075
BOULNOIS JAMES JOSEPH DE & SO	1826	SURDENT	2 COLLEGE GREEN	BRISTOL	D925 L075
BOULNOIS JOHN DE	1827	SURDENT	2 COLLEGE GREEN	BRISTOL	D926 L075
	1828	SURDENT	2 COLLEGE GREEN	BRISTOL	D927 L075
	1830	SURDENT	2 ST AUGUSTINE'S PL	BRISTOL	D928 L075
BOULTON	1855	DENT	CROCKHERBTOWN	CARDIFF (OCC)	DC46 L085
BOULTON R B	1855	DENT	63 CROCKHERBTOWN	CARDIFF	DC47 L085
BOWDEN (& SINGLETON&BROTHERS)	1833	SURDENT	17 LR MAUDLIN ST	BRISTOL	D931 L075
BOWDEN (&SINGLETON&BROTHERS)	1833	SURDENT	WELLINGTON PL	BRISTOL	D931 L075
BOWMER GEORGE	1844	DENT	KENDALL ST	NOTTINGHAM	D504 L023
BRADDOCK CHARLES	1849	DENT	140C VAUXHALL RD	LIVERPOOL	D413 L016
BRADLEY JOSEPH	1794	DENT		LEOMINSTER	D282 L011
BRADLEY T	1855	DENT	9 BOND ST	LONDON	D594 L046
BRADLEY T D	1854	DENT	9 BOND ST	BRIGHTON	D605 L047
BRADSHAW FRANCIS JONES	1835	DENT	GRANBY ST	LEICESTER	D007 L014
BRAE A E	1840	DENT	29 PARK SQ	LEEDS	D734 L063
	1841	DENT	29 PARK SQ	LEEDS	D241 L009
BRAE ANDREW E	1846	SURDENT	29 PARK ST	LEEDS	D713 L061
BRAE ANDREW EDMUND	1828	DENT	29 PARK SQ	LEEDS	D025 L020
	1830	SURDENT	29 PARK SQ	LEEDS	D256 L010
	1834	DENT	29 PARK SQ	LEEDS	D042 L015
	1834	DENT	29 PARK SQ	LEEDS (LATE JOSEPH M	D236 L009
	1837	DENT	29 PARK SQ	LEEDS	D566 L020
	1837	DENT	29 PARK SQ	LEEDS	D257 L010
	1839	SURDENT	29 PARK SQ	LEEDS	D082 L015
	1841	DENT	29 PARK SQ	LEEDS	D331 L016
	1842	SURDENT	29 PARK SQ	LEEDS	D060 L015
	1845	SURDENT	29 PARK SQ	LEEDS	D275 L015
	1846	DENT	29 PARK SQ	LEEDS	D879 L072
	1847	SURDENT	29 PARK SQ	LEEDS	D276 L015
	1849	DENT	29 PARK SQ	LEEDS	D277 L015
	1853	SURDENT	29 PARK SQ	LEEDS	D261 L010
BRAE ANDREW EDWARD	1848	DENT	29 PARK LANE	LEEDS	D332 L016
	1851	DENT	29 PARK SQ	LEEDS	D283 L015
	1852	DENT	29 PARK LANE	LEEDS	D216 L009
	1855	DENT	29 PARK LANE	LEEDS	D222 L009
BRENDON WILLIAM EDWARD	1844	DENT	15 DEVONSHIRE TCE	PLYMOUTH	D492 L022
	1844	DENT	15 DEVONSHIRE PL	PLYMOUTH	D144 L008
	1850	DENT	DEVONSHIRE TCE	PLYMOUTH	D147 L008
BRENNAN ANDREW	1842	SURDENT	PRINCE'S ST	NORWICH	D648 L051
	1845	DENT	ST ANDREW'S HALL PLAIN	NORWICH	D650 L051
	1850	DENT	PRINCES ST	NORWICH	DA91 L011
BREUER	1793	DENT APOTH	BROAD ST	BATH *	DB21 L011
	1794	SURDENT	BROAD ST	BATH	DB22 L011
	1796	SURDENT	BROAD ST	BATH	DB23 L011
	1801	DENT APOTH	39 BROAD ST	BATH *	DB49 L025
BREWER	1812	DENT	44 BROAD ST	BATH	D114 L007

BREWER (& FATH T)	1822	SURDENT	KINGSTON BDGS	BATH	D005 L020
BREWER JAMES	1826	SURDENT APOTH	2 ST ANDREWS TERR	BATH *	D117 L007
BREWER T	1819	SURDENT	6 BROAD ST	BATH	D115 L007
BREWER THEODORE	1800	SURDENT ETC MIDWIFE	39 BROAD ST	BATH *	D111 L007
	1805	SUR DENT	42 BROAD ST	BATH *	D112 L007
	1809	SUR DENT	42 BROAD ST	BATH *	D113 L007
	1809	SUR DENT	42 BROAD ST	BATH *	D046 L011
BREWER THEODORE & SON	1822	SURDENT	KINGSTON BDGS	BATH	D005 L020
BRIDGEMAN WILLIAM K	1854	DENT	50 HIGH ST	KING'S LYNN	D651 L051
BRIDGES THOMAS	1849	SURDENT	113 NORFOLK ST	SHEFFIELD	D756 L066
	1852	SURDENT	113 NORFOLK ST	SHEFFIELD	D260 L010
	1852	DENT	113 NORFOLK ST	SHEFFIELD	D216 L009
	1855	DENT	113 NORFOLK ST	SHEFFIELD	D222 L009
BRIDGES THOMAS BARTLETT	1854	DENT	113 NORFOLK ST	SHEFFIELD	D757 L066
BRIDGMAN WILLIAM K	1850	DENT	69 ST GILES ST	NORWICH	D652 L051
BRIDGMAN WILLIAM KEENELY	1850	DENT	69 ST GILES ST	NORWICH	DA91 L011
BRIDGMAN WILLIAM KENEELEY	1852	SURDENT	69 ST GILES ST	NORWICH	D653 L051
BRIDGMAN WILLIAM KENEELY	1845	DENT	WILLOW LANE	NORWICH	D650 L051
	1854	DENT	69 ST GILES ST	NORWICH	D651 L051
BROMLEY C	1834	SURDENT	1 PORTLAND PL	SOUTHAMPTON	D335 L017
	1836	SURDENT	1 PORTLAND TCE	SOUTHAMPTON	D336 L017
	1848	DENT	1 PORTLAND TCE	SOUTHAMPTON	D357 L017
	1849	DENT	1 PORTLAND TCE	SOUTHAMPTON	D341 L017
	1852	DENT	1 PORTLAND TCE	SOUTHAMPTON	DB72 L025
	1853	DENT	1 PORTLAND TCE	SOUTHAMPTON	D343 L017
	1855	SURDENT	1 PORTLAND TCE	SOUTHAMPTON	DA84 L011
	1855	DENT	1 PORTLAND TCE	SOUTHAMPTON	D344 L017
BROMLEY CHARLES	1823	DENT	9 HIGH ST	SOUTHAMPTON	D142 L017
	1830	DENT	31 HIGH ST	SOUTHAMPTON	D119 L020
	1839	SURDENT	1 PORTLAND TCE	SOUTHAMPTON	D337 L017
	1843	SURDENT	1 PORTLAND TCE	SOUTHAMPTON	D338 L017
	1844	DENT	1 PORTLAND TCE	SOUTHAMPTON	D144 L06B
	1845	DENT	1 PORTLAND TCE	SOUTHAMPTON	D339 L017
	1847	DENT	1 PORTLAND TCE	SOUTHAMPTON	D340 L017
	1849	DENT	1 PORTLAND TCE	SOUTHAMPTON	D345 L017
	1851	DENT	1 PORTLAND TCE	SOUTHAMPTON	D342 L017
	1852	DENT	1 PORTLAND TCE	SOUTHAMPTON	D346 L017
	1852	DENT	1 PORTLAND TCE	SOUTHAMPTON	D788 L020
BROOKES JOHN	1832	DENT	127 DUKE ST	LIVERPOOL	D445 L016
	1834	DENT	125 DUKE ST	LIVERPOOL	D405 L016
BROOKHOUSE ROBERT	1838	DENT	22 COOPER ST	MANCHESTER	D470 L020
	1840	DENT	24 PRINCESS ST	MANCHESTER	D471 L020
	1841	DENT	24 PRINCESS ST	MANCHESTER	D472 L020
	1841	DENT	24 PRINCES ST	MANCHESTER	D331 L016
	1843	DENT	24 PRINCESS ST	MANCHESTER	D473 L020
	1845	DENT	34 COOPER ST	MANCHESTER	D474 L020
	1846	DENT	40 & 68 MOSLEY ST	MANCHESTER	D879 L072
	1848	DENT	100 MOSLEY ST	MANCHESTER	D475 L020
	1848	DENT	100 MOSLEY ST	MANCHESTER	D332 L016
	1850	DENT	109 MOSLEY ST	MANCHESTER	D476 L020
	1851	DENT	109 MOSLEY ST	MANCHESTER	D567 L020
	1852	DENT	100 MOSLEY ST	MANCHESTER	D216 L009
	1852	DENT	109 MOSLEY ST	MANCHESTER	D477 L020
	1855	DENT	100 MOSLEY ST	MANCHESTER	D478 L020
BROOKS & ROSE	1834	DENT	126 DUKE ST	LIVERPOOL	D236 L009
BROOKS JOHN	1835	DENT	28 GT GEORGE ST	LIVERPOOL	D406 L016
	1837	DENT	28 GT GEORGE ST	LIVERPOOL	D407 L016

BROOKS JOHN	1837 DENT	GT GEORGE ST	LIVERPOOL	D566 L020
	1839 DENT	55 GT GEORGE ST	LIVERPOOL	D408 L016
	1841 DENT	55 GT GEORGE ST	LIVERPOOL	D409 L016
	1843 DENT	55 GT GEORGE ST	LIVERPOOL	D410 L016
	1843 DENT	55 GT GEORGE ST	LIVERPOOL	D434 L019
	1845 DENT	55 GT GEORGE ST	LIVERPOOL	D411 L016
	1846 DENT	55 GT GEORGE ST	LIVERPOOL	D303 L014
	1846 DENT	55 GT GEORGE ST	LIVERPOOL	DB79 L072
	1847 DENT	55 GT GEORGE ST	LIVERPOOL	D412 L016
	1848 DENT	55 GT GEORGE ST	LIVERPOOL	D332 L016
	1849 DENT	55 GT GEORGE ST	LIVERPOOL	D413 L016
	1851 DENT	55 GT GEORGE ST	LIVERPOOL	D414 L016
	1851 DENT	55 GT GEORGE ST	LIVERPOOL	D438 L020
	1852 DENT	55 GT GEORGE ST	LIVERPOOL	D216 L009
	1853 DENT	55 GT GEORGE ST	LIVERPOOL	D415 L016
BROOKS R	1854 DENT	WEST ST	BUCKINGHAM	DA71 L011
BROOKS ROBERT HEYGATE	1849 SURDENT	PARSONS ST	BANBURY	DA94 L011
	1850 SURDENT	PARSONS ST	BANBURY	DA95 L011
	1851 DENT	PARSON ST	BANBURY	DA42 L011
	1851 SURDENT	HIGH ST	BANBURY	DA96 L011
	1852 SURDENT	HIGH ST	BANBURY	DA97 L011
	1853 SURDENT	HIGH ST	BANBURY	DA98 L011
	1853 SURDENT	HIGH ST	BANBURY	DB80 L082
	1854 SURDENT	HIGH ST	BANBURY	D628 L049
	1854 SURDENT	HIGH ST	BANBURY	DA99 L011
	1855 SURDENT	HIGH ST	BANBURY	DB01 L011
BROOKSBANK MICHAEL	1853 SURDENT	64 MARKET ST	BRADFORD	D261 L010
	1855 SURDENT	64 MARKET ST	BRADFORD	D222 L009
BROOMFIELD GEORGE	1834 DENT	11 CASTLE GATE	YORK	D236 L009
	1837 DENT	10 NESSGATE	YORK	D257 L010
	1840 SURDENT	10 NEESGATE	YORK	D734 L063
	1840 DENT	10 NESSGATE	YORK	DB88 L006
	1841 SURDENT	10 NEES GATE	YORK	D241 L009
	1841 DENT	9 LONG ROOM ST	SCARBORO	D331 L016
	1855 DENT	9 ST NICHOLAS ST	SCARBORO	D262 L010
	1855 DENT	9 ST NICHOLAS ST	SCARBORO	D550 L031
BROTHERS (&SINGLETON&BOWDEN)	1833 SURDENT	17 LR MAUDLIN ST	BRISTOL	D931 L075
	1833 SURDENT	WELLINGTON PL	BRISTOL	D931 L075
BROWN	1809 SURDENT	TEMPLE ROW	BIRMINGHAM	D046 L002
	1817 DENT		HENLEY (EV FRIDAY LED323 L014
	1818 DENT		HENLEY (EV FRIDAY LED324 L014
	1822 DENT		HENLEY (EV FRIDAY LED321 L014
	1822 DENT		HENLEY (FRIDAY IN SED318 L014 NG
	1823 DENT		HENLEY (EV FRIDAY LED322 L014
	1824 DENT		HENLEY (FRIDAY IN SED319 L014 NG
	1825 DENT		HENLEY (EV FRIDAY LED325 L014
	1829 DENT		HENLEY (FRIDAY AT LED320 L014 W
	1840 SURDENT	PORTLAND ST	LEAMINGTON	D307 L014
	1841 SURDENT	PORTLAND ST	LEAMINGTON	D306 L014
	1842 SURDENT	59 PORTLAND ST	LEAMINGTON	D305 L014
	1845 SURDENT	59 PORTLAND ST	LEAMINGTON	D309 L014
	1848 SURDENT	59 PORTLAND ST	LEAMINGTON	D308 L014
BROWN C	1855 SURDENT	23 OLD STEYNE	BRIGHTON	D594 L046
BROWN CHARLES	1839 SURDENT	WILLIAM ST	WOOLWICH	D584 L020
	1845 DENT	WILLIAM ST	WOOLWICH	DA66 L011
	1847 DENT	WILLIAM ST	WOOLWICH	D586 L044
	1850 SURDENT	WILLIAM ST	WOOLWICH	DA75 L011

BROWN G	1832 DENT	CHURCH ST	LEAMINGTON	D315 L014
	1833 DENT	34 CHURCH ST	LEAMINGTON	D316 L014
	1837 DENT	2 UPPER PARADE	LEAMINGTON	D317 L014
	1845 DENT		LEAMINGTON	D077 L006
	1849 DENT	59 PORTLAND ST	LEAMINGTON	D310 L014
	1854 DENT	59 PORTLAND ST	LEAMINGTON	D015 L001
BROWN GEORGE	1833 SURDENT	34 CHURCH ST	LEAMINGTON	D312 L014
	1834 SURDENT	34 CHURCH ST	LEAMINGTON	D313 L014
	1835 DENT	2 UPPER PARADE	LEAMINGTON	D311 L014
	1835 DENT	2 UPPER UNION PARADE	LEAMINGTON	D007 L014
	1838 SURDENT	2 UPPER PARADE	LEAMINGTON	D314 L014
	1841 DENT	57 PORTLAND ST	LEAMINGTON	D028 L002
	1850 DENT	59 PORTLAND ST	LEAMINGTON	D013 L002
	1850 SURDENT	59 PORTLAND ST	LEAMINGTON	D063 L002
BROWN H	1845 DENT		WARWICK	D077 L006
	1854 DENT	WEST ST	WARWICK	D015 L001
BROWN H S	1845 DENT	STRATFORD	WARWICK	D077 L006
BROWN HENRY	1841 DENT	WEST ST	WARWICK	D028 L002
	1846 DENT	WEST ST	WARWICK	D303 L014
	1850 SURDENT	WEST ST	WARWICK	D063 L002
	1851 DENT	WEST ST	WARWICK	DA42 L011
BROWN JOHN CROW	1855 DENT	48 BRIGGATE	LEEDS	D222 L014
BROWN S	1822 DENT	BATH ST	LEAMINGTON	D005 L020
BROWN SAMUEL	1811 SURDENT		HENLEY IN ARDEN	D284 L011
BROWN W	1851 DENT	2 CAMDEN COTTAGES	HASTINGS	DA77 L011
BROWNE C	1851 DENT	12 SOUTHWOOD TCE	HIGHGATE	DA77 L011
BROWNE JOHN C	1851 DENT	48 BRIGGATE	LEEDS	D283 L015
BROWNE JOHN CROW	1849 DENT	48 BRIGGATE	LEEDS	D277 L015
	1853 DENT	48 BRIGGATE	LEEDS	D261 L010
BUCHANAN A D	1855 DENT	RED LION ST	BOSTON	D682 L056
BUCHANAN ALFRED DANIEL	1851 SURDENT	RED LION ST	BOSTON	DB54 L025
BUCK W	1855 DENT	28 HIGH ST	COLCHESTER	D594 L046
BUCK WILLIAM	1848 SURDENT	28 HIGH ST	COLCHESTER	DA53 L011
BUCKELL JOHN W	1852 DENT	2 JEWRY ST	WINCHESTER	D346 L017
BUCKELL W	1848 DENT	NEW ST	SALISBURY	D357 L011
	1855 DENT	NEW ST	SALISBURY	DA84 L011
BUCKELL WILLIAM	1852 DENT	NEW ST	SALISBURY	D346 L017
	1852 DENT	NEW ST	SALISBURY	D788 L020
BUCKLER C	1848 DENT	66 HIGH ST	NEWPORT I OF W	D357 L017
	1852 DENT	67 HIGH ST	NEWPORT (HANTS)	DB72 L025
	1855 DENT	166 HIGH ST	CHICHESTER	DA84 L011
BUCKNELL JOHN	1839 DENT	EAST ST	CHICHESTER	D584 L011
BUGGS LUKE	1850 DENT	MARKET ST	WISBEACH	DA91 L011
BULLOCK (& EVANS)	1840 DENT	SOMERSET ROW	SWANSEA	D143 L020
BUNTER G	1855 DENT	HIGH ST	MAIDSTONE	D594 L046
BUNTER GEORGE	1854 DENT	MIDDLE ROW	MAIDSTONE	DB82 L082
BURCH R	1855 DENT	HIGH ST	SAFFRON WALDEN	D594 L046
BURGESS	1839 DENT	2 VICTORIA TCE	LEAMINGTON	D326 L014
BURLEY JOHN	1850 SURDENT	GERARD ST	HALIFAX	D571 L041
	1853 SURDENT	25 LISTER LANE	HALIFAX	D261 L010
	1855 DENT	25 LISTER LANE	HALIFAX	D222 L009
BURTON T J	1851 DENT	95 CHURCH ST	CROYDON	D611 L048
	1853 DENT	4 CHURCH ST	CROYDON	D612 L048
	1855 SURDENT	15 SURREY ST	CROYDON	D594 L046
	1855 DENT	90 HIGH ST	CROYDON	D613 L048
BUTCHER RICHARD	1852 DENT	STANDISHGATE	WIGAN	D537 L029
	1854 DENT	STANDISHGATE	WIGAN	D439 L019

BUTCHER RICHARD	1855 DENT	STANDISHGATE	WIGAN	D732 L064
BUTTERS JAMES	1851 DENT	8 MORPETH ST	LIVERPOOL	D414 L016
	1853 DENT	8 MORPETH ST	LIVERPOOL	D415 L016
BUTTERS JAMES HALL	1855 DENT	8 MORPETH ST	LIVERPOOL	D416 L016
CAFFERATA	1844 DENT	21 BRIDGE ST	SUNDERLAND	D213 L009
CAFFERATA J	1816 DENT	CORNWALLIS ST	LIVERPOOL	D049 L016
	1818 DENT	CORNWALLIS ST	LIVERPOOL	D302 L002
	1819 DENT	CORNWALLIS ST	LIVERPOOL	D735 L064
CAFFERATA J L	1850 SURDENT	21 BRIDGE ST	SUNDERLAND	D214 L009
	1851 SURDENT	21 BRIDGE ST	SUNDERLAND	D215 L009
	1853 SURDENT	21 BRIDGE ST	SUNDERLAND	D243 L009
	1855 DENT	21 BRIDGE ST	SUNDERLAND	D223 L009
CAFFERATA JAMES L	1841 SURDENT	21 BRIDGE ST	SUNDERLAND	D241 L009
	1844 DENT	21 BRIDGE ST	SUNDERLAND	DB78 L081
	1854 SURDENT	23 BRIDGE ST	SUNDERLAND	D218 L009
CAFFERATA JAMES LEWIS	1847 DENT	21 BRIDGE ST	SUNDERLAND	D242 L009
	1851 SURDENT	21 BRIDGE ST	SUNDERLAND	D292 L013
CAFFERATA JAMES LOUIS	1834 DENT	BRIDGE ST	SUNDERLAND	D236 L009
	1848 DENT	21 BRIDGE ST	SUNDERLAND	D332 L016
	1855 DENT	19 BRIDGE ST	SUNDERLAND	D222 L009
CAFFERATA JOSEPH	1824 DENT	3 CORNWALLIS ST	LIVERPOOL	D401 L016
	1827 DENT	3 CORNWALLIS ST	LIVERPOOL	D402 L016
	1828 DENT	3 CORNWALLIS ST	LIVERPOOL	D025 L020
	1829 DENT	3 CORNWALLIS ST	LIVERPOOL	D404 L016
CALDCLEUGH J	1853 DENT	81 NEW ELVET	DURHAM	D243 L009
CALDCLEUGH JOHN	1852 SURDENT	32 CLAYPATH	DURHAM	D287 L013
	1853 SURDENT	81 NEW ELVET	DURHAM	D286 L013
	1854 SURDENT	81 NEW ELVET	DURHAM	D289 L013
	1855 SURDENT	81 NEW ELVET	DURHAM	DB76 L081
CALDCLOUGH JOHN	1855 DENT	81 NEW ELVET	DURHAM	D222 L009
CANTON	1851 SURDENT	HILL ST	RICHMOND	DA83 L011
CAPPER JOHN	1852 SURDENT	115 FITZWILLIAM ST	SHEFFIELD	D260 L010
	1855 DENT	115 FITZWILLIAM ST	SHEFFIELD	D222 L009
CARELLI J W	1832 SURDENT	66 COLLEGE ST	BRISTOL	D930 L075
	1833 SURDENT	66 COLLEGE ST	BRISTOL	D931 L075
CARR JOHN	1828 DENT	PINSTONE ST	SHEFFIELD	D750 L066
CARR JOHN WILLIAM	1828 DENT SUR	HUMBER ST	HULL *	D025 L020
CARSON M	1828 DENT	FLAT ST	SHEFFIELD	D750 L066
CARSON MATILDA	1839 DENT	17 FLAT ST	SHEFFIELD	D301 L002
	1840 DENT	17 FLAT ST	SHEFFIELD	D734 L063
	1841 DENT	17 FLAT ST	SHEFFIELD	D241 L009
CARTER	1839 SURDENT	55 ST GEORGE'S PL	CHELTENHAM	DB32 L069
CARTER JOHN HENRY	1846 DENT	22 MARKET ST	MANCHESTER	DB79 L072
	1851 DENTSUR	GEORGE ST	WAKEFIELD	DB54 L025
	1853 DENT	GEORGE ST	WAKEFIELD	D261 L010
CARTWRIGHT	1848 SURDENT	DIX'S FIELD	EXETER	D176 L008
	1849 SURDENT	NORTHERNHAY PL	EXETER	D177 L008
CARTWRIGHT & DAVIS	1850 DENT	7 POST OFFICE ST	NORWICH	DA91 L011
	1850 DENT	7 POST OFFICE ST	NORWICH	D652 L051
CARTWRIGHT E G	1851 SURDENT	SOUTHERNHAY	EXETER	D179 L008
CARTWRIGHT EDWARD	1850 DENT	23 DIX'S FIELD	EXETER	D147 L008
CARTWRIGHT EDWARD C	1848 DENT	5 NORTHERNHAY PL	EXETER	DA50 L011
CARTWRIGHT G	1850 SURDENT	NORTHERNHAY PL	EXETER	D178 L008
CATTLIN WILLIAM ALFRED	1845 DENT		NORTH HOLLOWAY	DA66 L011
CAUDLE WILLIAM	1826 DENT	7 RICHMOND ST	BRIGHTON	D597 L011
CAVE THOMAS	1851 DENT	HIGH ST	MAIDSTONE	DA77 L011
CAWLEY G	1847 DENT	COBOURG ST	EXETER	D152 L008

CAWLEY GEORGE	1844 DENT	DEVONSHIRE TCE	PLYMOUTH	D492 L022
	1844 DENT	DEVONSHIRE TCE	PLYMOUTH	D144 L008
	1850 DENT	DEVONSHIRE TCE	PLYMOUTH	D147 L008
	1852 DENT	3 DEVONSHIRE TCE	PLYMOUTH	D493 L022
	1852 DENT	3 DEVONSHIRE TCE	PLYMOUTH	D788 L020
	1852 DENT	3 DEVONSHIRE TCE	PLYMOUTH	D145 L008
CHAMBERLAIN & TAYLOR	1855 DENT	124 HIGH ST	SUNDERLAND	D223 L009
CHAMBERLAIN JOSEPH	1823 DENT	GEORGE LANE	IPSWICH	D142 L011
CHAMBERS THOMAS	1848 DENT	MOOR LANE	BOLTON	D332 L016
	1851 DENT	MOOR LANE	BOLTON	D438 L020
	1854 DENT	26 MOOR LANE	BOLTON	D439 L019
	1855 DENT	26 MOOR LANE	BOLTON	D732 L064
CHARLTON	1787 SURDENT	GROVE	BATH	D110 L007
	1793 SURDENT	4 LOWER CHURCH ST	BATH	DB21 L011
	1794 SURDENT	5 LOWER CHURCH ST	BATH	DB22 L011
	1796 SURDENT	5 LOWER CHURCH ST	BATH	DB23 L011
CHERRIMAN	1845 DENT	SHIP ST	BRIGHTON	DB70 L025
CHERRIMAN J	1851 DENT	26 SHIP ST	BRIGHTON	DA77 L011
	1855 SURDENT	26 SHIP ST	BRIGHTON	D594 L046
	1855 SURDENT	17 CLARENCE ST	BRIGHTON	D594 L046
CHERRIMAN J V	1843 SURDENT	26 SHIP ST	BRIGHTON	D600 L047
	1845 DENT	26 SHIP ST	BRIGHTON	D606 L047
CHERRIMAN JOHN	1846 DENT	SHIP ST	BRIGHTON	D601 L047
	1848 DENT	26 SHIP ST	BRIGHTON	D602 L047
	1850 DENT	26 SHIP ST	BRIGHTON	D603 L047
	1852 DENT	26 SHIP ST	BRIGHTON	D604 L047
	1854 DENT	26 SHIP ST	BRIGHTON	D605 L047
CHERRIMAN REUBEN	1845 DENT	26 SHIP ST	BRIGHTON	DA66 L011
CHILD WILLIAM	1853 DENT	24 NORTON ST	LIVERPOOL	D415 L016
	1853 SURDENT	4 PORTLAND CRESC	LEEDS	D261 L010
	1855 DENT	4 PORTLAND CRESC	LEEDS	D222 L009
CHURCH WILLIAM	1840 DENT	15 BLADUD'S BDGS	BATH	D143 L020
CLARK A	1851 DENT	FRIAR'S WALK	LEWES	DA77 L011
	1851 DENT	13 WARWICK ST	WORTHING	DA77 L011
	1855 SURDENT	67 MIDDLE ST	BRIGHTON	D594 L046
CLARK ANDREW	1852 DENT	8 NORTH ST	BRIGHTON	D604 L047
CLARK E	1851 DENT	33 NORTH ST	LEWES	DA77 L011
	1855 DENT	22 OLD STEYNE	BRIGHTON	D594 L046
CLARK EBENEZER	1839 DENT	19 OLD STEYNE	BRIGHTON	D584 L011
	1846 DENT	19 OLD STEINE	BRIGHTON	D601 L047
	1848 DENT	19 OLD STEINE	BRIGHTON	D602 L047
	1850 DENT	19 OLD STEINE	BRIGHTON	D603 L047
	1852 DENT	19 OLD STEINE	BRIGHTON	D604 L047
CLARK ISAIAH	1841 DENT	LOW PAVEMENT	NOTTINGHAM	D331 L016
CLARK JAMES	1832 DENT	127 ST JAMES ST	BRIGHTON	DB19 L011
CLARK WILLIAM	1835 DENT	PLEASANT ST	LEICESTER	D007 L014
CLARKE	1840 DENT	CARRINGTON ST	NOTTINGHAM	D503 L023
	1845 DENT	19 OLD STEINE	BRIGHTON	DB70 L025
CLARKE & SON	1846 DENT	SADLER GATE BRIDGE	DERBY	D693 L057
	1848 DENT	LOW PAVEMENT	NOTTINGHAM	D800 L020
	1848 DENT	LOW PAVEMENT	NOTTINGHAM	D506 L023
	1850 DENT	30 NORTH ST	BRISTOL	D960 L075
	1850 DENT	LOW PAVEMENT	NOTTINGHAM	D013 L020
	1851 SURDENT	30 NORTH ST	BRISTOL	D896 L075
	1852 SURDENT	30 NORTH ST	BRISTOL	D897 L075
	1853 DENT	30 NORTH ST	BRISTOL	D802 L020
	1853 DENT	30 NORTH ST	BRISTOL	D951 L075

CLARKE & SON	1853	SURDENT	12 NORTH ST	BRISTOL	D898 L075
	1853	DENT	CHURCH ST	MANSFIELD	D507 L023
	1854	DENT	LOW PAVEMENT	NOTTINGHAM	D510 L023
	1854	SURDENT	23 CUMBERLAND ST	BRISTOL	D899 L075
	1855	DENT	CHURCH ST	MANSFIELD	D511 L023
	1855	SURDENT	23 CUMBERLAND ST	BRISTOL	D947 L075
CLARKE & SONS	1853	SURDENT	LOW PAVEMENT	NOTTINGHAM	D507 L023
CLARKE (& FATH & BRO 1)	1853	SURDENT	LOW PAVEMENT	NOTTINGHAM	D507 L023
CLARKE (& FATH & BRO 2)	1853	SURDENT	LOW PAVEMENT	NOTTINGHAM	D507 L023
CLARKE (& FATH E)	1850	SURDENT	30 NORTH ST	BRISTOL	D946 L075
CLARKE (& FATH I)	1847	DENT	LOW PAVEMENT	NOTTINGHAM	D505 L023
	1855	DENT	LOW PAVEMENT	NOTTINGHAM	D511 L023
CLARKE (& FATH)	1846	DENT	SADLER GATE BRIDGE	DERBY	D693 L057
	1848	DENT	LOW PAVEMENT	NOTTINGHAM	D800 L020
	1848	DENT	LOW PAVEMENT	NOTTINGHAM	D506 L023
	1850	DENT	LOW PAVEMENT	NOTTINGHAM	D013 L020
	1850	DENT	30 NORTH ST	BRISTOL	D960 L075
	1851	SURDENT	30 NORTH ST	BRISTOL	D896 L075
	1852	SURDENT	30 NORTH ST	BRISTOL	D897 L075
	1853	DENT	CHURCH ST	MANSFIELD	D507 L023
	1853	DENT	30 NORTH ST	BRISTOL	D802 L020
	1853	SURDENT	12 NORTH ST	BRISTOL	D898 L075
	1853	DENT	30 NORTH ST	BRISTOL	D951 L075
	1854	DENT	LOW PAVEMENT	NOTTINGHAM	D510 L023
	1854	SURDENT	23 CUMBERLAND ST	BRISTOL	D899 L075
	1855	SURDENT	23 CUMBERLAND ST	BRISTOL	D947 L075
	1855	DENT	CHURCH ST	MANSFIELD	D511 L023
CLARKE ANDREW	1854	DENT	67 MIDDLE ST	BRIGHTON	D605 L047
CLARKE B J	1849	DENT	11 PITTVILLE ST	CHELTENHAM	D881 L082
CLARKE BENJAMIN	1854	DENT	22 OLD STEINE	BRIGHTON	D605 L047
CLARKE E & SON	1850	SURDENT	30 NORTH ST	BRISTOL	D946 L075
CLARKE EBENEZER	1839	DENT	19 OLD STEINE	BRIGHTON	D607 L047
	1843	SURDENT	19 OLD STEYNE	BRIGHTON	D600 L047
	1845	DENT	19 OLD STEINE	BRIGHTON	D606 L047
	1854	DENT	22 OLD STEINE	BRIGHTON	D605 L047
CLARKE I & SON	1855	DENT	LOW PAVEMENT	NOTTINGHAM	D511 L023
CLARKE ISAIAH	1828	DENT	BRIDLESMITH GATE	NOTTINGHAM	D025 L020
	1831	DENT	BRIDLESMITH GATE	NOTTINGHAM	D501 L024
	1834	DENT SUR	LOW PAVEMENT	NOTTINGHAM *	D502 L023
	1835	DENT	LOW PAVEMENT	NOTTINGHAM	D007 L014
	1840	DENT SUR	LOW PAVEMENT	NOTTINGHAM *	D503 L023
	1844	DENT	LOW PAVEMENT	NOTTINGHAM	D504 L023
	1844	DENT	LOW PAVEMENT	NOTTINGHAM	D509 L023
	1847	DENT	46 GALLOWTREEGATE	LEICESTER	D505 L025
CLARKE ISAIAH & SON	1847	DENT	LOW PAVEMENT	NOTTINGHAM	D505 L023
CLARKE ISAIAH WILLIAM	1832	DENT	32 BRIDLESMITH GATE	NOTTINGHAM	D508 L023
CLARKE J	1848	DENT	MARKET ST	NOTTINGHAM	D800 L020
CLARKE JAAMES	1840	DENT	127 ST JAMES ST	BRIGHTON	D585 L044
CLARKE JAMES	1833	DENT	127 ST JAMES ST	BRIGHTON	D583 L044
	1841	DENT	MARKET ST	NOTTINGHAM	D331 L016
	1844	DENT	MARKET ST	NOTTINGHAM	D504 L023
	1844	DENT	MARKET ST	NOTTINGHAM	D509 L023
	1847	DENT	MARKET ST	NOTTINGHAM	D505 L023
	1848	DENT	MARKET ST	NOTTINGHAM	D506 L023
	1850	DENT	3 MARKET ST	NOTTINGHAM	D013 L020
	1853	DENT	9 WESTGATE	MANSFIELD	D507 L023
	1853	SURDENT	BRIDLESMITH GATE	NOTTINGHAM	D507 L023

CLARKE JAMES	1854 DENT		BRIDLESMITH GATE	NOTTINGHAM	D510 L023
CLARKE JOHN EDWARD	1828 DENT		3 SUFFOLK ST	BIRMINGHAM	D025 L006
CLARKE JOHN.E	1829 DENT		3 SUFFOLK STREET	BIRMINGHAM	D055 L002
	1830 DENT		3 SUFFOLK STREET	BIRMINGHAM	D056 L002
CLARKE JOHN.EDWARD	1828 DENT		3 SUFFOLK STREET	BIRMINGHAM	D054 L002
CLARKE RICHARD	1791 DENT		BARTHOLOMEW YD	EXETER	D154 L008
	1794 DENT		BARTHOLOMEW YD	EXETER	D282 L011
	1796 DENT		BARTHOLOMEW YD	EXETER	D155 L008
	1807 DENT		BARTHOLOMEW YD	EXETER	DA50 L011
	1811 DENT		BARTHOLOMEW YD	EXETER	D284 L011
	1816 DENT		BARTHOLOMEW YD	EXETER	D156 L008
	1822 DENT		NEW BRIDGE ST	EXETER	D157 L008
	1825 DENT		NEW BRIDGE ST	EXETER	D158 L008
CLARKE ROBERT	1844 DENT		WEEKDAY CROSS	NOTTINGHAM	D504 L023
CLARKE T	1831 DENT		118 ST JAMES ST	BRIGHTON	D582 L044
CLARKE T M	1848 DENT CUPPER		MEDICAL HALL GEORGE ST	RICHMOND *	DB45 L011
	1851 SURDENT CUPPER		GEORGE ST	RICHMOND *	DA83 L011
	1855 DENT		GEORGE ST	RICHMOND	D594 L046
CLARKE THOMAS	1785 DENT		THE LEATHER BOTTLE DERITEND	BIRMINGHAM	D036 L002
	1787 DENT		THE LEATHER BOTTLE DERITEND	BIRMINGHAM	D037 L002
	1790 DENT		LEATHER BOTTLE DERITEND	BIRMINGHAM	D076 L002
	1791 DENT		THE LEATHER BOTTLE DERITEND	BIRMINGHAM	D039 L002
	1793 DENT		LEATHER BOTTLE DERITEND	BIRMINGHAM	D281 L011
CLAY BENNETT	1851 DENT		KING ST	MAIDSTONE	DA77 L011
CLIFTON JOHN	1826 DENT		HIGH ST	BOSTON	D864 L070
	1828 DENT		HIGH ST	BOSTON	D025 L020
	1841 DENT		SKIRBECK QUARTER	BOSTON	D331 L016
CLOUGH EDWARD	1848 DENT		NORTH PDE	HALIFAX	D332 L016
	1851 SURDENT		55 NEWLAND	LINCOLN	DB54 L025
COBB J S	1853 DENT		GEORGE ST	YARMOUTH	D655 L051
COCKS WILLIAM CARY	1847 DENT		MAN OF ROSS HOUSE	ROSS	D012 L001
COGAN DAVID	1850 DENT		3 ORIEL VILLAS	CHELTENHAM	DA74 L011
COGAN J D	1846 SURDENT		6 WALCOT TCE	BATH	D124 L007
	1849 SURDENT MED ELECTR		6 WALCOT TCE	BATH *	D126 L007
	1850 SURDENT		16 WALCOT TCE	BATH	D127 L007
	1852 DENT		6 WALCOT TCE	BATH	D128 L007
	1854 DENT		6 WALCOT TCE	BATH	D129 L007
COGAN JOHN	1840 DENT		PARAGON BDGS	BATH	D143 L020
COGAN JOHN D	1841 SURDENT		16 PARAGON BDGS	BATH	D122 L007
	1842 SURDENT		16 PARAGON BDGS	BATH	D123 L007
	1852 SURDENT		6 WALCOT TCE	BATH	D788 L020
COGAN JOHN DANIEL	1848 SURDENT		6 WALCOT TCE	BATH	D125 L007
COGAN SAMUEL W	1848 DENT		EAST REACH	TAUNTON	DA50 L011
COKER THOMAS	1840 DENT		HIGH ST	TAUNTON	D676 L055
	1840 DENT		HIGH ST	TAUNTON	D143 L020
	1852 DENT		BRIDGE ST	TAUNTON	D788 L020
COLEMAN A	1854 DENT		24 HARMER ST	GRAVESEND	DC35 L084
	1855 DENT		24 HARMER ST	GRAVESEND	D594 L046
	1855 DENT		24 HARMER ST	GRAVESEND	DC18 L084
COLES S J	1847 DENT		PRINCESS SQ	PLYMOUTH	D152 L008
COLES STRATTON	1844 DENT		20 PRINCESS SQ	PLYMOUTH	D144 L008
	1844 DENT		20 PRINCESS SQ	PLYMOUTH	D492 L022
	1852 DENT		10 PRINCESS SQ	PLYMOUTH	D145 L008
	1852 DENT		10 PRINCESS SQ	PLYMOUTH	D788 L020
COLES STRATTON J	1850 DENT		PRINCESS SQ	PLYMOUTH	D147 L008
	1852 DENT		10 PRINCESS SQ	PLYMOUTH	D493 L022
COLLER THOMAS	1848 DENT		TONBRIDGE	TAUNTON	DA50 L011

Name	Year/Type	Address	Town	Code
COMLEY W	1845 DENT	3 BRUNSWICK COTTAGES	SOUTH NEWINGTON RD	DA66 L011
	1851 DENT	3 BRUNSWICK COTTAGES	STOKE NEWINGTON RD	DA77 L011
	1855 DENT	STOKE NEWINGTON RD	LONDON	D594 L046
COMLEY WILLIAM	1839 DENT CUPPER	STOKE NEW'TON RD	STOKE NEWINGTON *	D584 L020
COMPTON SAMUEL	1852 DENT		PAINGTON	D145 L008
	1852 DENT	PAIGNTON	TORQUAY	D788 L020
COOPE THOMAS	1838 DENT	WHITWORTH NEW RD	ROCHDALE	D470 L020
COOPER & CO	1847 DENT	10 SLATER ST	LIVERPOOL	D412 L016
	1848 DENT	10 SLATER ST	LIVERPOOL	D332 L016
	1849 DENT	10 SLATER ST	LIVERPOOL	D413 L016
	1851 DENT	10 SLATER ST	LIVERPOOL	D438 L020
	1851 DENT	10 SLATER ST	LIVERPOOL	D414 L016
	1852 DENT	10 SLATER ST	LIVERPOOL	D216 L009
	1853 DENT	10 SLATER ST	LIVERPOOL	D415 L016
	1855 DENT	29 BOLD ST	LIVERPOOL	D416 L016
COOPER JOHN	1845 DENT	MANOR ST	CLAPHAM	DA66 L011
COOPER ROBERT	1845 DENT	SOUTH ST	EASTBOURNE	DA66 L011
	1846 DENT	10 SLATER ST	LIVERPOOL	D303 L014
COOPER ROBERT J	1845 DENT	10 SLATER ST	LIVERPOOL	D411 L016
COOPER S & CO	1846 DENT	10 SLATER ST	LIVERPOOL	DB79 L072
COOPER THOMAS	1841 DENT	WHITWORTH RD	ROCHDALE	D472 L020
COPPEL CHARLES	1837 DENT	51 LUNE ST	PRESTON	DB68 L078
	1841 DENT	51 LUNE ST	PRESTON	D534 L028
	1844 DENT	63 FISHERGATE	PRESTON	D436 L019
	1846 DENT	63 FISHERGATE	PRESTON	D713 L072
	1848 DENT	63 FISHERGATE	PRESTON	D332 L016
	1851 DENT	63 FISHERGATE	PRESTON	D727 L020
	1851 DENT	62 FISHERGATE	PRESTON	D438 L020
	1851 DENT	63 FISHERGATE	PRESTON	D437 L019
	1854 DENT	68 FISHERGATE	PRESTON	D439 L019
	1855 DENT	68 FISHERGATE	PRESTON	D732 L064
COPPELL CHARLES	1851 DENT	63 FISHERGATE	PRESTON	D673 L053
	1853 DENT	63 FISHERGATE	PRESTON	D533 L028
COREY CHARLES	1853 DENT	3 SLATER ST	LIVERPOOL	D415 L016
	1855 DENT	3 SLATER ST	LIVERPOOL	D416 L016
COREY WILLIAM	1850 DENT	40 DEVONSHIRE PL	BRIGHTON	D603 L047
CORNISH HENRY ROBERTS	1852 SURDENT	MARKET PL	PENZANCE	D788 L020
CORNWALL	1853 DENT	69 LONDON ST	READING	D627 L049
CORNWALL AUGUSTUS	1852 DENT	69 LONDON ST	READING	D788 L020
CORNWALL AUGUSTUS R	1854 DENT	38 BROAD ST	READING	D628 L049
COTTLE F J	1852 DENT	GRONEZ ST	ALDERNEY	DB72 L025
COX E	1840 DENT	BRIDGE ST	NOTTINGHAM	D503 L023
CRAWCORN	1853 DENT	BRUNSWICK TCE	WINDSOR	D627 L049
CRAWCOUR BARNETT	1822 SUR DENT	MAGDALEN ST	NORWICH *	D005 L020
CRAWCOUR BERNARD	1830 DENT	MAGDALEN ST	NORWICH	D119 L020
CRAWCOUR HENRY	1836 DENT	MAGDALEN ST	NORWICH	D649 L051
CRAWCOUR LINDSAY	1853 SURDENT	10 BRUNSWICK TCE	WINDSOR	DA47 L011
CRAWCOUR M	1816 SURDENT	NEW CRESCENT	EXETER	D156 L008
	1822 SURDENT	NEW CRESCENT	EXETER	D157 L008
CRAWSHAW HENRY	1855 DENT	171 WOODHOUSE LANE	LEEDS	D222 L009
CREED WILLIAM	1843 DENT	35 SIR THOMAS BDGS	LIVERPOOL	D434 L019
CREWE JAMES	1827 DENT	8 BEVINGTON BUSH RD	LIVERPOOL	D402 L016
CROCKER FREDERICK	1830 SURDENT	13 COOPER ST	MANCHESTER	D466 L020
	1832 SURDENT	13 COOPER ST	MANCHESTER	D467 L020
	1833 SURDENT	13 COOPER ST	MANCHESTER	D468 L020
CROCKER JONATHAN	1853 DENT	20 STOKES CROFT	BRISTOL	D802 L020
CROSS CHARLES	1810 DENT	BY MOUNTERGATE CHURCH	NORWICH	D875 L051

CROWTHER ISAAC	1840 DENT	14 BRIDGE END	LEEDS	D734 L063
	1841 DENT	14 BRIDGE END	LEEDS	D241 L009
CROXFORD G	1854 DENT	CHINNOR	TETSWORTH	DA71 L011
CULLIS	1839 SURDENT	CLARENCE ST	CHELTENHAM	D957 L068
CULLIS G	1849 SURDENT	PITTVILLE ST	CHELTENHAM	D842 L069
CULLIS G H	1840 SURDENT	11 CLARENCE ST	CHELTENHAM	D833 L069
	1841 SURDENT	5 REGENT ST	CHELTENHAM	D834 L069
	1848 DENT	2 PORTLAND ST	CHELTENHAM	D954 L069
	1849 DENT	2 PORTLAND ST	CHELTENHAM	D881 L082
	1850 DENT	33 CAMBRAY	CHELTENHAM	DA74 L011
	1850 SURDENT	33 CAMBRAY PL	CHELTENHAM	D843 L069
	1851 SURDENT	33 CAMBRAY PL	CHELTENHAM	D844 L069
	1851 DENT	33 CAMBRAY	CHELTENHAM	D953 L069
	1852 SURDENT	33 CAMBRAY PL	CHELTENHAM	D845 L069
	1853 SURDENT	33 CAMBRAY PL	CHELTENHAM	D846 L069
	1853 SURDENT	33 CAMBRAY PL	CHELTENHAM	D847 L069
CULLIS GEORGE H	1842 DENT	5 PITTVILLE ST	CHELTENHAM	D846 L049
	1844 SURDENT	REGENT ST	CHELTENHAM	D959 L069
CULLIS GEORGE HENRY	1847 DENT	2 PORTLAND ST	CHELTENHAM	D890 L068
	1852 DENT	33 CAMBRAY PL	CHELTENHAM	D788 L020
	1853 SURDENT	33 CAMBRAY	CHELTENHAM	D956 L068
CUMBER	1840 CUPPER DENT		GUERNSEY *	DA81 L011
CUMBER HENRY	1839 DENT CUPPER	44 FOUNTAIN ST	GUERNSEY *	D654 L011
CUNNINGHAM P G	1839 DENT	WINCHESTER ST	SALISBURY	D654 L068
	1848 DENT	ENDLESS ST	SALISBURY	D357 L011
	1855 DENT	BLUE BOAR ROW	SALISBURY	DA84 L011
CUNNINGHAM PATRICK GREGSON	1842 DENT	EXETER ST	SALISBURY	DB46 L049
	1852 DENT	ENDLESS ST	SALISBURY	D346 L017
	1852 DENT	ENDLESS ST	SALISBURY	D788 L020
CURPHEY W	1844 DENT	DUKE ST	DOUGLAS I OF M	DB52 L025
	1848 DENT	41 DUKE ST	DOUGLAS I OF M	DB24 L011
	1852 DENT	41 DUKE ST	DOUGLAS I OF M	DB73 L079
CURPHEY WILLIAM	1837 WATCHMAK DENT	DUKE ST	DOUGLAS I OF M *	D566 L020
	1843 DENT	FORT ST	DOUGLAS I OF M	DC55 L087
	1847 DENT	FORT ST	DOUGLAS I OF MAN	D505 L025
	1852 DENT	FORT ST	DOUGLAS I OF M	DC56 L087
CURSON BENJAMIN	1824 SURDENT	144 CHAPEL ST	SALFORD	D401 L019
CURTIS W B	1834 SURDENT	20 PARK ST	BRISTOL	D932 L075
	1835 SURDENT	20 PARK ST	BRISTOL	D820 L002
	1836 SURDENT	13 PARK ST	BRISTOL	D933 L075
	1837 SURDENT	13 PARK ST	BRISTOL	D934 L075
	1838 SURDENT	13 PARK ST	BRISTOL	D935 L075
	1839 SUR DENT	13 PARK ST	BRISTOL *	D654 L068
	1839 SURDENT	13 PARK ST	BRISTOL	D936 L075
	1839 SURDENT	9 RICHMOND TCE	CLIFTON	D654 L068
	1840 DENT	9 RICHMOND TCE	CLIFTON	D143 L020
	1840 DENT	13 PARK ST	BRISTOL	D143 L020
	1840 SURDENT	9 RICHMOND TCE	BRISTOL	D945 L075
	1841 SURDENT	9 RICHMOND TCE	BRISTOL	D937 L075
	1842 SURDENT	9 RICHMOND TCE	BRISTOL	D938 L075
	1843 SURDENT	9 RICHMOND TCE	BRISTOL	D939 L075
	1844 SURDENT	9 RICHMOND TCE	BRISTOL	D940 L075
	1845 SURDENT	9 RICHMOND TCE	BRISTOL	D822 L002
	1846 SURDENT	9 RICHMOND TCE	BRISTOL	D941 L075
	1846 SURDENT	9 RICHMOND TCE	BRISTOL	D879 L072
	1847 SURDENT	9 RICHMOND TCE	BRISTOL	D942 L075
	1848 SURDENT	9 RICHMOND TCE	BRISTOL	D943 L075

CURTIS W B	1849	SURDENT	9 RICHMOND TCE	BRISTOL	D944 L075
	1850	SURDENT	9 RICHMOND TCE	BRISTOL	D946 L075
	1851	SURDENT		BRISTOL	D896 L075
	1852	SURDENT	50 ROYAL YORK CRESC	BRISTOL	D897 L075
	1853	SURDENT	50 ROYAL YORK CRESC	BRISTOL	D898 L075
	1854	SURDENT	50 ROYAL YORK CRESC	BRISTOL	D899 L075
	1855	SURDENT	50 ROYAL YORK CRESC	BRISTOL	D947 L075
CURTIS WILLIAM	1852	DENT	9 RICHMOND TCE CLIFTON	BRISTOL	D788 L020
CURTIS WILLIAM B	1848	DENT	9 RICHMOND TCE	BRISTOL	DA50 L011
	1848	DENT	9 RICHMOND TCE	BRISTOL	D125 L075
	1849	DENT	9 RICHMOND TCE	BRISTOL	D891 L068
	1850	DENT	9 RICHMOND TCE	BRISTOL	D960 L075
	1853	DENT	RICHMOND TCE	BRISTOL	D951 L075
CURZON BENJAMIN	1829	SURDENT	1 ST STEPHEN'S ST	SALFORD	D565 L020
CUTTRISS W	1854	DENT	HIGH ST	BEDFORD	DA71 L011
DALE	1842	SURDENT	4 LOWER PARADE	LEAMINGTON	D305 L014
	1845	SURDENT	107 WARWICK ST	LEAMINGTON	D309 L014
	1848	SURDENT	107 WARWICK ST	LEAMINGTON	D308 L014
DALE & LEVASON	1838	SURDENT	4 UNION PARADE	LEAMINGTON	D314 L014
	1839	DENT	4 LOWER PARADE	LEAMINGTON	D326 L014
	1839	DENT	4 LOW UNION PDE	LEAMINGTON	D301 L002
	1840	SURDENT	4 LOWER PARADE	LEAMINGTON	D307 L014
	1841	SURDENT	4 LOWER PARADE	LEAMINGTON	D306 L014
DALE & MORGAN	1854	DENT	107 WARWICK ST	LEAMINGTON	D015 L001
DALE (& LEVASON)	1835	DENT	4 UNION PARADE	LEAMINGTON	D311 L014
	1837	DENT	4 LOWER PARADE	LEAMINGTON	D317 L014
DALE H	1846	DENT	107 WARWICK ST	LEAMINGTON	D303 L014
DALE HENRY	1841	DENT	4 LOWER PARADE	LEAMINGTON	D028 L002
	1849	DENT	107 WARWICK ST	LEAMINGTON	D310 L014
	1850	DENT	107 WARWICK ST	LEAMINGTON	D013 L002
DALES HENRY	1850	SURDENT	107 WARWICK ST	LEAMINGTON	D063 L002
DARLEY GEORGE	1854	DENT	MILL LANE	NORWICH	D651 L051
DASH J	1855	SURDENT	37 QUEEN'S RD	BRIGHTON	D594 L046
DASH JAMES	1854	DENT	37 QUEEN'S RD	BRIGHTON	D605 L047
DAVENPORT & ROBB	1855	DENT	27 WHITEFRIARGATE	HULL	D222 L009
DAVENPORT & ROWNEY	1855	DENT	27 WHITEFRIARS' GATE	HULL	D682 L056
	1855	DENT	CHEQUERGATE	LOUTH	D682 L056
DAVENPORT J W	1848	DENT	46 GEORGE ST	HULL	D378 L018
DAVENPORT JOSEPH W	1851	SURDENT	46 GEORGE ST	HULL	D259 L010
	1851	DENT	46 GEORGE ST	HULL	D379 L018
DAVIDSON WILLIAM	1855	DENT	130 QUEEN ST	WHITEHAVEN	D222 L020
DAVIES ALBERT & J	1852	DENT	40 PARADISE STREET	BIRMINGHAM	D078 L002
DAVIES JOHN (& A)	1852	DENT	40 PARADISE STREET	BIRMINGHAM	D078 L002
DAVIS (& CARTWRIGHT)	1850	DENT	7 POST OFFICE ST	NORWICH	DA91 L011
	1850	DENT	7 POST OFFICE ST	NORWICH	D652 L051
DAVIS J O (JUN)	1855	SURDENT	TONTINE ST	FOLKESTONE	D594 L046
DAVIS SAMUEL	1853	DENT	55 BOLD ST	LIVERPOOL	D415 L016
DAWSON E	1855	DENT	EASTGATE	LOUTH	D682 L056
DE BERRI & SON	1837	DENT	17 EASY ROW	BIRMINGHAM	D566 L020
DE BERRI (& FATH)	1837	DENT	17 EASY ROW	BIRMINGHAM	D566 L020
DE BERRY (& FATH)	1839	SURDENT	17 EASY ROW	BIRMINGHAM	D083 L002
DE BERRY (& FATHER S)	1839	SURDENT	17 EASY ROW	BHAM	D083 L002
DE BERRY SAMUEL AND SON	1839	SURDENT	17 EASY ROW	BIRMINGHAM	D083 L002
DE BOULNOIS JAMES JOSEPH	1822	SURDENT	59 QUEEN ST	BRISTOL	D005 L020
DE BOULNOIS JOHN	1829	SURDENT	2 HANMER'S BDGS PARK ST	BRISTOL	D821 L002
DE LA BARRE ANTHONY B	1846	DENT	156 BRIGGATE	LEEDS	D879 L072
DE LESSERT C	1854	DENT	DARLINGTON ST	WOLVERHAMPTON	D015 L001

Name	Year/Type	Address	City	Ref
DE LESSERT CHARLES G	1850 DENT	DARLINGTON ST	WOLVERHAMPTON	D013 L001
	1851 DENT	DARLINGTON ST	WOLVERHAMPTON	D104 L006
	1855 SURDENT	DARLINGTON ST	WOLVERHAMPTON	D064 L011
	1855 SURDENT	DARLINGTON ST	WOLVERHAMPTON	D098 L006
DE LESSERT CHARLES GRIERSON	1846 DENT	ST JOHN'S SQ	WOLVERHAMPTON	D713 L061
	1851 SURDENT	DARL'GTON ST	WOLVERHAMPTON	D699 L059
DE LOUDE & SON	1851 SURDENT	ST JOHN'S SQ	WOLVERHAMPTON	D699 L059
DE LOUDE (& FATH C L)	1850 DENT	85 GROSVENOR ST	CHORLTON	D476 L020
DE LOUDE (& FATH)	1851 SURDENT	ST JOHNS SQUARE	WOLVERHAMPTON	D699 L059
DE LOUDE CHARLES	1834 DENT	39 WINDSOR ST	LIVERPOOL	D405 L016
	1835 DENT	40 WINDSOR ST	LIVERPOOL	D406 L016
DE LOUDE CHARLES LOUIS & SON	1850 DENT	85 GROSVENOR ST	CHORLTON	D476 L020
DE LOUDE L C	1838 DENT		WOLVERHAMPTON	D696 L058
	1846 SUR DENT	CHURCH ST	WOLVERHAMPTON *	D713 L061
DE LOUDE LOUIS CHARLES	1841 DENT	CHURCH ST	WOLVERHAMPTON	D028 L002
	1845 SURDENT	CHURCH ST	WOLVERHAMPTON	D077 L002
DE LOUDE THOMAS C	1832 DENT	7 CLAYTON SQ 20 DEVONSHIRE PL	LIVERPOOL	D445 L016
DE RAYMOND G	1855 DENT	HILL ST	POOLE	DA84 L011
DEAN (& IMRIE)	1845 DENT	75 PICCADILLY	MANCHESTER	D474 L020
DEANE HENRY EDWARD	1846 DENT	75 PICCADILLY	MANCHESTER	DB79 L072
	1848 DENT	75 PICCADILLY	MANCHESTER	D475 L020
	1848 DENT	75 PICCADILLY	MANCHESTER	D332 L016
	1850 DENT	26 PICCADILLY	MANCHESTER	D476 L020
	1851 DENT	26 PICCADILLY	MANCHESTER	D567 L020
	1852 DENT	26 PICCADILLY	MANCHESTER	D477 L020
	1852 DENT	26 PICCADILLY	MANCHESTER	D216 L009
	1855 DENT	23 LEVER ST	MANCHESTER	D478 L020
DEARLE G	1853 DENT	PRINCE'S ST	NORWICH	D655 L051
DEARLE GEORGE	1852 SURDENT	PRINCE'S ST	NORWICH	D653 L051
DEBERE & SON	1839 DENT	17 EASY ROW	BHAM	D301 L002
DEBERE (& FATHER)	1839 DENT	17 EASY ROW	BHAM	D301 L002
DELABARRE ANT BERNASCONI	1853 SURDENT	9 ST PAUL'S ST	HUDDERSFIELD	D261 L010
DELABARRE ANTHONY BERNASCONI	1842 SURDENT	51 BRIGGATE	LEEDS	D060 L015
	1847 SURDENT	56 BRIGGATE	LEEDS	D276 L015
DELABARRE MONSIEUR	1840 DENT	1 MILL HILL	LEEDS	D734 L063
	1841 DENT	1 MILL HILL	LEEDS	D241 L009
	1855 DENT	9 ST PAUL'S ST	HUDDERSFIELD	D222 L009
DEMPSTER H	1855 DENT	4 PARK TCE HAMMERSMITH	LONDON	D594 L046
DEVEY J.E (?F)	1842 DENT	18 ST MARTINS STREET	BIRMINGHAM	D075 L002
DEVONPORT J W	1845 SURDENT	MR BROADBENT'S BROAD ST	HALIFAX	D570 L041
DEVONPORT JOSEPH WILDE	1852 DENT	46 GEORGE ST	HULL	D216 L009
DICK	1845 SURDENT	64 NORFOLK ST	SHEFFIELD	D755 L066
DICKER W J	1847 DENT	15 UNION ST	PLYMOUTH	D152 L008
DICKER WILLIAM J	1852 DENT CUPPER	17 PRINCESS ST	PLYMOUTH *	D493 L022
DICKER WILLIAM JOSEPH	1844 DENT CUPPER	15 UNION PL	PLYMOUTH *	D492 L022
	1844 DENT CUPPER	15 UNION PL	PLYMOUTH *	D144 L008
	1850 DENT	PRINCESS SQ	PLYMOUTH	D147 L008
	1852 DENT CUPPER	17 PRINCESS ST	PLYMOUTH *	D788 L020
	1852 DENT CUPPER	17 PRINCESS ST	PLYMOUTH *	D145 L008
DICKIN JOSEPH PEARSON	1848 DENT	YORKSHIRE ST	ROCHDALE	D332 L016
	1851 DENT	54 CHEETHAM ST	ROCHDALE	D438 L020
DINSDALE C	1850 DENT MECH	1 ALBION ST	NEWCASTLE*	D214 L009
	1851 SURDENT	1 ALBION ST	NEWCASTLE	D215 L009
	1853 DENT	1 ALBION ST	NEWCASTLE	D243 L009
	1855 DENT	1 ALBION ST	NEWCASTLE	D219 L009
DINSDALE CUTHBERT	1848 DENT	25 NELSON ST	NEWCASTLE	D332 L016
	1852 DENT	1 ALBION ST	NEWCASTLE	D216 L009

DINSDALE CUTHBERT	1855 DENT	1 ALBION ST	NEWCASTLE	D222 L009
DINSDALE T C	1855 DENT	2 ALBION ST	NEWCASTLE	D223 L009
DIXON	1846 SURDENT	TONTINE SQ	HANLEY	D109 L006
DIXON & PICNOT	1846 DENT	13 WELLINGTON ST	LEEDS	D879 L072
	1847 SURDENT	13 WELLINGTON ST	LEEDS	D276 L015
	1848 DENT	13 WELLINGTON ST	LEEDS	D332 L016
	1849 DENT	13 WELLINGTON ST	LEEDS	D277 L015
	1851 DENT	13 WELLINGTON ST	LEEDS	D283 L015
	1852 DENT	13 WELLINGTON ST	LEEDS	D216 L009
	1855 DENT	13 WELLINGTON ST	LEEDS	D222 L009
DIXON DR	1846 SURDENT	TONTINE SQ	HANLEY	D713 L061
DIXON J P	1854 DENT	PICCADILLY	SHELTON	D015 L001
DIXON JAMES B	1851 SURDENT	MARKET SQ	HANLEY	D104 L006
DIXON JAMES BROWNE	1850 DENT	TONTINE SQ	HANLEY	D013 L001
DIXON JOHN	1828 DENT	125 EAST ST	LEEDS	D025 L020
	1830 SURDENT	125 EAST ST	LEEDS	D256 L010
	1834 DENT	10 PARK ROW	LEEDS	D042 L015
	1837 DENT	10 PARK ROW	LEEDS	D257 L010
	1839 SURDENT	10 PARK ROW	LEEDS	D082 L015
	1840 DENT	10 PARK ROW	LEEDS	D734 L063
	1841 DENT	10 PARK ROW	LEEDS	D241 L009
	1841 DENT	10 PARK ROW	LEEDS	D331 L016
DIXON RUTH	1842 SURDENT	10 PARK ROW	LEEDS	D060 L015
	1845 SURDENT	10 PARK ROW	LEEDS	D275 L015
	1846 SURDENT	10 PARK ROW	LEEDS	D713 L061
DIXON THOMAS	1840 DENT	BOND ST	LEEDS	D734 L063
	1840 DENT	5 INFIRMARY ST	LEEDS	D734 L063
	1841 DENT	BOND ST	LEEDS	D241 L009
	1841 DENT	20 BOND ST	LEEDS	D331 L016
	1841 DENT	5 INFIRMARY ST	LEEDS	D331 L016
	1841 DENT	5 INFIRMARY ST	LEEDS	D241 L009
	1842 SURDENT	5 INFIRMARY ST	LEEDS	D060 L015
	1845 SURDENT	20 BOND ST	LEEDS	D275 L015
	1846 SURDENT	20 BOND ST	LEEDS	D713 L061
	1846 DENT	20 BOND ST	LEEDS	D879 L072
	1847 SURDENT	5 INFIRMARY ST	LEEDS	D276 L015
	1847 SURDENT	20 BOND ST	LEEDS	D276 L015
	1848 DENT	20 BOND ST	LEEDS	D332 L016
	1848 DENT	5 INFIRMARY ST	LEEDS	D332 L016
	1849 DENT	5 INFIRMARY ST	LEEDS	D277 L015
	1851 DENT	27 EAST PDE	LEEDS	D283 L015
	1852 DENT	5 INFIRMARY ST	LEEDS	D216 L009
	1852 DENT	27 EAST PDE	LEEDS	D216 L009
	1853 SURDENT	27 EAST PDE	LEEDS	D261 L010
	1855 DENT	27 EAST PDE	LEEDS	D222 L009
DOLEMAN JOHN	1828 DENT	BRIDLESMITH GATE	NOTTINGHAM	D025 L020
DON B	1853 MECH DENT	4 EAST CROSS ST	SUNDERLAND	D243 L009
	1855 MECH DENT	4 EAST CROSS ST	SUNDERLAND	D223 L009
DOWNES E Y	1852 CHEM DENT	MEDICAL HALL	ABERGAVENNY *	D476 L011
DOWNING & DOWNING	1838 SURDENT	ELDON SQ	NEWCASTLE	D239 L009
	1847 SURDENT	9 NORTHUMBERLAND ST	NEWCASTLE	D242 L009
	1847 SURDENT	17 ELDON SQ	NEWCASTLE	D242 L009
DOWNING (& DOWNING)	1838 SURDENT	ELDON SQ	NEWCASTLE	D239 L009
	1847 SURDENT	17 ELDON SQ	NEWCASTLE	D242 L009
	1847 SURDENT	9 NORTHUMBERLAND ST	NEWCASTLE	D242 L009
DOWNING (& FATH R & BRO 1)	1841 DENT	17 ELDON SQ	NEWCASTLE	D241 L009
DOWNING (& FATH R & BRO 2)	1841 DENT	17 ELDON SQ	NEWCASTLE	D241 L009

DOWNING B	1853 DENT	9 ELDON SQ	NEWCASTLE	D243 L009
DOWNING E	1850 DENT	9 NORTHUMBERLAND PL	NEWCASTLE	D214 L009
	1851 SURDENT	9 NORTHUMBERLAND PL	NEWCASTLE	D215 L009
	1853 DENT	9 NORTHUMBERLAND ST	NEWCASTLE	D243 L009
	1855 DENT	9 NORTHUMBERLAND PL	NEWCASTLE	D219 L009
	1855 DENT	30 NORTHUMBERLAND ST	NEWCASTLE	D223 L009
DOWNING EDWARD	1844 DENT	9 NORTHUMBERLAND PL	NEWCASTLE	D213 L009
	1848 DENT	9 NORTHUMBERLAND ST	NEWCASTLE	D332 L016
	1852 DENT	9 NORTHUMBERLAND ST	NEWCASTLE	D216 L009
	1855 DENT	9 NORTHUMBERLAND ST	NEWCASTLE	D222 L009
DOWNING M	1853 DENT	ORCHARD ST	BRISTOL	D802 L020
	1853 DENT	ORCHARD ST	BRISTOL	D951 L075
DOWNING MESSRS	1836 DENT	ELDON SQ	NEWCASTLE	DB34 L011
DOWNING R	1847 DENT	30 OLD ELVET	DURHAM ALT MON & TUED297 L013
	1850 DENT	9 ELDON SQ	NEWCASTLE	D214 L009
	1851 SURDENT	9 ELDON SQ	NEWCASTLE	D215 L009
	1855 DENT	9 ELDON SQ	NEWCASTLE	D223 L009
	1855 DENT	9 ELDON SQ	NEWCASTLE	D219 L009
DOWNING RICHARD	1827 DENT SUR	2 SAVILLE ROW	NEWCASTLE*	D211 L009
	1828 DENT	48 NORTHUMBERLAND PL	NEWCASTLE	D025 L020
	1829 DENT	48 NORTHUMBERLAND PL	NEWCASTLE	D212 L009
	1833 DENT	17 ELDON SQ	NEWCASTLE	D246 L009
	1834 DENT	17 ELDON SQ	NEWCASTLE	D236 L009
	1837 DENT	17 ELDON SQ	NEWCASTLE	D566 L020
	1848 DENT	17 ELDON SQ	NEWCASTLE	D332 L016
	1852 DENT	9 ELDON SQ	NEWCASTLE	D216 L009
DOWNING RICHARD & R	1839 SURDENT	ELDON SQ	NEWCASTLE	D240 L009
DOWNING RICHARD & SONS	1841 DENT	17 ELDON SQ	NEWCASTLE	D241 L009
DOWNING RICHARD (& FATHER R)	1839 SURDENT	ELDON SQ	NEWCASTLE	D240 L009
DOWNING WILLIAM	1844 DENT	17 ELDON SQ	NEWCASTLE	D213 L009
DOWNINGS (& MAWN)	1820 SURDENT	NORTHUMBERLAND PL	NEWCASTLE	D787 L020
	1821 SURDENT	NORTHUMBERLAND PL	NEWCASTLE	D210 L009
DRABBLE ROBERT CHARLES	1852 SURDENT	95 FITZWILLIAM ST	SHEFFIELD	D260 L010
	1854 DENT	45 FITZWILLIAM ST	SHEFFIELD	D757 L066
DRAKE (& DUTTON)	1848 DENT	3 WHITEFRIARGATE	HULL	D332 L016
	1848 DENT	3 WHITEFRIARGATE	HULL	D378 L018
DRAKE (& MOSELEY)	1855 SURDENT	HIGH ST	WOLVERHAMPTON	D098 L006
DRAKE (& MOSELY)	1854 DENT	48 HIGH ST	NEWCASTLE UNDER LYMED015 L001
	1854 DENT		WOLVERHAMPTON	D015 L001
	1855 SURDENT	HIGH ST	WOLVERHAMPTON	D064 L011
DRESCHFELD LEOPOLD	1855 DENT	4 CAVENDISH ST	CHORLTON	D478 L020
DREWEATT THOMAS & CO	1852 DENT	84 HIGH ST	PORTSMOUTH	D346 L017
DRUMMOND & CO	1837 DENT	2 PORTLAND BDGS	MANCHESTER	D566 L020
DRURY ALEX RUPERT O'BRIAN	1850 SURDENT	FERGUSON ST	HALIFAX	D571 L041
DRURY RUPERT ALEXANDER	1850 DENT	45 NORTH PDE MANN'M LANE	BRADFORD	DB35 L078
DUFF JOHN	1850 DENT	10 SOUTHWELL ST	BRISTOL	D960 L075
	1852 DENT	COTHAM GATE COTHAM RD	BRISTOL	D788 L020
	1853 DENT	16 SOUTHWELL ST	BRISTOL	D951 L075
DUNCAN RICHARD	1852 DENT	P O COURT	CARLISLE	D216 L009
	1855 DENT	32 SCOTCH ST	CARLISLE	D222 L020
DUNSFORD & SUGGETT	1850 DENT	17 ST GILES ST	NORWICH	D652 L051
	1852 SURDENT	ST GILES ST	NORWICH	D653 L051
	1853 DENT	17 ST GILES ST	NORWICH	D655 L051
	1854 DENT	70 HIGH ST	KING'S LYNN	D651 L051
	1854 DENT	17 ST GILES ST	NORWICH	D651 L051
DURANT E	1855 SURDENT	HIGH ST	DORKING	D594 L046
DURLACHER	1812 CORN CUTTER DENT	2 ABBEY PLACE	BATH *	D114 L007

DURLACHER	1819	SURDENT CORN OPERATO7 YORK ST	BATH *	D115 L007
	1824	SURDENT CORN OPERATO7 YORK ST	BATH *	D116 L007
	1839	SURDENT CORNOPERATOR83 WINCHCOMB ST	CHELTENHAM *	D957 L068
DURLACHER ABRAHAM	1822	SURDENT 7 YORK ST	BATH	D005 L020
	1830	DENT 83 WINCHCOMBE ST	CHELTENHAM	D119 L020
DUTTON & DRAKE	1848	DENT 3 WHITEFRIARGATE	HULL	D378 L018
	1848	DENT 3 WHITEFRIARGATE	HULL	D332 L016
DUTTON WILLIAM HENRY	1846	SURDENT 5 GEORGE ST	HULL	D258 L010
	1851	SURDENT 4 WHITEFRIARGATE	HULL	D259 L010
	1851	DENT 4 WHITEFRIARGATE	HULL	D379 L018
	1852	DENT 3 WHITEFRIARGATE	HULL	D216 L009
	1855	DENT 20 CHARLOTTE ST	HULL	D222 L009
DYASON C	1851	DENT SAXON ST	DOVER	DA77 L011
DYASON T	1847	DENT 4 SAXON ST	DOVER	D586 L044
DYASON TASSEL	1849	DENT 4 SAXON ST	DOVER	D587 L011
DYASON TASSELL	1845	DENT 185 SNARGATE ST	DOVER	DA66 L011
	1855	SURDENT 4 SAXON ST	DOVER	D594 L046
EBDON E	1822	SURDENT PEMBROKE ST	PLYMOUTH	D877 L022
EDEN T E	1855	SURDENT 26 OLD STEYNE	BRIGHTON	D594 L046
EDEN THOMAS E	1852	DENT 30 CANNON PL	BRIGHTON	D604 L047
EDEN THOMAS EDWARD	1854	DENT 26 OLD STEINE	BRIGHTON	D605 L047
EDWARDS E	1846	SURDENT 26 MILSOM ST	BATH	D124 L007
EDWARDS EDWARD	1848	SURDENT 26 MILSOM ST	BATH	D125 L007
	1849	SURDENT 26 MILSOM ST	BATH	D126 L007
	1850	SURDENT 13 ABBEY CHURCHYARD	BATH	D127 L007
	1853	SURDENT WEARFIELD PL	EXETER	D153 L008
	1854	SURDENT 1 BARING TCE	EXETER	DB71 L025
EDWARDS H	1852	DENT SHIRE HALL LANE	DORCHESTER	D788 L020
	1855	DENT 27 SOUTH ST	DORCHESTER	DA84 L011
EDWARDS JAMES	1848	SURDENT 18 GAY ST	BATH	D125 L007
	1849	SURDENT 18 GAY ST	BATH	D126 L007
	1850	SURDENT 18 GAY ST	BATH	D127 L007
	1852	DENT 18 GAY ST	BATH	D128 L007
	1852	SURDENT 18 GAY ST	BATH	D788 L020
	1854	DENT 18 GAY ST	BATH	D129 L007
ELLIOTT JOHN	1844	DENT FORE ST	KINGSBRIDGE	D144 L008
ELLIS THOMAS SUR	1830	DENT ACC SUR AND APO25 DIGBETH	BIRMINGHAM *	D056 L002
EMANUEL JAMES.M	1852	DENT 19 NEWHALL STREET	BIRMINGHAM	D078 L002
ENGLISH	1847	DENT 23 COLMORE ROW	BIRMINGHAM	D061 L002
ENGLISH & SON	1842	DENT 23 COLMORE ROW	BIRMINGHAM	D075 L002
	1847	DENT 23 COLMORE ROW	BIRMINGHAM	D061 L002
ENGLISH (& FATH T)	1841	DENT 23 COLMORE ROW	BIRMINGHAM	D058 L002
	1842	DENT 23 COLMORE ROW	BIRMINGHAM	D075 L002
	1845	DENT 23 COLMORE ROW	BIRMINGHAM	D077 L002
	1846	DENT 23 COLMORE ROW	BIRMINGHAM	D879 L072
	1847	DENT 23 CLOMORE ROW	BIRMINGHAM	D061 L002
ENGLISH THOMAS	1818	DENT SUR COLMORE ROW	BHAM *	D302 L002
	1818	SURDENT COLMORE ROW	BIRMINGHAM	D050 L002
	1821	SURDENT COLMORE ROW	BIRMINGHAM	D051 L002
	1822	SUR DENT COLMORE ROW	BIRMINGHAM *	D005 L020
	1823	SURDENT 23 COLMORE ROW	BIRMINGHAM	D052 L002
	1825	SURDENT 23 COLMORE ROW	BIRMINGHAM	D053 L002
	1828	DENT 23 COLMORE ROW	BIRMINGHAM	D054 L002
	1828	DENT 23 COLMORE ROW	BIRMINGHAM	D025 L006
	1829	DENT 23 COLMORE ROW	BIRMINGHAM	D055 L002
	1830	DENT 23 COLMORE ROW	BIRMINGHAM	D056 L002
	1833	SURDENT 23 COLMORE ROW	BIRMINGHAM	D079 L002

ENGLISH THOMAS	1835 DENT	23 COLMORE ROW	BIRMINGHAM	D057 L002
	1837 DENT	23 COLMORE ROW	BIRMINGHAM	D566 L020
ENGLISH THOMAS & SON	1845 DENT	23 COLMORE·ROW	BIRMINGHAM	D077 L002
	1846 DENT	23 COLMORE ROW	BIRMINGHAM	D879 L072
ENGLISH THOMAS & SON.	1841 DENT	23 COLMORE ROW	BIRMINGHAM	D058 L002
ENGLISH THOMAS ROBERT	1850 DENT	23 COLMORE ROW	BHAM	D013 L002
ENGLISH THOMAS ROBERT.	1852 DENT	HOME 12 GEORGE STREET	BIRMINGHAM	D078 L002
	1852 DENT	233 COLMORE ROW	BIRMINGHAM	D078 L002
ENGLISH THOMAS.ROBERT	1849 SURDENT	HOME 11 GEORGE ST ISLINGTON RW	BHM	D062 L002
	1849 SURDENT	23 COLMORE ROW	BIRMINGHAM	D062 L002
	1850 SURDENT	23 COLMORE ROW	BIRMINGHAM	D063 L002
	1850 SURDENT	HOME 11 GEORGE ST ISLINGTON RW	BHM	D063 L002
	1855 SURDENT	HOME 12 GEORGE ST EDGBASTON	BHAM	D064 L002
	1855 SURDENT	23 COLMORE ROW	BIRMINGHAM	D064 L002
ENSOR EDWARD (& W)	1846 DENT	40 SEEL ST	LIVERPOOL	D303 L014
ENSOR S	1816 DENT	NAVIGATION ST	BIRMINGHAM	D049 L016
	1818 DENT	NAVIGATION ST	BHAM	D302 L002
ENSOR S (ILAS)	1816 DENT DRUG SUR AP	NAVIGATION ST	BHAM *	D049 L002
ENSOR SILAS	1822 DENT	NAVIGATION ST	BIRMINGHAM	D005 L020
ENSOR WILLIAM	1837 DENT	64 SEEL ST	LIVERPOOL	D407 L016
	1841 DENT	40 SEEL ST	LIVERPOOL	D409 L016
	1843 DENT	40 SEEL ST	LIVERPOOL	D410 L016
	1845 DENT	40 SEEL ST	LIVERPOOL	D411 L016
	1847 DENT	40 SEEL ST	LIVERPOOL	D412 L016
	1849 DENT	40 SEEL ST	LIVERPOOL	D413 L016
	1851 DENT	40 SEEL ST	LIVERPOOL	D414 L016
	1853 DENT	40 SEEL ST	LIVERPOOL	D415 L016
	1855 DENT	51 RODNEY ST	LIVERPOOL	D416 L016
ENSOR WILLIAM & E	1846 DENT	40 SEEL ST	LIVERPOOL	D303 L014
ENSOR WILLIAM EDWARD	1843 DENT	40 SEEL ST	LIVERPOOL	D434 L019
	1846 DENT	40 SEEL ST	LIVERPOOL	D879 L072
	1848 DENT	40 SEEL ST	LIVERPOOL	D332 L016
	1851 DENT	40 SEEL ST	LIVERPOOL	D438 L020
	1852 DENT	40 SEEL ST	LIVERPOOL	D216 L009
ESKELL & SONS	1841 DENT	CHESTER GATE	MACCLESFIELD	D472 L020
ESKELL (& FATH & BRO 1)	1841 DENT	CHESTER GATE	MACCLESFIELD	D472 L020
ESKELL (& FATH & BRO 2)	1841 DENT	CHESTER GATE	MACCLESFIELD	D472 L020
ESKELL A	1850 DENT	BENNETTS HILL	BHAM	D013 L002
ESKELL ABRAHAM	1849 SURDENT	3 CHURCH ST	SHEFFIELD	D756 L066
	1852 DENT	3 BENNETTS HILL	BIRMINGHAM	D078 L002
	1854 DENT	23 COLMORE ROW	BIRMINGHAM	D069 L002
	1855 SURDENT	39 BENNETTS HILL	BIRMINGHAM	D064 L002
ESKELL ALBERT	1845 DENT	74 SEEL ST	LIVERPOOL	D411 L016
	1851 DENT	55 GEORGE ST	MANCHESTER	D567 L020
	1851 SURDENT	23 HIGH PETERGATE	YORK	D259 L010
	1852 DENT	35 GEORGE ST	MANCHESTER	D477 L020
	1853 SURDENT	3 COOKRIDGE ST	LEEDS	D261 L010
	1855 DENT	3 COOKRIDGE ST	LEEDS	D222 L009
ESKELL FRANCIS	1848 DENT	32 COOPER ST	MANCHESTER	D332 L016
	1848 DENT	NORFOLK ST	SHEFFIELD	D332 L016
ESKELL FREDERICK	1843 DENT	28 COOPER ST	MANCHESTER	D473 L020
	1845 DENT	28 COOPER ST	MANCHESTER	D474 L020
	1846 DENT	28 COOPER ST	MANCHESTER	D879 L072
	1848 DENT	32 COOPER ST	MANCHESTER	D475 L020
	1850 DENT	52 COOPER ST	MANCHESTER	D476 L020
	1851 DENT	32 COOPER ST	MANCHESTER	D567 L020
	1852 DENT	32 COOPER ST	MANCHESTER	D477 L020

ESKELL FREDERICK A	1851 DENT	2 ST PETER'S SQ	MANCHESTER	D567 L020
	1852 DENT	2 ST PETER'S SQ	MANCHESTER	D216 L009
	1852 DENT	2 ST PETER'S SQ	MANCHESTER	D477 L020
	1855 DENT	2 ST PETER'S SQ	MANCHESTER	D478 L020
ESKELL LOUIS	1847 DENT		HALIFAX	D276 L015
	1847 DENT	DARLEY ST	BRADFORD	D276 L015
	1848 DENT	SQUARE	HALIFAX	D332 L016
	1853 SURDENT	DARLEY ST	BRADFORD	D261 L010
	1855 DENT	DARLEY ST	BRADFORD	D222 L009
ESKELL PHILIP	1837 DENT	40 NORFOLK ST	SHEFFIELD	D566 L020
	1852 SURDENT	39 CHURCH ST	SHEFFIELD	D260 L010
	1852 DENT	3 CHURCH ST	SHEFFIELD	D216 L009
	1854 DENT	39 CHURCH ST	SHEFFIELD	D757 L066
	1855 DENT	3 CHURCH ST	SHEFFIELD	D222 L009
ESKELL PHILIPPUS	1837 DENT	40 NORFOLK ST	SHEFFIELD	D257 L010
	1839 DENT	99 NORFOLK ST	SHEFFIELD	D301 L002
	1840 DENT	99 NORFOLK ST	SHEFFIELD	D734 L063
	1841 DENT	99 NORFOLK ST	SHEFFIELD	D753 L066
	1845 SURDENT	209 GLOSSOP RD	SHEFFIELD	D755 L066
	1846 DENT	209 GLOSSOP RD	SHEFFIELD	D879 L072
	1849 SURDENT	205 BATH BDGS	SHEFFIELD	D756 L066
ESKELL PHILLIPUS	1841 DENT	99 NORFOLK ST	SHEFFIELD	D241 L009
	1841 DENT	90 NORFOLK ST	SHEFFIELD	D754 L066
	1841 DENT	99 NORFOLK ST	SHEFFIELD	D331 L016
ESKILL A	1851 SURDENT	HIGH ST	DONCASTER	D259 L056
EVANS & BULLOCK	1840 DENT	SOMERSET ROW	SWANSEA	D143 L020
EVANS JOHN ROBERTS	1846 DENT	HIGH ST	LEICESTER	D658 L024
EVANS THOMAS	1844 DENT	OXFORD ST	SWANSEA	D144 L078
EVATT H R	1839 DENT	56 QUEEN ST	SHEFFIELD	D301 L002
	1840 DENT	56 QUEEN ST	SHEFFIELD	D734 L063
	1841 DENT	56 QUEEN ST	SHEFFIELD	D241 L009
EVATT HENRY R	1837 DENT	15 QUEEN ST	SHEFFIELD	D566 L020
	1841 DENT	56 QUEEN ST	SHEFFIELD	D754 L066
EVATT HENRY ROYLE	1837 DENT	15 QUEEN ST	SHEFFIELD	D257 L010
	1841 DENT	56 QUEEN ST	SHEFFIELD	D753 L066
	1846 DENT	QUEEN ST	SHEFFIELD	D879 L072
EVATT HENRY ROYLES	1845 SURDENT	54 QUEEN ST	SHEFFIELD	D755 L066
EVATT JAMES	1849 DENT	13 TRAFALGAR ST	LEEDS	D277 L015
EVATT WILIAM	1822 DENT	QUEEN ST	SHEFFIELD	D005 L020
EVATT WILLIAM	1811 DENT RAZORMAKER	LAMBERT ST	SHEFFIELD *	D284 L011
	1817 DENT	NORTH ST	SHEFFIELD	D747 L066
	1821 DENT	5 QUEEN ST	SHEFFIELD	D748 L066
	1822 DENT	15 QUEEN ST	SHEFFIELD	D255 L010
	1825 DENT	15 QUEEN ST	SHEFFIELD	D749 L066
	1828 DENT	5 QUEEN ST	SHEFFIELD	D025 L011
	1828 DENT	QUEEN ST	SHEFFIELD	D750 L066
	1828 SURGICAL DENT	5 QUEEN ST	SHEFFIELD	D025 L020
	1830 DENT	5 QUEEN ST	SHEFFIELD	D751 L066
	1833 DENT	15 QUEEN ST	SHEFFIELD	D752 L066
	1834 DENT	QUEEN ST	SHEFFIELD	D236 L009
	1841 DENT	QUEEN ST	SHEFFIELD	D331 L016
FARTHING	1848 SURDENT	UPPER SOUTHERNHAY	EXETER	D176 L009
	1849 SURDENT	UPPER SOUTHERNHAY	EXETER	D177 L008
	1850 SURDENT	UPPER SOUTHERNHAY	EXETER	D178 L008
	1851 SURDENT	UPPER SOUTHERNHAY	EXETER	D179 L008
FARTHING & BLACKMORE	1840 DENT	TANCRED ST	TAUNTON	D676 L055
FARTHING JOHN	1843 SURDENT	11 PORTLAND ST	SOUTHAMPTON	D338 L017

FARTHING JOHN	1844 DENT	12 PORTLAND ST	SOUTHAMPTON	D144 L068
	1845 DENT	3 TUNS GATE	GUILDFORD	DA66 L011
	1847 DENT	35 ABOVE BAR	SOUTHAMPTON	D340 L017
	1848 DENT	1 SOUTHERNHAY PL	EXETER	DA50 L011
	1850 DENT	UPPER SOUTHERNHAY	EXETER	D147 L008
	1852 SURDENT	UPPER SOUTHERNHAY	EXETER	D180 L008
	1855 DENT	26 GEORGE ST	CARDIFF	DC46 L085
FARTHING WILLIAM	1845 SURDENT	12 PORTLAND ST	SOUTHAMPTON	D339 L017
FAULKNER & PIERPOINT	1840 DENT	18 OLDHAM ST	MANCHESTER	D471 L020
	1841 DENT	18 OLDHAM ST	MANCHESTER	D472 L020
	1841 DENT	18 OLDHAM ST	MANCHESTER	D331 L016
FAULKNER & PIERREPOINT	1843 DENT	18 OLDHAM ST	MANCHESTER	D473 L020
FAULKNER & SON	1815 SURDENT	11 OLDHAM ST	MANCHESTER	D459 L020
	1817 SURDENT	11 OLDHAM ST	MANCHESTER	D460 L020
	1822 DENT	2 LEVER ST	MANCHESTER	D005 L020
	1824 SURDENT	2 LEVER ST	MANCHESTER	D463 L020
	1828 SURDENT	2 LEVER ST	MANCHESTER	D025 L020
	1828 SURDENT	2 LEVER ST	MANCHESTER	D464 L020
	1829 SURDENT	2 LEVER ST	MANCHESTER	D565 L020
	1829 SURDENT	2 LEVER ST	MANCHESTER	D465 L020
	1836 DENT	3 LEVER ST	MANCHESTER	D469 L020
	1837 DENT	3 LEVER ST	MANCHESTER	D566 L020
	1838 DENT	3 LEVER ST	MANCHESTER	D470 L020
FAULKNER (& FATH J)	1824 DENT	2 LEVER ST	MANCHESTER	D401 L019
	1830 SURDENT	2 LEVER ST	MANCHESTER	D466 L020
	1832 SURDENT	3 LEVER ST	MANCHESTER	D467 L020
	1833 SURDENT	3 LEVER ST	MANCHESTER	D468 L020
	1834 DENT	3 LEVER ST	MANCHESTER	D236 L009
FAULKNER (& FATH T)	1818 DENT	11 OLDHAM ST	MANCHESTER	D302 L002
	1819 DENT	11 OLDHAM ST	MANCHESTER	D735 L064
FAULKNER (& FATH)	1815 SURDENT	11 OLDHAM ST	MANCHESTER	D459 L020
	1817 SURDENT	11 OLDHAM ST	MANCHESTER	D460 L020
	1822 DENT	2 LEVER ST	MANCHESTER	D005 L020
	1824 SURDENT	2 LEVER ST	MANCHESTER	D463 L020
	1828 SURDENT	2 LEVER ST	MANCHESTER	D464 L020
	1828 SURDENT	2 LEVER ST	MANCHESTER	D025 L020
	1829 SURDENT	2 LEVER ST	MANCHESTER	D465 L020
	1829 SURDENT	2 LEVER ST	MANCHESTER	D565 L020
	1836 DENT	3 LEVER ST	MANCHESTER	D469 L020
	1837 DENT	3 LEVER ST	MANCHESTER	D566 L020
	1838 DENT	3 LEVER ST	MANCHESTER	D470 L020
FAULKNER J (JUN)	1816 DENT	11 OLDHAM ST	MANCHESTER	D049 L016
FAULKNER J (SEN)	1816 DENT	14 OLDHAM ST	MANCHESTER	D049 L016
	1818 DENT	14 OLDHAM ST	MANCHESTER	D302 L002
	1819 DENT	14 OLDHAM ST	MANCHESTER	D735 L064
FAULKNER JOHN	1811 DENT	LLOYD ST	MANCHESTER	D525 L020
	1813 DENT	215 DEANSGATE	MANCHESTER	D458 L020
	1815 DENT	14 OLDHAM ST	MANCHESTER	D459 L020
	1819 SURDENT	11 OLDHAM ST	MANCHESTER	D461 L020
	1821 SURDENT	2 LEVER ST	MANCHESTER	D462 L020
	1824 SURDENT	100 OLDHAM ST	MANCHESTER	D463 L020
	1828 SURDENT	100 OLDHAM ST	MANCHESTER	D464 L020
	1828 SURDENT	100 OLDHAM ST	MANCHESTER	D025 L020
	1829 SURDENT	100 OLDHAM ST	MANCHESTER	D565 L020
	1829 SURDENT	100 OLDHAM ST	MANCHESTER	D465 L020
	1830 SURDENT	100 OLDHAM ST	MANCHESTER	D466 L020
	1832 SURDENT	100 OLDHAM ST	MANCHESTER	D467 L020

FAULKNER JOHN	1833 SURDENT	100 OLDHAM ST	MANCHESTER	D468 L020
	1836 DENT	18 OLDHAM ST	MANCHESTER	D469 L020
	1837 DENT	18 OLDHAM ST	MANCHESTER	D566 L020
	1838 DENT	18 OLDHAM ST	MANCHESTER	D470 L020
	1841 DENT	NEW WISDOR	SALFORD	D331 L016
	1843 DENT	3 LEVER ST	MANCHESTER	D473 L020
	1845 DENT	ARLINGTON PL	GREENWICH	DA66 L011
	1849 DENT	ARLINGTON PL	GREENWICH	D587 L011
	1850 DENT	ARLINGTON PL	GREENWICH	DA75 L011
FAULKNER JOHN & SON	1824 SURDENT	2 LEVER ST	MANCHESTER	D401 L019
	1830 SURDENT	2 LEVER ST	MANCHESTER	D466 L020
	1832 SURDENT	3 LEVER ST	MANCHESTER	D467 L020
	1833 SURDENT	3 LEVER ST	MANCHESTER	D468 L020
	1834 DENT	3 LEVER ST	MANCHESTER	D236 L009
FAULKNER JOHN (SEN)	1817 SURDENT	14 OLDHAM ST	MANCHESTER	D460 L020
	1819 SURDENT	14 OLDHAM ST	MANCHESTER	D461 L020
	1821 SURDENT	14 OLDHAM ST	MANCHESTER	D462 L020
	1822 DENT	14 OLDHAM ST	MANCHESTER	D005 L020
	1824 SURDENT	100 OLDHAM ST	MANCHESTER	D401 L019
	1834 DENT	18 OLDHAM ST	MANCHESTER	D236 L009
FAULKNER T & SON	1818 DENT	11 OLDHAM ST	MANCHESTER	D302 L002
	1819 DENT	11 OLDHAM ST	MANCHESTER	D735 L064
FAULKNER THOMAS	1788 FUSTIAN CUTT TDRAWER TURNER ST	MANCHESTER *	D450 L020
	1794 DENT	OLDHAM ST	MANCHESTER	D282 L011
	1797 DENT	12 OLDHAM ST	MANCHESTER	D452 L020
	1804 DENT	12 OLDHAM ST	MANCHESTER	D455 L020
	1808 DENT	4 OLDHAM ST	MANCHESTER	D456 L020
	1811 DENT	OLDHAM ST	MANCHESTER	D284 L011
	1811 DENT	4 OLDHAM ST	MANCHESTER	D525 L020
	1811 DENT	4 OLDHAM ST	MANCHESTER	D457 L020
	1813 DENT	4 OLDHAM ST	MANCHESTER	D458 L020
	1815 DENT	HOUSE 10 ANCOATS PL	MANCHESTER	D459 L020
	1817 DENT	10 ANCOATS PL	MANCHESTER	D460 L020
	1840 DENT	3 LEVER ST	MANCHESTER	D471 L020
	1841 DENT	3 LEVER ST	MANCHESTER	D472 L020
	1841 DENT	3 LEVER ST	MANCHESTER	D331 L016
FAULKNER THOMAS JOHN	1845 DENT	12 OXFORD ST	MANCHESTER	D474 L020
	1846 DENT	12 OXFORD ST	MANCHESTER	D879 L072
	1848 DENT	12 OXFORD ST	MANCHESTER	D475 L020
	1848 DENT	12 OXFORD ST	MANCHESTER	D332 L016
	1850 DENT	12 OXFORD ST	MANCHESTER	D476 L020
	1851 DENT	12 OXFORD ST	MANCHESTER	D567 L020
	1852 DENT	12 OXFORD ST	MANCHESTER	D477 L020
	1852 DENT	18 OXFORD ST	MANCHESTER	D216 L009
	1855 DENT	180 OXFORD ST	MANCHESTER	D478 L020
FAWSSETT T	1855 DENT	BROOK GREEN LANE HAMERSMITH	LONDON	D594 L046
FAY	1838 DENT	7 DOCK ST	HULL	D375 L018
	1839 SUR DENT	7 DOCK ST	HULL *	D376 L018
FAY TULLIUS PRIEST	1839 DENT	159 DUKE ST	LIVERPOOL	D408 L016
	1841 DENT	3 NELSON ST	LIVERPOOL	D409 L016
	1843 DENT	3 NELSON ST	LIVERPOOL	D410 L016
	1843 DENT	3 NELSON ST	LIVERPOOL	D434 L019
	1845 DENT	3 NELSON ST	LIVERPOOL	D411 L016
	1846 DENT	3 NELSON ST	LIVERPOOL	D303 L014
	1846 DENT	3 NELSON ST	LIVERPOOL	D879 L072
	1847 DENT	3 NELSON ST	LIVERPOOL	D412 L016
	1848 DENT	3 NELSON ST	LIVERPOOL	D332 L016

FAY TULLIUS PRIEST	1849 DENT	3 NELSON ST	LIVERPOOL	D413 L016
	1851 DENT	2 ST JAMES ST	LIVERPOOL	D414 L016
	1851 DENT	2 ST JAMES RD	LIVERPOOL	D438 L020
	1852 DENT	2 ST JAMES RD	LIVERPOOL	D216 L009
	1853 DENT	2 ST JAMES ST	LIVERPOOL	D415 L016
	1855 DENT	2 ST JAMES ST	LIVERPOOL	D416 L016
FELTHAM	1852 SURDENT	OXFORD PL ST MARK'S	ST HELIER	DC61 L088
	1853 SURDENT	OXFORD PL	ST HELIER	DB75 L080
	1854 SURDENT	BATH ST	ST HELIER	DC62 L088
	1855 SURDENT	BATH ST	ST HELIER	DC63 L088
FELTHAM R	1852 DENT	1 OXFORD PL	ST HELIER	DB72 L025
FERGUSON RALPH	1848 DENT	CLARENCE TCE	STOCKTON ON TEES	D332 L016
FERGUSON RALPH HODGSON	1847 DENT	14 CLARENCE TCE	STOCKTON	D242 L009
FIELDING FREDERICK W	1845 DENT	HIGH ST	CROYDON	DA66 L011
FISHER & BLUNDELL	1845 DENT	9 SHIP ST	BRIGHTON	DA66 L011
	1845 DENT	9 SHIP ST	BRIGHTON	D606 L047
	1846 DENT	9 SHIP ST	BRIGHTON	D601 L047
FISHER (& G CUPPER)	1845 DENT	9 SHIP ST	BRIGHTON	DB70 L025
FISHER F	1824 DENT	60 EAST ST	BRIGHTON	D599 L047
	1826 DENT	54 OLD STEYNE	BRIGHTON	D597 L011
	1831 DENT	58 OLD STEYNE	BRIGHTON	D582 L044
	1833 DENT	58 OLD STEYNE	BRIGHTON	D583 L044
FISHER FREDERICK	1832 DENT	59 OLD STEYNE	BRIGHTON	D819 L011
	1839 DENT CUPPER	9 SHIP ST	BRIGHTON *	D607 L047
	1839 DENT	59 OLD STEYNE	BRIGHTON	D584 L011
	1840 DENT	58 OLD STEYNE	BRIGHTON	D585 L044
	1843 SURDENT	SHIP ST	BRIGHTON	D600 L047
	1848 DENT	9 SHIP ST	BRIGHTON	D602 L047
FISHER GEORGE	1839 DENT CUPPER	SHIP ST	BRIGHTON *	D607 L047
	1850 DENT	10 SHIP ST	BRIGHTON	D603 L047
	1852 DENT	59 QUEEN'S RD	BRIGHTON	D604 L047
FISHER GEORGE & CO	1839 DENT	9 SHIP ST	BRIGHTON	D584 L011
FLEMING JAMES	1843 DENT	32 CLARENDON ST	CHORLTON	D473 L020
FLETCHER	1818 SURDENT CHIROP	3 UPPER SHIP ST	BRIGHTON *	DB26 L011
	1822 DENT	20 KING'S RD	BRIGHTON	DA68 L011
	1822 DENT	15 BROAD ST	BRIGHTON	D598 L047
	1823 DENT	20 KING'S RD	BRIGHTON	D142 L011
	1824 DENT	15 BROAD ST	BRIGHTON	D599 L047
FLINT PETER	1811 DENT ETC		BURTON ON TRENT *	D284 L011
FORBES JOHN LUKE	1832 DENT BLEEDER	10 OLIVE YD	NOTTINGHAM *	D508 L023
FORT WILLIAM	1851 DENT	2 WINCKLEY ST	PRESTON	D437 L019
	1851 DENT	WINCKLEY ST	PRESTON	D673 L053
	1851 DENT	2 WINCKLEY ST	PRESTON	D727 L020
	1851 DENT	2 WINCKLEY ST	PRESTON	D438 L020
	1853 DENT	WINCKLEY ST	PRESTON	D533 L028
	1854 DENT	5 WINCKLEY ST	PRESTON	D439 L019
	1855 DENT	5 WINCKLEY ST	PRESTON	D732 L064
FOTHERGILL A (& W)	1855 DENT	99 HIGH ST	STOCKTON	D223 L009
FOTHERGILL ALEXANDER & W	1851 SURDENT	72 NORTHGATE	DARLINGTON	D215 L009
FOTHERGILL ALEXANDER (& W)	1851 SURDENT	72 NORTHGATE	DARLINGTON	D292 L013
FOTHERGILL W & A	1855 DENT	99 HIGH ST	STOCKTON	D223 L009
FOTHERGILL WILLIAM	1855 DENT	NORTHGATE	DARLINGTON	D222 L009
FOTHERGILL WILLIAM & A	1851 SURDENT	72 NORTHGATE	DARLINGTON	D292 L013
FOTHERGILL WILLIAM (&A)	1851 SURDENT	72 NORTHGATE	DARLINGTON	D215 L009
FOTHERGILL WM	1847 SURDENT	72 NORTHGATE	DARLINGTON	D242 L009
FOX & SON	1855 SURDENT	7 SOUTHERNHAY PL	EXETER	D183 L008
FOX (& FATH)	1855 SURDENT	7 SOUTHERNHAY PL	EXETER	D183 L008

FOX C W	1847 DENT	PRINCESS SQ	PLYMOUTH	D152 L008
FOX CHARLES PRIDEAUX	1844 DENT	17 VICTORIA PDE	TORQUAY	D144 L008
FOX CORNELIUS WILLS	1844 DENT	12 PRINCESS SQ	PLYMOUTH	D492 L022
	1844 DENT	12 PRINCESS SQ	PLYMOUTH	D144 L008
FOX GEORGE	1839 SURDENT	37 PARADISE STREET	BIRMINGHAM	D083 L002
	1841 DENT	7 EASY ROW	BIRMINGHAM	D058 L002
	1844 DENT	33 BLACKETT ST	NEWCASTLE	D213 L009
	1850 DENT		KINGSBRIDGE	D147 L008
	1852 DENT	DUNCOMBE ST	KINGSBRIDGE	D788 L020
FOX GEORGE F	1849 DENT	22 BRUNSWICK SQ	GLOUCESTER	D891 L068
	1853 DENT	4 MONTPELIER PL	GLOUCESTER	D951 L075
FOX R W	1838 SURDENT	55 PARK ST	BRISTOL	D935 L075
	1839 SURDENT	55 PARK ST	BRISTOL	D936 L075
	1839 SUR DENT	PARK ST	BRISTOL *	D654 L068
	1840 SURDENT	13 PARK ST	BRISTOL	D945 L075
	1840 DENT	PARK ST	BRISTOL	D143 L020
	1840 DENT	7 SOUTHERNHAY PL	EXETER	D143 L008
	1841 SURDENT	14 PARK ST	BRISTOL	D937 L075
	1842 SURDENT	14 PARK ST	BRISTOL	D938 L075
	1843 SURDENT	14 PARK ST	BRISTOL	D939 L075
	1844 SURDENT	14 PARK ST	BRISTOL	D940 L075
	1845 SURDENT	14 PARK ST	BRISTOL	D822 L002
	1846 SURDENT	14 PARK ST	BRISTOL	D941 L075
	1847 SURDENT	14 PARK ST	BRISTOL	D942 L075
	1848 SURDENT	14 PARK ST	BRISTOL	D943 L075
	1849 SURDENT	14 PARK ST	BRISTOL	D944 L075
	1850 SURDENT	14 PARK ST	BRISTOL	D946 L075
	1851 SURDENT	14 PARK ST	BRISTOL	D896 L075
	1852 SURDENT	14 PARK ST	BRISTOL	D897 L075
	1853 SURDENT	14 PARK ST	BRISTOL	D898 L075
	1854 SURDENT	14 PARK ST	BRISTOL	D899 L075
	1855 SURDENT	14 PARK ST	BRISTOL	D947 L075
FOX R WERE	1844 SURDENT	7 SOUTHERNHAY PL	EXETER	D172 L008
	1845 SURDENT	7 SOUTHERNHAY PL	EXETER	D173 L008
	1846 SURDENT	7 SOUTHERNHAY PL	EXETER	D174 L008
	1847 SURDENT	7 SOUTHERNHAY PL	EXETER	D175 L008
	1848 SURDENT	7 SOUTHERNHAY	EXETER	D176 L008
	1849 SURDENT	7 SOUTHERNHAY PL	EXETER	D177 L008
	1850 SURDENT	7 SOUTHERNHAY PL	EXETER	D178 L008
	1851 SURDENT	7 SOUTHERNHAY	EXETER	D179 L008
	1852 SURDENT	7 SOUTHERNHAY	EXETER	D180 L008
	1853 SURDENT	7 SOUTHERNHAY	EXETER	D181 L008
	1854 SURDENT	7 SOUTHERNHAY	EXETER	D182 L008
FOX ROBERT W	1830 DENT	17 DIX'S FIELD	EXETER	D160 L008
	1831 DENT	17 DIX'S FIELD	EXETER	D161 L008
	1832 DENT	17 DIX'S FIELD	EXETER	D162 L008
	1833 DENT	17 DIX'S FIELD	EXETER	D163 L008
	1834 DENT	7 SOUTHERNHAY PL	EXETER	D164 L008
	1836 DENT	7 SOUTHERNHAY PL	EXETER	D165 L008
	1837 DENT	7 SOUTHERNHAY PL	EXETER	D166 L008
	1838 DENT	7 SOUTHERNHAY PL	EXETER	D167 L008
	1839 DENT	7 SOUTHERNHAY PL	EXETER	D151 L008
	1840 DENT	7 SOUTHERNHAY PL	EXETER	D168 L008
	1853 SURDENT	7 SOUTHERNHAY PL	EXETER	D153 L008
	1854 SURDENT	7 SOUTHERNHAY PL	EXETER	D871 L025
FOX ROBERT WEIR	1830 DENT	11 DIX'S FIELD	EXETER	D119 L008
FOX ROBERT WERE	1828 SURDENT	19 HIGH ST	EXETER	D150 L008

FOX ROBERT WERE	1841 SURDENT	7 SOUTHERNHAY PL	EXETER	D169 L008
	1842 DENT	14 PARK ST	BRISTOL	DB46 L049
	1842 SURDENT	7 SOUTHERNHAY PL	EXETER	D170 L008
	1843 SURDENT	7 SOUTHERNHAY PL	EXETER	D171 L008
	1844 DENT	7 SOUTHERNHAY	EXETER	D144 L008
	1846 SURDENT	14 PARK ST	BRISTOL	DB79 L072
	1848 DENT	14 PARK ST	BRISTOL	D125 L075
	1848 DENT	7 SOUTHERNHAY	EXETER	DA50 L011
	1848 DENT	14 PARK ST	BRISTOL	DA50 L011
	1849 DENT	14 PARK ST	BRISTOL	D891 L068
	1850 DENT	14 PARK ST	BRISTOL	D960 L075
	1850 DENT	7 SOUTHERNHAY	EXETER	D147 L008
	1852 DENT	14 PARK ST	BRISTOL	D788 L020
	1852 DENT	7 HIGHER SOUTHERNHAY	EXETER	D145 L008
	1852 DENT	7 HIGHER SOUTHERNHAY	EXETER	D788 L020
	1853 DENT	14 PARK ST	BRISTOL	D802 L020
	1853 DENT	14 PARK ST	BRISTOL	D951 L075
FOX THOMAS	1836 DENT	PRINCESS SQ	PLYMOUTH	DA44 L011
FRANCIS RICHARD	1850 DENT	LONGBRIDGE	SHEPTON MALLET	DA78 L011
FULLER EDWARD	1839 DENT	3 VERULAM PL	HASTINGS	D584 L011
FULLER FRANCIS	1835 DENT	KING ST	LEICESTER	D007 L014
	1841 DENT	KING ST	LEICESTER	D028 L002
GABRIEL ARNOLD	1853 DENT	9 MT PLEASANT	LIVERPOOL	D415 L016
GABRIEL J	1838 DENT	21 GEORGE ST	HULL	D375 L018
GABRIEL JOHN	1839 DENT	21 GEORGE ST	HULL	D376 L018
GABRIEL L	1840 SURDENT	21 GEORGE ST	HULL	D888 L006
GABRIEL LION	1846 DENT	14 UPPER NEWINGTON ST	LIVERPOOL	D303 L014
GABRIEL LYON	1841 DENT	21 GEORGE ST	HULL	D241 L009
	1843 DENT	21 BROWNLOW ST	LIVERPOOL	D434 L019
	1843 DENT	21 BROWNLOW ST	LIVERPOOL	D410 L016
	1845 DENT	14 UPPER NEWINGTON	LIVERPOOL	D411 L016
	1846 DENT	14 UPPER NEWINGTON	LIVERPOOL	DB79 L072
	1847 DENT	14 UPPER NEWINGTON	LIVERPOOL	D412 L016
GABRIEL LYON (LION)	1841 DENT	21 GEORGE ST	HULL	D331 L016
GABRIEL MESSRS	1855 DENT	28 HIGH ST	CROYDON	D613 L048
GACHES D	1853 DENT	NORTHGATE ST	IPSWICH	D655 L051
GACHES DANIEL	1844 DENT	NORTHGATE ST	IPSWICH	D667 L052
	1850 DENT	NORTHGATE ST	IPSWICH	DA91 L011
	1855 DENT	NORTHGATE ST	IPSWICH	D668 L052
GALLEN J J	1847 SURDENT	33 BELGRAVE TCE	LEEDS	D276 L015
GALLEN JARDINE JOHN	1846 DENT MD	33 BELGRAVE PL	LEEDS	D879 L072
GALLEN JOHN	1838 DENT	74 GEORGE ST	MANCHESTER	D470 L020
GALLEN JOHN GORDON	1851 DENT	223 OXFORD ST	MANCHESTER	D567 L020
	1852 DENT	223 OXFORD ST	MANCHESTER	D477 L020
GALLEN JOHN J	1847 SURDENT	WADE LANE	LEEDS	D280 L015
GALLEN JOHN JARDINE	1848 DENT MA	BELGRAVE HO WADE LANE	LEEDS	D332 L016
	1848 DENT MA	33 DARLEY ST	BRADFORD	D332 L016
	1849 DENT	BELGRAVE HO WADE LANE	LEEDS	D277 L015
	1850 DENT MD	DREWTON ST	BRADFORD (THURS)	DB35 L078
	1852 DENT	238 OXFORD ST	MANCHESTER	D216 L009
GAMBLE J G	1854 DENT	ROTHER ST	STRATFORD ON AVON	D015 L001
GAWTHERRY ROBERT	1855 DENT	55 GT GEORGE ST	LIVERPOOL	D416 L016
GARDENER W	1854 DENT		FENNY STRATFORD	DA71 L011
GARNER EDWARD	1849 DENT	CHURCHYARD	BOSTON	D870 L056
GARNER J	1849 DENT	CHURCH YARD	BOSTON	D681 L056
GARNER JOSEPH SAMUEL	1849 DENT	ST BOTOLPH'S CHURCHYARD	BOSTON	D333 L016
	1850 DENT	ST BOTOLPH'S CHURCHYARD	BOSTON	D013 L020

GARNET HENRY WILLIAM	1855 DENT	FERNLEY PL	SHEFFIELD	D222 L009
GARNETT GEORGE BELK	1850 DENT	38 WEST PDE	HUDDERSFIELD	D539 L030
	1853 SURDENT	TRINITY ST	HUDDERSFIELD	D261 L010
GARNETT GEORGE BELT	1855 DENT	TRINITY ST	HUDDERSFIELD	D222 L009
GARNETT HENRY WILLIAM	1845 SURDENT	FERNLEY PL	SHEFFIELD	D755 L066
	1846 DENT	FERNLEY PL	SHEFFIELD	D879 L072
	1848 DENT	FERNLEY PL	SHEFFIELD	D332 L016
	1849 SURDENT	FERNLEY PL	SHEFFIELD	D756 L066
	1852 DENT	FERNLEY PL	SHEFFIELD	D216 L009
	1852 SURDENT	FERNLEY PL	SHEFFIELD	D260 L010
	1854 DENT	298 GLOSSOP RD	SHEFFIELD	D757 L066
GARNIER MICHAEL	1848 DENT	EAST COTTAGE EAST TCE	CARDIFF	DC49 L085
GARRETT L	1852 DENT	ATHOLL ST	DOUGLAS I OF M	DB73 L079
GARRETT PHILLIP L	1852 DENT	56 ATHOLL ST	DOUGLAS I OF M	DC56 L087
GARRY WILLIAM	1830 DENT	223 DEANSGATE	MANCHESTER	D466 L020
	1832 SURDENT	223 DEANSGATE	MANCHESTER	D467 L020
	1833 SURDENT	223 DEANSGATE	MANCHESTER	D468 L020
	1834 DENT	223 DEANSGATE	MANCHESTER	D236 L009
GEDGE WILLIAM EDWARD	1852 DENT	5 TORWOOD ROW	TORQUAY	D788 L020
	1852 DENT	5 TORWOOD ROW	TORQUAY	D145 L008
GIDNEY E	1832 SURDENT	100 OLDHAM ST	MANCHESTER (ADV)	D467 L020
GIDNEY ELEAZER	1834 DENT	29 PICCADILLY	MANCHESTER	D236 L009
	1840 DENT	43 PICCADILLY	MANCHESTER	D471 L020
	1841 DENT	43 PICCADILLY	MANCHESTER	D472 L020
	1841 DENT	41 PICCADILLY	MANCHESTER	D331 L016
	1843 DENT	41 PICCADILLY	MANCHESTER	D473 L020
	1848 DENT	6 AYTOUN ST	MANCHESTER	D475 L020
	1848 DENT	6 AYTOUN ST	MANCHESTER	D332 L016
	1850 DENT	6 AYTOUN ST	MANCHESTER	D476 L020
	1851 DENT	5 AYTOUN ST	MANCHESTER	D567 L020
	1852 DENT	5 AYTOUN ST	MANCHESTER	D477 L020
	1852 DENT	6 AYTOUN ST	MANCHESTER	D216 L009
	1855 DENT	6 AYTOUN ST	MANCHESTER	D478 L020
GILBARD JAMES	1851 SURDENT	DISPENSARY QUEEN ST	EXETER	D179 L008
	1852 DENT	DISPENSARY QUEEN ST	EXETER	D788 L020
	1852 DENT	DISPENSARY QUEEN ST	EXETER	D145 L008
	1852 SURDENT	DISPENSARY QUEEN ST	EXETER	D180 L008
	1853 SURDENT	DISPENSARY QUEEN ST	EXETER	D181 L008
	1853 SURDENT	DISPENSARY QUEEN ST	EXETER	D153 L008
	1854 SURDENT	DISPENSARY QUEEN ST	EXETER	DB71 L025
	1854 SURDENT	DISPENSARY QUEEN ST	EXETER	D182 L008
	1855 SURDENT	DISPENSARY QUEEN ST	EXETER	D183 L008
GILBERT G	1855 SURDENT	15 BUTCHER ST	PORTSEA	DA84 L011
GILBERT GEORGE	1852 DENT	BUTCHER ST	PORTSEA	D346 L017
GILL SETH	1855 DENT	76 ISLINGTON	LIVERPOOL	D416 L016
GOEPEL JOHN ROBERT	1847 DENT	86 CROSSHALL ST	LIVERPOOL	D412 L016
	1848 DENT	86 CROSSHALL ST	LIVERPOOL	D332 L016
	1849 DENT	86 CROSSHALL ST	LIVERPOOL	D413 L016
	1851 DENT	86 CROSSHALL ST	LIVERPOOL	D414 L016
	1851 DENT	86 CROSSHALL ST	LIVERPOOL	D430 L020
	1852 DENT	86 CROSSHALL ST	LIVERPOOL	D216 L009
	1853 DENT	86 CROSSHALL ST	LIVERPOOL	D415 L016
	1855 DENT	86 CROSSHALL ST	LIVERPOOL	D416 L016
GOLDSTONE	1793 DENT APOTH	43 BROAD ST	BATH *	DB21 L011
	1794 DENT APOTH	43 BROAD ST	BATH *	DB22 L011
	1796 DENT APOTH	43 BROAD ST	BATH *	DB23 L011
	1801 DENT APOTH	7 NORTHUMBERLAND BDG	BATH *	DB49 L025

GOLDSTONE	1809	SUR DENT	7 NORTHUMBERLAND BUILDINGS	BATH *	D113 L007
GOLDSTONE A	1841	SURDENT	11 WELLINGTON PL CLIFTON	BRISTOL	D937 L075
	1842	SURDENT	8 GRANBY HILL	BRISTOL	D938 L075
	1843	SURDENT	8 GRANBY HILL	BRISTOL	D939 L075
	1844	SURDENT	8 GRANBY HILL	BRISTOL	D940 L075
	1847	SURDENT	4 NELSON PL CLIFTON	BRISTOL	D942 L075
	1848	SURDENT	NELSON BDGS CLIFTON	BRISTOL	D943 L075
	1849	SURDENT	NELSON BDGS CLIFTON	BRISTOL	D944 L075
GOLDSTONE ALFRED	1848	DENT	3 NELSON PL CLIFTON	BRISTOL	DA50 L011
	1848	DENT	3 NELSON PL CLIFTON	BRISTOL	D125 L075
	1849	DENT	3 NELSON PL CLIFTON	BRISTOL	D891 L068
GOLDSTONE C	1793	DENT APOTH	NR LANSDOWN PL	BATH *	DB21 L011
	1794	DENT APOTH	43 BROAD ST	BATH *	DB22 L011
	1794	DENT APOTH	NR LANSDOWN PL	BATH *	DB22 L011
	1796	DENT APOTH	NR LANSDOWN PL	BATH *	DB23 L011
	1796	DENT APOTH	43 BROAD ST	BATH *	DB23 L011
GOLDSTONE EDWARD	1842	SURDENT		DEVIZES	DB46 L049
GOLDSTONE GEORGE	1800	SURDENT ETC	43 BROAD ST	BATH *	D111 L007
GOODLING GEORGE	1823	DENT	ST HELEN'S	IPSWICH	D142 L011
GOODMAN JAMES	1852	DENT	EAST REACH	TAUNTON	D788 L020
GOODMAN SAMUEL	1854	DENT	6 QUIET ST	BATH	D129 L007
GORDEN JAMES	1840	DENT	46 PARK ST	BRISTOL	D143 L020
GORDON J	1833	SURDENT	22 COLLEGE GREEN	BRISTOL	D931 L075
	1834	SURDENT	46 PARK ST	BRISTOL	D932 L075
	1835	SURDENT	46 PARK ST	BRISTOL	D820 L002
	1836	SURDENT	46 PARK ST	BRISTOL	D933 L075
	1837	SURDENT	46 PARK ST	BRISTOL	D934 L075
	1838	SURDENT	46 PARK ST	BRISTOL	D935 L075
	1839	SURDENT	46 PARK ST	BRISTOL	D936 L075
	1840	SURDENT	46 PARK ST	BRISTOL	D945 L075
	1841	SURDENT	46 PARK ST	BRISTOL	D937 L075
	1842	SURDENT	46 PARK ST	BRISTOL	D938 L075
	1843	SURDENT	46 PARK ST	BRISTOL	D939 L075
	1844	SURDENT	46 PARK ST	BRISTOL	D940 L075
	1845	SURDENT	46 PARK ST	BRISTOL	D822 L002
	1846	SURDENT	46 PARK ST	BRISTOL	D941 L075
	1847	SURDENT	46 PARK ST	BRISTOL	D942 L075
	1848	SURDENT	46 PARK ST	BRISTOL	D943 L075
	1849	SURDENT	46 PARK ST	BRISTOL	D944 L075
	1850	SURDENT	46 PARK ST	BRISTOL	D946 L075
	1851	SURDENT	46 PARK ST	BRISTOL	D896 L075
	1852	SURDENT	46 PARK ST	BRISTOL	D897 L075
	1853	SURDENT	46 PARK ST	BRISTOL	D898 L075
	1854	SURDENT	46 PARK ST	BRISTOL	D899 L075
	1855	SURDENT	46 PARK ST	BRISTOL	D947 L075
GORDON JAMES	1828	SURDENT	22 COLLEGE GREEN	BRISTOL	D927 L075
	1829	SURDENT	22 COLLEGE GREEN	BRISTOL	DB21 L002
	1830	SURDENT	22 COLLEGE GREEN	BRISTOL	D119 L020
	1830	SURDENT	22 COLLEGE GREEN	BRISTOL	D928 L075
	1831	SURDENT	22 COLLEGE GREEN	BRISTOL	D929 L075
	1832	SURDENT	22 COLLEGE GREEN	BRISTOL	D930 L075
	1839	SUR DENT	46 PARK ST	BRISTOL *	D654 L068
	1842	DENT	46 PARK ST	BRISTOL	DB46 L049
	1846	SURDENT	46 PARK ST	BRISTOL	DB79 L072
	1848	DENT	46 PARK ST	BRISTOL	D125 L075
	1848	DENT	46 PARK ST	BRISTOL	DA50 L011
	1849	DENT	46 PARK ST	BRISTOL	D891 L068

GORDON JAMES	1850 DENT	46 PARK ST	BRISTOL	D960 L075
	1852 DENT	46 PARK ST	BRISTOL	D788 L020
	1853 DENT	46 PARK ST	BRISTOL	D802 L020
	1853 DENT	46 PARK ST	BRISTOL	D951 L075
GOULD FREDERIC	1845 DENT	MARKET PL	KINGSTON	DA66 L011
GOULD FREDERICK	1851 CHEM DENT	MARKET PL	KINGSTON ON THAMES	*DA83 L011
GOULSON BENJAMIN	1804 BLEEDER TDRAWER	1 LOMAX'S BDGS	MANCHESTER *	D455 L020
GRAVES H S	1840 SURDENT	NORTH PDE	BRADFORD	D734 L063
	1840 SURDENT	NORTH PARK	HALIFAX	D734 L063
	1841 SURDENT	NORTH PDE	BRADFORD	D241 L009
	1841 SURDENT	NORTH PARK	HALIFAX	D241 L009
GRAVES HENRY	1841 DENT	KING CROSS LANE	HALIFAX	D331 L016
GRAVES HENRY SWAN	1837 DENT	33 CONEY ST	YORK	D257 L010
	1842 SURDENT	2 HORTON ST	HALIFAX	D060 L015
	1845 SURDENT	6 CLARE HALL RD	HALIFAX	D570 L041
	1847 SURDENT	6 CLARE HALL RD	HALIFAX	D276 L015
GRAY JOHN	1845 SURDENT	14 HOWARD ST	SHEFFIELD	D755 L066
	1846 DENT	14 HOWARD ST	SHEFFIELD	D879 L072
	1848 DENT	14 HOWARD ST	SHEFFIELD	D332 L016
	1849 SURDENT	14 HOWARD ST	SHEFFIELD	D756 L066
	1852 DENT	14 HOWARD ST	SHEFFIELD	D216 L009
	1852 SURDENT	14 HOWARD ST	SHEFFIELD	D260 L010
	1854 DENT	14 HOWARD ST	SHEFFIELD	D757 L066
	1855 DENT	14 HOWARD ST	SHEFFIELD	D222 L009
GRAYSON JOHN	1848 DENT	HIGHGATE	KENDAL	D332 L016
	1849 DENT	HIGHGATE	KENDAL	D441 L019
	1851 DENT	HIGHGATE	KENDAL	D437 L019
	1855 DENT	HIGHGATE	KENDAL	D222 L020
GREEN THOMAS	1800 DENT	22 STEELHOUSE LANE	BIRMINGHAM	D041 L002
	1803 DENT	22 STEELHOUSE LANE	BIRMINGHAM	D043 L002
	1808 DENT	22 STEELHOUSE LANE	BIRMINGHAM	D045 L002
	1811 DENT	22 STEELHOUSE LANE	BIRMINGHAM	D284 L011
	1812 DENT	STEELHOUSE LANE	BIRMINGHAM	D047 L002
	1815 DENT BLEEDER	STEELHOUSE LANE	BIRMINGHAM *	D048 L002
	1816 DENT	22 STEELHOUSE LANE	BIRMINGHAM	D049 L002
	1816 DENT	22 STEELHOUSE LANE	BIRMINGHAM	D049 L016
	1818 DENT	22 STEELHOUSE LANE	BHAM	D302 L002
	1818 DENT	STEELHOUSE LANE	BIRMINGHAM	D050 L002
	1821 DENT	STEELHOUSE LANE	BIRMINGHAM	D051 L002
	1823 DENT	30 STEELHOUSE LANE	BIRMINGHAM	D052 L002
	1825 DENT	30 STEELHOUSE LANE	BIRMINGHAM	D053 L002
GREEN THOS.	1809 DENT	22 STEELHOUSE LANE	BIRMINGHAM	D046 L002
GREENSILL EDWARD	1850 DENT	SOHO ST	BHAM	D013 L002
	1852 DENT	SOHO STREET HANDSWORTH	BIRMINGHAM	D078 L002
GREGORY E J	1849 DENT	189 HIGH ST	CHELTENHAM	D881 L082
GREGORY EDWARD JAMES	1853 SURDENT	189 HIGH ST	CHELTENHAM	D956 L068
GROVES	1814 SURDENT	DURNFORD ST	STONEHOUSE	D876 L022
GROVES & GROVES	1850 DENT	2 EAST SOUTHERNHAY	EXETER	D147 L008
	1853 SURDENT	1 EAST SOUTHERNHAY	EXETER	D153 L008
GROVES (& BRO)	1850 DENT	2 EAST SOUTHERNHAY	EXETER	D147 L008
	1853 SURDENT	1 EAST SOUTHERNHAY	EXETER	D153 L008
GROVES A N	1828 DENT	13 BEDFORD CIRCUS	EXETER	D150 L008
	1830 DENT	13 BEDFORD CIRCUS	EXETER	D160 L008
GROVES ANTHONY A	1825 DENT	NORTHERNHAY	EXETER	D158 L008
GROVES ANTHONY N	1822 DENT	NORTHERNHAY	EXETER	D157 L008
	1823 DENT	NORTHERNHAY	EXETER	D142 L008
	1827 DENT	NORTHERNHAY	EXETER	D149 L008

GROVES ANTHONY N & I	1828 DENT	NORTHERNHAY	EXETER	D159 L008
GROVES BROTHERS	1854 SURDENT	1 EAST SOUTHERNHAY	EXETER	DB71 L025
GROVES E	1843 SURDENT	CATHEDRAL YD	EXETER	D171 L008
	1844 SURDENT	CATHEDRAL YD	EXETER	D172 L008
	1845 SURDENT	CATHEDRAL YD	EXETER	D173 L008
	1846 SURDENT	CATHEDRAL YD	EXETER	D174 L008
	1847 SURDENT	CATHEDRAL YD	EXETER	D175 L008
	1848 SURDENT	CATHEDRAL YD	EXETER	D176 L008
	1849 SURDENT	2 EAST SOUTHERNHAY	EXETER	D177 L008
	1850 SURDENT	2 EAST SOUTHERNHAY	EXETER	D178 L008
	1851 SURDENT	2 EAST SOUTHERNHAY	EXETER	D179 L008
	1852 SURDENT	2 EAST SOUTHERNHAY	EXETER	D180 L008
GROVES EDWARD	1852 DENT	EAST SOUTHERNHAY	EXETER	D788 L020
GROVES EDWIN	1837 DENT	12 CASTLE ST	EXETER	D166 L008
	1838 DENT	12 CASTLE ST	EXETER	D167 L008
	1839 DENT	12 CASTLE ST	EXETER	D151 L008
	1844 DENT	CATHEDRAL YD	EXETER	D144 L008
	1852 DENT	EAST SOUTHERNHAY	EXETER	D145 L008
	1853 SURDENT	2 EAST SOUTHERNHAY	EXETER	D181 L008
	1854 SURDENT	2 EAST SOUTHERNHAY	EXETER	D182 L008
	1855 SURDENT	2 EAST SOUTHERNHAY	EXETER	D183 L008
GROVES EDWIN (& J)	1848 DENT	1 EAST SOUTHERNHAY	EXETER	DA50 L011
GROVES I	1827 DENT	NORTHERNHAY	EXETER	D149 L008
	1830 DENT	13 BEDFORD CIRCUS	EXETER	D160 L008
GROVES I (& A N)	1828 DENT	NORTHERNHAY	EXETER	D159 L008
GROVES J	1828 DENT	13 BEDFORD CIRCUS	EXETER	D150 L008
GROVES JOHN	1830 DENT	13 BEDFORD CIRCUS	EXETER	D119 L008
	1831 DENT	13 BEDFORD CIRCUS	EXETER	D161 L008
	1832 DENT	13 BEDFORD CIRCUS	EXETER	D162 L008
	1833 DENT	13 BEDFORD CIRCUS	EXETER	D163 L008
	1834 DENT	13 BEDFORD CIRCUS	EXETER	D164 L008
	1836 DENT	13 BEDFORD CIRCUS	EXETER	D165 L008
GROVES JOHN & E	1848 DENT	1 EAST SOUTHERNHAY	EXETER	DA50 L011
GUNTON ALFRED	1854 DENT	LOWER GOAT LANE	NORWICH	D651 L051

HAGREEN J	1853 DENT	1 ST ANDREW'S ST	CAMBRIDGE	D655 L051
HAGREEN JAMES	1851 DENT	ST ANDREW ST	CAMBRIDGE	DA48 L011
HAGREEN JAMES THOMAS	1850 DENT	1 ST ANDREW ST	CAMBRIDGE	DA91 L011
	1855 SURDENT	ST ANDREW'S ST	CAMBRIDGE	DA45 L011
HAIR Q B	1845 DENT	CHAPEL PL	TUNBRIDGE WELLS	DB69 L025
	1845 DENT	CHAPEL PL	TUNBRIDGE WELLS	DA66 L011
	1849 SURDENT	CHAPEL PL	TUNBRIDGE WELLS	DA69 L011
	1850 DENT	WEEK ST	MAIDSTONE	D592 L045
	1850 SURDENT	BEDFORD HOUSE	TUNBRIDGE WELLS	DA52 L011
	1851 DENT	WEEK ST	MAIDSTONE	DA77 L011
	1855 SURDENT	CHAPEL ST	TUNBRIDGE WELLS	D594 L046
HAIR QUINTIN	1839 SURDENT	NEVILL ST	TONBRIDGE WELLS	D584 L020
	1839 DENT	MRS HOBSON'S HIGH ST	MAIDSTONE	D591 L045
	1854 DENT	WEEK ST	MAIDSTONE	DB82 L0B2
HALL WILLIAM	1850 DENT	PRINCES END	TIPTON	D013 L001
HAMILTON H	1855 DENT	HIGH ST	POOLE	DA84 L011
HAMILTON HORATIO	1852 DENT	HIGH ST	POOLE	D788 L020
HAMMILL WILLIAM	1840 DENT	ST ANDREW'S ST	PLYMOUTH	D143 L008
HAMMOND T C	1840 DENT	NORTH ST	RIPON	D734 L063
	1841 SURDENT	NORTH ST	RIPON	D241 L009
	1851 SURDENT	NORTH ST	BOROUGHBRIDGE	DB54 L025
HAMMOND THOMAS CUNDALE	1841 DENT	NORTH ST	RIPON	D331 L016
HAMPSON ELIJAH	1843 DENT	7 BEVINGTON HILL	LIVERPOOL	D410 L016
	1845 DENT	11 BEVINGTON HILL	LIVERPOOL	D411 L016
	1847 DENT	11 BEVINGTON HILL	LIVERPOOL	D412 L016
HAMSON HENRY	1855 DENT	5 NORTH RD	LEEDS	D222 L009
HANNAH JAMES	1843 DENT	32 MT PLEASANT	LIVERPOOL	D410 L016
	1843 DENT	32 PLEASANT ST	LIVERPOOL	D434 L019
	1845 DENT	32 PLEASANT ST	LIVERPOOL	D411 L016
	1846 DENT	32 PLEASANT ST	LIVERPOOL	D303 L014
	1847 DENT	32 MT PLEASANT	LIVERPOOL	D412 L016
	1849 DENT	32 PLEASANT ST	LIVERPOOL	D413 L016
	1851 DENT	32 PLEASANT ST	LIVERPOOL	D414 L016
	1853 DENT	32 PLEASANT ST	LIVERPOOL	D415 L016
HANSON THOMAS	1824 SURDENT	50 BRIDGE ST	MANCHESTER	D401 L019
HARCOURT J H	1836 SURDENT	22 COLLEGE GREEN	BRISTOL	D933 L075
HARDING G	1851 DENT	ST JOHN'S ST	CHICHESTER	DA77 L011
HARDING GEORGE	1855 DENT	EAST ST	CHICHESTER	D594 L046
HARDING J	1846 SURDENT	14 AXFORD BDGS	BATH	D124 L007
HARDING THOMAS HENRY	1851 CHEM DENT	GEORGE ST	RICHMOND *	DA83 L011
HARGREAVES CHARLES	1855 DENT	34 SIDNEY ST	CHORLTON	D478 L020
HARRINGTON G F	1848 DENT	84 ST THOMAS ST	PORTSMOUTH	D357 L017
	1855 SURDENT	84 ST THOMAS'S ST	PORTSMOUTH	DA84 L011
HARRINGTON GEORGE FELLOWES	1852 DENT	84 ST THOMAS ST	PORTSMOUTH	D346 L017
	1852 DENT	ST THOMAS ST	PORTSMOUTH	D788 L020
HARRIS	1822 DENT	CLEMENS ST	LEAMINGTON	D005 L020
	1822 DENT	CLEMENS ST	LEAMINGTON	D321 L014
	1825 DENT	CLEMENS ST	LEAMINGTON	D325 L014
HARRIS JOSEPH	1831 DENT	FRIAR LANE	LEICESTER	D501 L024
	1831 DENT	SNARGATE ST	DOVER	D582 L044
	1833 DENT	SNARGATE ST	DOVER	D583 L044
	1835 DENT	FRIAR LANE	LEICESTER	D007 L014
	1839 DENT	38 SNARGATE ST	DOVER	D584 L011
	1840 DENT	SNARGATE ST	DOVER	D585 L044
	1841 DENT	FRIAR'S LANE	LEICESTER	D028 L002
HARRISON EUNSON (& R)	1855 DENT	35 GEORGE ST	HULL	D222 L009
HARRISON HENRY	1853 SURDENT	5 NORTH ROW	LEEDS	D261 L010

HARRISON MESSRS	1848 DENT	36 GEORGE ST	HULL	D378 L018
HARRISON ROBERT	1848 DENT	36 GEORGE ST	HULL	D332 L016
HARRISON ROBERT & E	1855 DENT	35 GEORGE ST	HULL	D222 L009
HARRISON ROBERT & R E	1852 DENT	36 GEORGE ST	HULL	D216 L009
HARRISON ROBERT EUNSON (& R)	1852 DENT	36 GEORGE ST	HULL	D216 L009
HARRISON WILLIAM	1804 TDRAWER	1 CROWN ST	MANCHESTER	D455 L020
HARRISON WILLIAM RICHARD	1846 DENT	31 RICHMOND PL	BRIGHTON	D601 L047
HARRISONS MESSRS	1851 SURDENT	36 GEORGE ST	HULL	D259 L010
HART	1824 SURDENT	GREEN ST	BATH	D116 L007
	1850 SURDENT	PARK ST	BRISTOL	D946 L075
	1851 SURDENT	PARK ST	BRISTOL	D896 L075
	1852 SURDENT	PARK ST	BRISTOL	D897 L075
	1853 SURDENT	PARK ST	BRISTOL	D898 L075
	1854 SURDENT	PARK ST	BRISTOL	D899 L075
	1855 SURDENT	PARK ST	BRISTOL	D947 L075
HART A S (& J)	1848 DENT	68 COLLEGE ST	BRISTOL	D125 L075
	1848 DENT	68 COLLEGE ST	BRISTOL	DA50 L011
	1849 DENT	68 COLLEGE ST	BRISTOL	D891 L068
HART HAMMETT	1793 DENT	AVON ST	BRISTOL	D893 L075
	1795 DENT	AVON ST	BRISTOL	D894 L075
	1797 DENT	24 COLLEGE ST	BRISTOL	D895 L075
	1798 DENT	24 COLLEGE ST	BRISTOL	D900 L075
	1799 DENT	24 COLLEGE ST	BRISTOL	D901 L075
	1801 DENT	24 COLLEGE ST	BRISTOL	D902 L075
	1803 DENT	24 COLLEGE ST	BRISTOL	D903 L075
	1805 DENT	24 COLLEGE ST	BRISTOL	D904 L075
	1806 SURDENT	24 COLLEGE ST	BRISTOL	D905 L075
	1807 SURDENT	24 COLLEGE ST	BRISTOL	D906 L075
	1808 SURDENT	24 COLLEGE ST	BRISTOL	D907 L075
	1809 SURDENT	24 COLLEGE ST	BRISTOL	D908 L075
	1810 SURDENT	24 COLLEGE ST	BRISTOL	D909 L075
	1811 SURDENT	24 COLLEGE ST	BRISTOL	D910 L075
	1812 SURDENT	24 COLLEGE ST	BRISTOL	D911 L075
	1813 SURDENT	24 COLLEGE ST	BRISTOL	D912 L075
	1814 SURDENT	24 COLLEGE ST	BRISTOL	D913 L075
	1815 SURDENT	24 COLLEGE ST	BRISTOL	D914 L075
	1816 SURDENT	24 COLLEGE ST	BRISTOL	D915 L075
	1817 SURDENT	24 COLLEGE ST	BRISTOL	D916 L075
	1818 SURDENT	24 COLLEGE ST	BRISTOL	D917 L075
	1819 SURDENT	24 COLLEGE ST	BRISTOL	D918 L075
HART J & A S	1848 DENT	68 COLLEGE ST	BRISTOL	DA50 L011
	1848 DENT	68 COLLEGE ST	BRISTOL	D125 L075
	1849 DENT	68 COLLEGE ST	BRISTOL	D891 L068
HART JOSEPH	1830 SURDENT	68 COLLEGE ST	BRISTOL	D119 L020
	1839 DENT	68 COLLEGE ST	BRISTOL	D654 L068
	1840 DENT	68 COLLEGE ST	BRISTOL	D143 L020
	1842 DENT	68 COLLEGE ST	BRISTOL	DB46 L049
	1846 SURDENT	68 COLLEGE ST	BRISTOL	D879 L072
	1850 DENT	50 PARK ST	BRISTOL	D960 L075
	1852 DENT	50 PARK ST	BRISTOL	D788 L020
	1853 DENT	50 PARK ST	BRISTOL	D951 L075
	1853 DENT	50 PARK ST	BRISTOL	D802 L020
HART MESSRS	1822 SURDENT	24 COLLEGE ST	BRISTOL	D921 L075
	1823 SURDENT	24 COLLEGE ST	BRISTOL	D922 L075
	1824 SURDENT	24 COLLEGE ST	BRISTOL	D923 L075
	1825 SURDENT	68 COLLEGE GREEN	BRISTOL	D924 L075
	1826 SURDENT	68 COLLEGE GREEN	BRISTOL	D925 L075

HART MESSRS	1827 SURDENT	68 COLLEGE GREEN	BRISTOL	D926 L075
	1828 SURDENT	68 COLLEGE GREEN	BRISTOL	D927 L075
	1829 SURDENT	68 COLLEGE ST	BRISTOL	D821 L002
	1830 SURDENT	68 COLLEGE ST	BRISTOL	D928 L075
	1831 SURDENT	68 COLLEGE ST	BRISTOL	D929 L075
	1832 SURDENT	68 COLLEGE ST	BRISTOL	D930 L075
	1833 SURDENT	68 COLLEGE ST	BRISTOL	D931 L075
	1834 SURDENT	68 COLLEGE ST	BRISTOL	D932 L075
	1835 SURDENT	68 COLLEGE ST	BRISTOL	D820 L002
	1836 SURDENT	68 COLLEGE ST	BRISTOL	D933 L075
	1837 SURDENT	68 COLLEGE ST	BRISTOL	D934 L075
	1838 SURDENT	68 COLLEGE ST	BRISTOL	D935 L075
	1839 SURDENT	68 COLLEGE ST	BRISTOL	D936 L075
	1840 SURDENT	68 COLLEGE ST	BRISTOL	D945 L075
	1841 SURDENT	69 COLLEGE ST	BRISTOL	D937 L075
	1842 SURDENT	68 COLLEGE ST	BRISTOL	D938 L075
	1843 SURDENT	68 COLLEGE ST	BRISTOL	D939 L075
	1844 SURDENT	68 COLLEGE ST	BRISTOL	D940 L075
	1845 SURDENT	68 COLLEGE ST	BRISTOL	D822 L002
	1846 SURDENT	68 COLLEGE ST	BRISTOL	D941 L075
	1847 SURDENT	68 COLLEGE ST	BRISTOL	D942 L075
	1848 SURDENT	68 COLLEGE ST	BRISTOL	D943 L075
	1849 SURDENT	68 COLLEGE ST	BRISTOL	D944 L075
HART MR & MRS	1816 DENT	24 COLLEGE ST	BRISTOL	D948 L075
	1817 DENT	24 COLLEGE ST	BRISTOL	D949 L075
	1818 DENT	24 COLLEGE ST	BRISTOL	D950 L075
HART MRS	1820 SURDENT	24 COLLEGE ST	BRISTOL	D919 L075
	1821 SURDENT	24 COLLEGE ST	BRISTOL	D920 L075
	1822 SURDENT	24 COLLEGE ST	BRISTOL	D005 L020
HART MRS (& MR)	1816 DENT	24 COLLEGE ST	BRISTOL	D948 L075
	1817 DENT	24 COLLEGE ST	BRISTOL	D949 L075
	1818 DENT	24 COLLEGE ST	BRISTOL	D950 L075
HARTLEY FRANCIS WILLIAM	1840 DENT	NORTH BRIDGE	HALIFAX	D734 L063
	1841 DENT	NORTH BRIDGE	HALIFAX	D241 L009
HARTLEY WILLIAM	1847 SURDENT	4 TRAFALGAR ST	LEEDS	D276 L015
HARVEY CHARLES GREAVES	1844 DENT	BROAD ST	NOTTINGHAM	D509 L023
HARVEY CHRISTOPHER GEORGE	1844 CUPPER DENT	BROAD ST	NOTTINGHAM *	D504 L023
HASLAM SIMEON	1850 SURDENT CHEM	OLD CROSS	HERTFORD *	DA75 L011
HAWKER HENRY	1851 DENT	54 RODNEY ST	LIVERPOOL	D438 L020
	1852 DENT	54 RODNEY ST	LIVERPOOL	D216 L009
	1853 DENT	17 RODNEY ST	LIVERPOOL	D415 L016
	1855 DENT	17 RODNEY ST	LIVERPOOL	D416 L016
HAWKER ROBERT	1830 DENT	14 WELLINGTON ST	DEVONPORT	D119 L020
HAWKES WILLIAM	1822 DENT	39 SCALE LANE	HULL	D255 L010
	1822 DENT	39 SCALE LANE	HULL	D005 L030
	1823 DENT	39 SCALE LANE	HULL	D369 L018
	1826 DENT	39 SCALE LANE	HULL	D374 L018
HAY (& JORDAN)	1852 DENT	13 BRAZENOSE ST	MANCHESTER	D216 L009
HAY JOHN	1838 DENT	PARIS ST	EXETER	D167 L008
	1839 DENT	9 BEDFORD CIRCUS	EXETER	D151 L008
	1840 DENT	9 BEDFORD CIRCUS	EXETER	D168 L008
	1840 DENT	BEDFORD ST	EXETER	D143 L008
	1841 SURDENT	BEDFORD ST	EXETER	D169 L008
	1842 SURDENT	3 CHAPEL ROW	BATH	D123 L007
	1842 SURDENT	BEDFORD ST	EXETER	D170 L008
	1846 SURDENT	5 GAY ST	BATH	D124 L007
	1848 SURDENT	5 GAY ST	BATH	D125 L007

HAY JOHN	1849 SURDENT	10 FOUNTAIN BDGS	BATH	D126 L007
	1850 SURDENT	17 RUSSELL ST	BATH	D127 L007
	1852 DENT	17 RUSSELL ST	BATH	D128 L007
	1852 SURDENT	17 RUSSELL ST	BATH	D788 L020
	1854 DENT	BENNETT ST	BATH	D129 L007
HAYCROFT D	1840 DENT	44 CASTLE ST	READING	D143 L020
HAYMAN & LITTLE	1850 SURDENT	CUMBERLAND ST	BRISTOL	D946 L075
	1850 DENT	4 CUMBERLAND ST	BRISTOL	D960 L075
	1851 SURDENT	CUMBERLAND ST	BRISTOL	D896 L075
	1852 SURDENT	CUMBERLAND ST	BRISTOL	D897 L075
	1853 DENT	4 CUMBERLAND ST	BRISTOL	D802 L020
	1853 SURDENT	CUMBERLAND ST	BRISTOL	D898 L075
	1853 DENT	4 CUMBERLAND ST	BRISTOL	D951 L075
	1854 SURDENT	CUMBERLAND ST	BRISTOL	D899 L075
	1855 SURDENT	CUMBERLAND ST	BRISTOL	D947 L075
HAYWOOD JAMES DANIEL	1850 DENT	32 NEW ST	BHAM	D013 L002
HEARNE EDWARD	1847 DENT MB	21 BARNARD ST	SOUTHAMPTON +	D340 L017
HEATH	1827 DENT		LEICESTER	D663 L024
HEATH & WINCKWORTH	1822 SURDENT	8 EDGAR BDGS	BATH	D005 L020
HEATH C	1830 SURDENT	UNION ST	PLYMOUTH	D491 L022
HEATH GEORGE	1830 DENT	9 DEVONSHIRE PL	PLYMOUTH	D119 L008
	1836 DENT	PRINCESS SQ	PLYMOUTH	DA44 L011
	1840 DENT	PRINCESS SQ	PLYMOUTH	D143 L008
HEATHCOAT JOSEPH	1849 SURDENT	FREESTON GALLOWTREEGATE	LEICESTER	D661 L024
HEATHCOTE J	1852 DENT	TOWER ST	WINCHESTER	D872 L025
HEATHCOTE JOSEPH F	1852 DENT	THE SQUARE	WINCHESTER	D346 L017
HELE SAMUEL	1838 SURDENT	FRIERNHAY ST	EXETER	D167 L008
	1839 SURDENT	FRIERNHAY ST	EXETER	D151 L008
	1840 SURDENT	FRIERNHAY ST	EXETER	D168 L008
	1840 DENT	FRIERNHAY	EXETER	D143 L008
	1841 SURDENT	FRIERNHAY	EXETER	D169 L008
	1842 SURDENT	DISPENSARY QUEEN ST	EXETER	D170 L008
	1843 SURDENT	DISPENSARY QUEEN ST	EXETER	D171 L008
	1844 SURDENT	DISPENSARY QUEEN ST	EXETER	D172 L008
	1845 SURDENT	DISPENSARY QUEEN ST	EXETER	D173 L008
	1846 SURDENT	DISPENSARY QUEEN ST	EXETER	D174 L008
	1847 SURDENT	DISPENSARY QUEEN ST	EXETER	D175 L008
	1848 SURDENT	DISPENSARY QUEEN ST	EXETER	D176 L008
	1849 SURDENT	DISPENSARY QUEEN ST	EXETER	D177 L008
	1850 SURDENT	DISPENSARY QUEEN ST	EXETER	D178 L008
	1850 DENT	DISPENSARY QUEEN ST	EXETER	D147 L008
HELSBY CHARLES	1850 DENT	102 MOSLEY ST	MANCHESTER	D476 L020
HELSBY CHARLES & R	1852 DENT	102 MOSLEY ST	MANCHESTER	D216 L009
HELSBY CHARLES (& R)	1846 DENT	80 GEORGE ST	MANCHESTER	D879 L072
	1848 DENT	80 GEORGE ST	MANCHESTER	D475 L020
	1848 DENT	80 GEORGE ST	MANCHESTER	D332 L016
	1855 SURDENT	102 MOSLEY ST	MANCHESTER	D478 L020
HELSBY RICHARD	1828 SURDENT	29 GEORGE ST	MANCHESTER	D025 L020
	1828 SURDENT	29 GEORGE ST	MANCHESTER	D464 L020
	1829 SURDENT	29 GEORGE ST	MANCHESTER	D565 L020
	1829 SURDENT	29 GEORGE ST	MANCHESTER	D465 L020
	1830 SURDENT	29 GEORGE ST	MANCHESTER	D466 L020
	1832 SURDENT	80 GEORGE ST	MANCHESTER	D467 L020
	1833 SURDENT	80 GEORGE ST	MANCHESTER	D468 L020
	1834 DENT	80 GEORGE ST	MANCHESTER	D236 L009
	1836 DENT	80 GEORGE ST	MANCHESTER	D469 L020
	1837 DENT	80 GEORGE ST	MANCHESTER	D566 L020

HELSBY RICHARD	1838 DENT	80 GEORGE ST	MANCHESTER	D470	L020
	1840 DENT	80 GEORGE ST	MANCHESTER	D471	L020
	1841 DENT	80 GEORGE ST	MANCHESTER	D472	L020
	1841 DENT	80 GEORGE ST	MANCHESTER	D331	L016
	1843 DENT	80 GEORGE ST	MANCHESTER	D473	L020
	1845 DENT	89 GEORGE ST	MANCHESTER	D474	L020
	1850 DENT	102 MOSLEY ST	MANCHESTER	D476	L020
HELSBY RICHARD & C	1846 DENT	80 GEORGE ST	MANCHESTER	D879	L072
	1848 DENT	80 GEORGE ST	MANCHESTER	D332	L016
	1848 DENT	80 GEORGE ST	MANCHESTER	D475	L020
	1855 SURDENT	102 MOSLEY ST	MANCHESTER	D478	L020
HELSBY RICHARD & CO	1851 DENT	102 MOSLEY ST	MANCHESTER	D567	L020
	1852 DENT	102 MOSLEY ST	MANCHESTER	D477	L020
HELSBY RICHARD (& C)	1852 DENT	102 MOSLEY ST	MANCHESTER	D216	L009
HENNEY WALTER	1842 SURDENT	PRINCE'S ST	NORWICH	D648	L051
	1846 DENT	19 MILL ST	LIVERPOOL	D879	L072
	1846 DENT	4 GT GEORGE ST	LIVERPOOL	D303	L014
	1847 DENT	4 GT GEORGE ST	LIVERPOOL	D412	L016
	1848 DENT	2 GT GEORGE ST	LIVERPOOL	D332	L016
	1849 DENT	2 GT GEORGE ST	LIVERPOOL	D413	L016
	1851 DENT	2 GT GEORGE ST	LIVERPOOL	D414	L016
	1853 DENT	2 GT GEORGE ST	LIVERPOOL	D415	L016
HEPBURN (& THOMPSON)	1853 SURDENT	LOW PAVEMENT	NOTTINGHAM	D507	L023
HEPBURN D D	1855 DENT	LOW PAVEMENT	NOTTINGHAM	D511	L023
HEPBURN DUNCAN D	1854 DENT	HIGH PAVEMENT	NOTTINGHAM	D510	L023
HESKETH BIRCH	1767 OP FOR THE TEETH	COOK ST	LIVERPOOL	D030	L016
	1769 OP FOR THE TEETH	COOK ST	LIVERPOOL	D029	L016
	1772 OP FOR THE TEETH	COOK ST	LIVERPOOL	D059	L016
	1774 DENT	12 COOK ST	LIVERPOOL	D105	L016
	1777 DENT	12 COOK ST	LIVERPOOL	D327	L016
	1781 OP FOR THE TEETH	10 COOK ST	LIVERPOOL	D328	L016
	1787 DENT	DALE ST	LIVERPOOL	D329	L016
HESLOP RICHARD	1845 SURDENT	5 KING ST	HUDDERSFIELD	D538	L030
	1850 DENT	5 KING ST	HUDDERSFIELD	D539	L030
	1855 DENT	9 KING ST	HUDDERSFIELD	D222	L009
HEYWOOD JAMES.DANIEL	1849 SURDENT	98 SUFFOLK STREET	BIRMINGHAM	D062	L002
	1850 SURDENT	98 SUFFOLK STREET	BIRMINGHAM	D063	L002
HIAM C	1854 DENT	BEARWARD ST	NORTHAMPTON	D471	L011
HICKMAN HENRY	1851 SURDENT	QUEEN ST	WOLVERHAMPTON	D699	L059
HIGGINBOTTOM JOHN	1835 DENT	63 GT CROSSHALL ST	LIVERPOOL	D406	L016
	1839 DENT	56 GT CROSSHALL ST	LIVERPOOL	D408	L016
	1841 DENT	56 GT CROSSHALL ST	LIVERPOOL	D409	L016
	1843 DENT	56 GT CROSSHALL ST	LIVERPOOL	D410	L016
	1843 DENT	56 GT CROSSHALL ST	LIVERPOOL	D434	L019
	1845 DENT	56 GT CROSSHALL ST	LIVERPOOL	D411	L016
	1846 DENT	56 GT CROSSHLL ST	LIVERPOOL	D879	L072
	1846 DENT	CROSSHALL ST	LIVERPOOL	D303	L014
	1847 DENT	74 GT CROSSHALL ST	LIVERPOOL	D412	L016
	1848 DENT	74 GT CROSSHALL ST	LIVERPOOL	D332	L016
	1849 DENT	74 GT CROSSHALL ST	LIVERPOOL	D413	L016
	1851 DENT	74 GT CROSSHALL ST	LIVERPOOL	D438	L020
	1851 DENT	74 GT CROSSHALL ST	LIVERPOOL	D414	L016
	1852 DENT	74 CROSSHALL ST	LIVERPOOL	D216	L009
	1853 DENT	74 GT CROSSHALL ST	LIVERPOOL	D415	L016
	1855 DENT	74 GT CROSSHALL ST	LIVERPOOL	D416	L016
HIGGINS	1846 SURDENT	LANSDOWN TCE CLIFTON	BRISTOL	D879	L072
HIGGINS E	1845 SURDENT	8 LANSDOWN PL	CLIFTON	D822	L002

HIGGINS E	1846 SURDENT	8 LANSDOWN PL	CLIFTON	BRISTOL	D941 L075
	1847 SURDENT	8 LANSDOWN PL	CLIFTON	BRISTOL	D942 L075
HIGMAN H R	1853 DENT	76A BOLD ST		LIVERPOOL	D415 L016
	1855 DENT	78 BOLD ST		LIVERPOOL	D416 L016
HILDYARD CHARLES	1853 SURDENT	WEST PDE		HUDDERSFIELD	D261 L010
	1855 DENT	WEST PDE		HUDDERSFIELD	D222 L009
HILLYARD CHARLES	1855 DENT	6 ST ANNE ST		LIVERPOOL	D416 L016
HITCHCOCK WILLIAM RICHARD	1840 DENT	FORE ST		TAUNTON	D676 L055
HOCKLEY ANTHONY	1853 DENT	2 HIGH ST		CROYDON	D612 L048
HODGSON JOSEPH	1855 DENT	26 GT BRIDGEWATER ST		MANCHESTER	D478 L020
HOGARTH THOMAS	1848 DENT	41 GT GEORGE ST		LIVERPOOL	D332 L016
HOOTON JONATHAN	1855 DENT	80 GT DUCIE ST		MANCHESTER	D478 L020
HOPKINSON WILLIAM	1848 DENT	46 BROUGHTON RD		SALFORD	D332 L016
	1848 DENT	46 BROUGHTON RD		SALFORD	D475 L020
	1850 DENT	36 BROUGHTON RD		MANCHESTER	D476 L020
	1852 DENT	36 BROUGHTON RD		MANCHESTER	D216 L009
	1855 DENT	34 BROUGHTON RD		MANCHESTER	D478 L020
HOPTON & CO	1855 DENT SUCC TO BALL	31 CARLIOL ST		NEWCASTLE	D223 L009
HORDEN J	1845 DENT			LEAMINGTON	D077 L006
HORDERN	1839 DENT	CLEMENS ST		LEAMINGTON	D326 L014
	1840 DENT	CLEMENS ST		LEAMINGTON	D307 L014
	1841 DENT	CLEMENS ST		LEAMINGTON	D306 L014
	1842 SURDENT	7 CLEMENS ST		LEAMINGTON	D305 L014
	1845 SURDENT	SPENCER ST		LEAMINGTON	D309 L014
	1848 SURDENT	SPENCER ST		LEAMINGTON	D308 L014
HORDERN J	1839 DENT	7 CLEMENS ST		LEAMINGTON	D301 L002
	1839 DENT	BAILEY LANE		COVENTRY	D301 L002
	1846 DENT	3 SPENCER ST		LEAMINGTON	D303 L014
	1849 DENT	3 SPENCER ST		LEAMINGTON	D310 L014
	1854 DENT	1 EUSTON PL		LEAMINGTON	D015 L001
HORDERN JOHN	1850 SURDENT	1 EUSTON PL		LEAMINGTON	D063 L002
	1850 DENT	3 SPENCER ST		LEAMINGTON	D013 L002
HORDERN JOHN JAMES	1841 DENT	7 CLEMENS ST		LEAMINGTON	D028 L002
HORNER & KING	1837 DENT	43 CONEY ST		YORK	D257 L010
HORNER & TURNER	1822 DENT	CONEY ST		YORK	D255 L010
HORNER BENJAMIN	1828 DENT	43 CONEY ST		YORK	D025 L010
HORNOR	1809 SURDENT	CONEY ST		YORK	D046 L010
	1811 SURDENT	CONEY ST		YORK	D284 L011
HORNOR BENJAMIN	1800 DENT	20 LORD ST		LIVERPOOL	D389 L016
	1803 SURDENT	20 LORD ST		LIVERPOOL	D390 L016
	1830 DENT	43 CONEY ST		YORK	D256 L010
	1834 DENT	CONEY ST		YORK	D236 L009
	1834 DENT	FULFORD GRANGE		YORK	D236 L009
HOSKINS FRANCIS	1847 DENT	MIDDLE PAVEMENT		NOTTINGHAM	D505 L023
	1848 DENT	CARLTON ST		NOTTINGHAM	D506 L023
HOWARD G	1851 DENT	ROYAL HILL		GREENWICH	DA77 L011
HOWARD J	1844 SURDENT	83 PARROCK ST		GRAVESEND	DC14 L084
	1846 SURDENT	83 PARROCK ST		GRAVESEND	DC34 L084
	1847 SURDENT	83 PARROCK ST		GRAVESEND	DC15 L084
HOWARD JOHN	1841 SUR DENT	PARROCK ST		GRAVESEND *	DC12 L084
	1842 SURDENT	83 PARROCK ST		GRAVESEND	DC13 L084
	1845 DENT	PARROCK ST		GRAVESEND	DA66 L011
HOWATT JOHN	1849 DENT	7 MILL ST		LIVERPOOL	D413 L016
HUDSON T	1853 DENT	23 LONG ROW		S SHIELDS	D243 L009
HUDSON T & CO	1855 DENT	CAMDEN ST		N SHIELDS	D223 L009
HUGGINS J	1848 DENT	BROAD ST		NEW ALRESFORD	D357 L017
	1852 DENT	BROAD ST		NEW ALRESFORD	DB72 L025

HUGHES J A	1854 DENT	CHESTER ST	BIRKENHEAD	D967 L076
HUGHES JAMES	1849 DENT	26A CHESTER ST	BIRKENHEAD	D413 L016
	1850 DENT	CHESTER ST	BIRKENHEAD	D709 L034
HUGHES JAMES A	1851 DENT	CHESTER ST	BIRKENHEAD	D966 L076
	1851 DENT	23 CHESTER ST	BIRKENHEAD	D414 L016
	1853 DENT	24 CHESTER ST	BIRKENHEAD	D415 L016
	1855 DENT	25 CHESTER ST	BIRKENHEAD	D416 L016
HUGHES JOSEPH	1848 DENT	CHESTER ST	BIRKENHEAD	D332 L016
HUGO M	1848 SURDENT	BELMONT RD	ST HELIER	DC59 L088
	1849 SURDENT	BELMONT ROW	ST HELIER	DC60 L088
	1852 SURDENT	BELMONT RD	ST HELIER	DC61 L088
	1853 SURDENT	BELMONT RD	ST HELIER	DB75 L080
	1854 SURDENT	BELMONT RD	ST HELIER	DC62 L088
	1855 SURDENT	BELMONT RD	ST HELIER	DC63 L089
HUGO S	1853 DENT	ALLEZ ST	GUERNSEY	DC68 L088
HULME J HUGHES	1852 SURDENT	ST ANDREW'S HALL PLAIN	NORWICH	D653 L051
HULSTON JAMES	1820 APOTH DENT	BROAD STREET	WORCESTER*	D004 L001
	1822 PHY SUR APOTH DENT	BROAD STREET	WORCESTER*	D005 L001
	1828 SUR SURDENT	33 BROAD STREET	WORCESTER*	D025 L002
	1830 DENT APOTH	33 BROAD STREET	WORCESTER*	D006 L001
	1835 DENT APOTH	33 BROAD STREET	WORCESTER*	D007 L001
	1837 DENT APOTH	33 BROAD STREET	WORCESTER*	D009 L001
	1837 DENT APOTH	33 BROAD STREET	WORCESTER*	D008 L001
	1838 SURDENT	33 BROAD STREET	WORCESTER	D032 L005
	1840 DENT APOTH	33 BROAD STREET	WORCESTER*	D010 L001
	1840 DENT	33 BROAD STREET	WORCESTER	D011 L001
	1841 DENT	33 BROAD STREET	WORCESTER	D028 L002
HUME W	1849 SURDENT MATERIAL MAN	34 HAMPTON ST	BIRMINGHAM *	D062 L002
	1850 SURDENT MATERIAL MAN	34 HAMPTON ST	BIRMINGHAM *	D063 L002
HUMPHREY G E	1849 DENT	20 PORTLAND ST	SOUTHAMPTON	D341 L017
	1851 DENT	20 PORTLAND ST	SOUTHAMPTON	D342 L017
	1852 DENT	20 PORTLAND ST	SOUTHAMPTON	DB72 L025
	1853 DENT	20 PORTLAND ST	SOUTHAMPTON	D343 L017
	1855 SURDENT	7 PORTLAND TCE	SOUTHAMPTON	DA84 L011
	1855 DENT	7 PORTLAND TCE	SOUTHAMPTON	D344 L017
HUMPHREY GEORGE	1847 DENT	20 PORTLAND ST	SOUTHAMPTON	D340 L017
	1852 DENT	20 PORTLAND ST	SOUTHAMPTON	D346 L017
HUMPHREY GEORGE EDWARD	1845 SURDENT	20 PORTLAND ST	SOUTHAMPTON	D339 L017
HUMPHRY G	1848 DENT	20 PORTLAND ST	SOUTHAMPTON	D357 L017
HUMPHRY G E	1849 DENT	20 PORTLAND ST	SOUTHAMPTON	D345 L017
HUNT W	1855 DENT	CHEAP ST	SHERBORNE	DA84 L011
HUNT WILLIAM	1840 DENT	HENDFORD	YEOVIL	D143 L020
	1850 DENT	PEN HILL	YEOVIL	DA78 L011
	1852 DENT	PEN HILL	YEOVIL	D788 L020
HUNTER JAMES	1844 DENT	ST LEONARD'S CHURCHYARD	LUDLOW	D576 L002
HUNTLEY F H	1853 SURDENT	BARNFIELD PL	EXETER	D153 L008
	1854 SURDENT	BARNFIELD PL	EXETER	DB71 L025
HUNTLEY HENRY	1847 SURDENT	HIGH ST	EXETER	D175 L008
	1848 SURDENT	HIGH ST	EXETER	D176 L008
	1849 SURDENT	HIGH ST	EXETER	D177 L008
	1850 SURDENT	BARNFIELD	EXETER	D178 L008
	1851 SURDENT	BARNFIELD HOUSE	EXETER	D179 L008
	1852 SURDENT	BARNFIELD HOUSE	EXETER	D180 L008
	1853 SURDENT	BARNFIELD HOUSE	EXETER	D181 L008
	1854 SURDENT	BARNFIELD HOUSE	EXETER	D182 L008
	1855 SURDENT	BARNFIELD HOUSE	EXETER	D183 L008
HUNTLEY HENRY F	1848 DENT	19 HIGH ST	EXETER	DA50 L011

HUNTLEY HENRY FREDERICK	1850 DENT	11 HIGH ST	EXETER	D147 L008
	1852 DENT	BARNFIELD HO SOUTHERNHAY	EXETER	D145 L008
	1852 DENT	SOUTHERNHAY	EXETER	D788 L020
HUSSEY E W	1854 DENT	SMITHFORD ST	COVENTRY	D015 L001
HUSSEY EDWARD W	1850 SURDENT	FLEET ST	COVENTRY	D063 L002
HUSSEY EDWARD WILLIAM	1850 SURDENT	SMITHFORD ST	COVENTRY	D714 L002
HUTCHINSON J	1848 DENT	CHANDLER'S LANE	NOTTINGHAM	D800 L020
HUTCHINSON JAMES	1835 DENT	HAYWOOD ST	NOTTINGHAM	D007 L014
	1844 DENT	2 GREYHOUND YD	NOTTINGHAM	D509 L023
	1847 DENT	CHANDLER'S LANE	NOTTINGHAM	D505 L023
	1850 DENT	BRIDLESMITH GATE	NOTTINGHAM	D013 L020
HUTCHINSON MASSEY	1855 DENT	NEW NORTH RD	HUDDERSFIELD	D222 L009
HUTCHINSON MATILDA	1844 DENT	DRURY HILL	NOTTINGHAM	D504 L023
HUTCHINSON MATTHEW	1853 SURDENT	NEW NORTH RD	HUDDERSFIELD	D261 L010
HUTCHINSON T	1840 DENT CUPP BLEEDER	BRIDLESMITH GATE	NOTTINGHAM *	D503 L023
	1848 DENT	CLAYTON'S YD	NOTTINGHAM	D800 L020
	1855 DENT	CLAYTON'S YD	NOTTINGHAM	D511 L023
HUTCHINSON THOMAS	1828 DENT	BROAD ST	NOTTINGHAM	D025 L020
	1831 DENT PHLEBOTOMIST	BROAD ST	NOTTINGHAM *	D501 L024
	1832 DENT CUPPER ETC	11 BROAD ST	NOTTINGHAM *	D508 L023
	1834 DENT CUP BLEED	BRIDLESMITH GATE	NOTTINGHAM *	D502 L023
	1835 DENT	BRIDLESMITH GATE	NOTTINGHAM	D007 L014
	1841 DENT	CLAYTON'S YD	NOTINGHAM	D331 L016
	1844 DENT	BRIDLESMITHGATE	NOTTINGHAM	D504 L023
	1847 DENT	CLAYTON'S YD	NOTTINGHAM	D505 L023
	1854 DENT	BRIDLESMITH GATE	NOTTINGHAM	D510 L023
HYDEN DANIEL	1808 HD DENT	9 CHURCH ST	MANCHESTER *	D456 L020
	1811 HD DENT	9 CHURCH ST	MANCHESTER *	D457 L020
IMRIE & DEAN	1845 DENT	75 PICCADILLY	MANCHESTER	D474 L020
IMRIE R M	1834 DENT	109 DUKE ST	LIVERPOOL	D236 L009
IMRIE ROBERT MARSHALL	1834 DENT	6 FALKNER ST	MANCHESTER	D236 L009
	1836 DENT	6 FALKNER ST	MANCHESTER	D469 L020
	1838 DENT	75 PICCADILLY	MANCHESTER	D470 L020
	1840 DENT	75 PICCADILLY	MANCHESTER	D471 L020
	1841 DENT	75 PICCADILLY	MANCHESTER	D331 L016
	1841 DENT	75 PICCADILLY	MANCHESTER	D472 L020
IMRIE ROBERT MARSHALL & CO	1843 DENT	75 PICCADILLY	MANCHESTER	D473 L020
JACKSON C	1855 DENT	2 CASTLE PL	HASTINGS	D594 L046
JACKSON CHARLES	1852 SURDENT	9 YORK BDGS	HASTINGS	DA54 L011
JACOB HENRY LONG	1848 DENT	CORNHILL	BRIDGEWATER	DA50 L011
JAMES J	1850 DENT	TYTHING	WORCESTER	D099 L011
JAMES JAMES	1840 DENT	TYTHING	WORCESTER	D011 L001
JAMES JOHN	1847 DENT	TYTHING	WORCESTER	D012 L001
	1851 SURDENT CUP	8 FOREGATE STREET	WORCESTER*	D014 L001
	1853 DENT	9 FOREGATE STREET	WORCESTER	D031 L004
	1854 DENT	9 FOREGATE STREET	WORCESTER	D015 L001
	1855 SURDENT	9 FOREGATE STREET	WORCESTER	D016 L001
JAMES THOMAS	1840 DENT	TYTHING	WORCESTER	D734 L063
	1840 DENT	TYTHING	WORCESTER	D010 L001
	1841 DENT	TYTHING	WORCESTER	D028 L002
JARDINE J	1847 DENT	WELL ST	BRADFORD	D276 L015
JARDINE MARSH RBT	1850 DENT	42 CHEAPSIDE	BHAM	D013 L002
JARDINE MARSH.ROBERT	1849 SURDENT DRUGGIST	42 CHEAPSIDE	BIRMINGHAM *	D062 L002
	1850 SURDENT DRUGGIST	42 CHEAPSIDE	BIRMINGHAM *	D063 L002
JARRITT	1851 SURDENT	HILL ST	RICHMOND	DA83 L011
JAY THOMAS.EDWARD	1854 DENT	HIGH STREET	EVESHAM	D015 L001
JEFFERIES T	1855 DENT	335 HIGH ST	LINCOLN	D682 L056

JEFFERSON WILLIAM	1853 SURDENT	26 ELMWOOD ST	LEEDS	D261 L010
	1855 DENT	26 ELMWOOD ST	LEEDS	D222 L009
JENKINS H M	1855 DENT	HIGH ST	CHICHESTER	DA84 L011
JENKINS PERCIVAL	1846 DENT	16 HOUGHTON ST	LIVERPOOL	D303 L014
	1847 DENT	7 SLATER ST	LIVERPOOL	D412 L016
JEWERS FREDERICK	1844 DENT	8 UNION ST	PLYMOUTH	D492 L022
	1844 DENT	8 UNION ST	PLYMOUTH	D144 L008
	1850 DENT	42 UNION ST	STONEHOUSE	D147 L008
	1852 DENT	4 FLORA PL	PLYMOUTH	D493 L022
JEWERS FREDERICK ARTHUR	1852 DENT	4 FLORA PL	PLYMOUTH	D788 L020
	1852 DENT	4 FLORA PL	PLYMOUTH	D145 L008
JOEL E G	1850 SURDENT	37 VILLIERS ST	SUNDERLAND	D214 L009
	1851 SURDENT	37 VILLIERS ST	SUNDERLAND	D215 L009
	1853 SURDENT	27 VILLIERS ST	SUNDERLAND	D243 L009
	1855 DENT	27 VILLIERS ST	SUNDERLAND	D223 L009
JOEL EDWARD	1855 DCNT	27 VILLIERS ST	SUNDERLAND	D222 L009
JOEL EDWARD G	1851 SURDENT	37 VILLIERS ST	SUNDERLAND	D292 L013
JOHNSON G F	1855 DENT	144 NORTH ST	BRIGHTON	D594 L046
JOHNSON GEORGE F	1854 DENT	144 NORTH ST	BRIGHTON	D605 L047
JONES	1831 DENT	155 SNARGATE	DOVER	D582 L044
	1833 DENT	155 SNARGATE ST	DOVER	D583 L044
	1840 DENT	155 SNARGATE ST	DOVER	D585 L044
	1854 DENT	71 HIGH ST	WINCHESTER	D489 L021
JONES & BELL	1849 DENT	BRIDGE ST	CANTERBURY	D587 L011
	1850 DENT	WEEK ST	MAIDSTONE	D592 L045
	1850 SURDENT	CHAPEL PL	TUNBRIDGE WELLS	DA52 L011
	1851 DENT	BRIDGE ST	CANTERBURY	DA77 L011
	1851 DENT	WEEK ST	MAIDSTONE	DA77 L011
	1854 DENT	WEEK ST	MAIDSTONE	DB82 L082
	1855 DENT	12 LOWER BRIDGE ST	CANTERBURY	D594 L046
JONES (& ALEX)	1850 DENT	9 SHIP ST	BRIGHTON	D603 L047
	1851 DENT	9 SHIP ST	BRIGHTON	DA77 L011
	1852 DENT	9 SHIP ST	BRIGHTON	D604 L047
	1854 DENT	9 SHIP ST	BRIGHTON	D605 L047
	1855 DENT	9 SHIP ST	BRIGHTON	D594 L046
JONES (& NELSON)	1846 DENT	13 MT PLEASANT	LIVERPOOL	D303 L014
JONES C	1846 SURDENT	63 TRUMPINGTON ST	CAMBRIDGE	DA85 L011
JONES CHARLES JOHN	1830 DENT	JESUS LANE	CAMBRIDGE	D119 L020
JONES E	1850 DENT	9 EASY ROW	BIRMINGHAM	D099 L011
	1854 DENT	9 EASY ROW	BIRMINGHAM	D069 L002
JONES EDWARD	1839 DENT	9 EASY ROW	BHAM	D301 L002
	1847 DENT	9 EASY ROW	BIRMINGHAM	D061 L002
	1850 DENT	9 EASY ROW	BHAM	D013 L002
JONES EDWIN	1841 DENT	9 EASY ROW	BIRMINGHAM	D058 L002
	1842 DENT	9 EASY ROW	BIRMINGHAM	D075 L002
	1845 DENT	9 EASY ROW	BIRMINGHAM	D077 L002
	1846 DENT	9 EASY ROW	BIRMINGHAM	D879 L072
	1849 SURDENT	9 EASY ROW	BIRMINGHAM	D062 L002
	1850 SURDENT	9 EASY ROW	BIRMINGHAM	D063 L002
	1852 DENT	9 EASY ROW	BIRMINGHAM	D078 L002
	1855 SURDENT	37 BENNETTS HILL	BIRMINGHAM	D064 L002
JONES F	1855 DENT	MERCER ROW	LOUTH	D682 L056
JONES GRENVILLE	1834 DENT	WHITEFRIARS	CHESTER	D236 L009
	1840 DENT	MARDOL HEAD	SHREWSBURY	D734 L063
	1841 DENT	MARDOL HEAD	SHREWSBURY	D241 L009
	1842 SURDENT	3 UPPER PARADE	LEAMINGTON	D305 L014
	1842 SURDENT	MARDOL HEAD	SHREWSBURY	D123 L043

JONES GRENVILLE	1844 SURDENT	ST JOHN'S HILL	SHREWSBURY	D576 L002
JONES H M	1827 DENT	2 CRESCENT ROW	EXETER	D149 L008
	1828 DENT	HIGHER SOUTHERNHAY	EXETER	D150 L008
	1828 DENT	2 CRESCENT ROW	EXETER	D159 L008
	1830 DENT	16 PARIS ST	EXETER	D160 L008
	1840 DENT	NICHOLAS ST	CHESTER	D734 L063
JONES HENRY	1838 SURDENT	KINGSBRIDGE HOUSE	CANTERBURY	DB48 L025
	1839 SURDENT	109 WEEK ST	MAIDSTONE	D584 L020
	1839 DENT	MR BARTLETT'S WEEK ST	MAIDSTONE	D591 L045
	1845 DENT	109 WEEK ST	MAIDSTONE	DA66 L011
	1845 DENT	12 BRIDGE ST	CANTERBURY	DA66 L011
JONES HENRY M	1830 DENT	2 CRESCENT ROW	EXETER	D119 L008
	1834 DENT	NICHOLAS ST	CHESTER	D236 L009
JONES HENRY NICHOLLS	1843 DENT	20 NICHOLAS ST	CHESTER	D434 L019
JONES HENRY NICHOLS	1840 DENT	NICHOLAS ST	CHESTER	D718 L061
JONES HENRY NICHOLLS	1846 DENT	NICHOLAS ST	CHESTER	D713 L061
	1846 DENT	NICHOLAS ST	CHESTER	D303 L014
	1850 DENT	MARDOL HEAD	SHREWSBURY	D013 L043
	1851 SURDENT	MARDOL HEAD	SHREWSBURY	D780 L043
JONES HORATIO	1850 DENT	3 ST JOHN'S HILL	SHREWSBURY	D013 L043
	1851 SURDENT	ST JOHN'S HILL	SHREWSBURY	D780 L043
JONES ISAIAH	1830 DENT	ST GILES BROAD ST	NORWICH	D119 L020
JONES J	1853 DENT	63 TRUMPINGTON ST	CAMBRIDGE	D655 L051
JONES JAMES.GIBBS	1847 DENT	37 TYTHING	WORCESTER	D012 L001
JONES JOHN	1823 DENT	BRENT GOVELL ST	BURY ST EDMUNDS	D142 L011
	1824 SURDENT	230 GT ANCOATS ST	MANCHESTER	D401 L019
	1828 DRUGG CUPP DENT	41 GT ANCOATS ST	MANCHESTER *	D464 L020
	1839 DENT	TRUMPINGTON ST	CAMBRIDGE	D584 L020
	1850 DENT	63 TRUMPINGTON ST	CAMBRIDGE	DA91 L011
	1851 DENT	65 CHRISTIAN ST	LIVERPOOL	D414 L016
	1851 DENT	28 CHADDOCK ST	PRESTON	D438 L020
	1851 DENT	28 CHADDOCK ST	PRESTON	D727 L020
	1851 DENT	28 CHADDOCK ST	PRESTON	D437 L019
	1851 DENT HERBALIST	101 MILL ST	LIVERPOOL *	D438 L020
	1852 DENT HERBALIST	101 MILL ST	LIVERPOOL *	D216 L009
	1852 DENT HERBALIST	282 BRADFORD STREET	BIRMINGHAM *	D078 L002
	1855 SURDENT	TRUMPINGTON ST	CAMBRIDGE	DA45 L011
JONES MORRIS	1851 DENT	14 ST JAMES ST	LEEDS	D283 L015
	1852 DENT	14 ST JAMES ST	LEEDS	D216 L009
JONES ROBERT	1851 DENT	28 CHADDOCK ST	PRESTON	D673 L053
	1853 DENT	28 CHADDOCK ST	PRESTON	D533 L028
JONES S	1852 DENT	31 PORTLAND ST	SOUTHAMPTON	DB72 L025
	1855 SURDENT	71 HIGH ST	WINCHESTER	DA84 L011
JONES S A	1849 DENT	31 PORTLAND ST	SOUTHAMPTON	D341 L017
	1849 DENT	PORTLAND ST	SOUTHAMPTON	D345 L017
	1851 DENT	31 PORTLAND ST	SOUTHAMPTON	D342 L017
	1853 DENT	31 PORTLAND ST	SOUTHAMPTON	D343 L017
	1855 SURDENT	31 PORTLAND ST	SOUTHAMPTON	DA84 L011
JONES SAMUEL	1845 SURDENT	22 KING ST	KING'S LYNN	D650 L011
	1845 DENT	79 ST GILES ST	NORWICH	D650 L051
	1852 DENT	31 PORTLAND ST	SOUTHAMPTON	D346 L017
JONES SAMUEL A	1855 DENT	31 PORTLAND ST	SOUTHAMPTON	D344 L017
JONES SAMUEL AARON	1842 SURDENT	79 BROAD ST	NORWICH	D648 L051
JONES WILLIAM	1839 DENT	25 LONDON ST	NORWICH	D654 L011
JONES WILLIAM JOSEPH	1839 DENT	HIGH ST	CANTERBURY	D584 L011
JORDAN & HAY	1852 DENT	13 BRAZENOSE ST	MANCHESTER	D216 L009
JORDAN CHARLES	1840 DENT	57 LEVER ST	MANCHESTER	D471 L020

JORDAN CHARLES	1841 DENT	57 LEVER ST	MANCHESTER	D472 L020
	1843 DENT	23 ST JAMES PL	LIVERPOOL	D410 L016
	1849 DENT	33 BLOOM ST	LIVERPOOL	D413 L016
JORDAN H	1848 DENT	CORN MARKET	DERBY	D800 L020
JORDAN H E	1840 DENT		READING	DC05 L049
	1840 DENT	2 DUKE ST	READING	D143 L020
	1842 DENT	2 DUKE ST	READING	D625 L049
	1843 DENT		READING	DB96 L049
	1844 DENT	2 DUKE ST	READING	D626 L049
	1845 DENT		READING	DB97 L049
	1846 DENT		READING	DC06 L049
	1847 DENT	2 DUKE ST	READING	D815 L011
	1847 DENT	2 DUKE ST	READING	DB84 L049
	1847 DENT		READING	DC07 L049
	1848 DENT		READING	DC08 L049
	1853 DENT	3 FORBURY	READING	D627 L049
	1855 DENT		READING	DA90 L011
JORDAN H J	1841 DENT		READING	DA87 L011
	1844 DENT		READING	DA88 L011
	1852 DENT		READING	DA89 L011
JORDAN HENRY	1846 DENT	4 VICTORIA ST	DERBY	D693 L057
	1847 DENT	7 CORN MARKET	DERBY	D505 L025
	1849 DENT	7 CORN MARKET	DERBY	D803 L057
	1850 DENT	CORN MKT	DERBY	D013 L020
	1850 DENT	7 CORN MARKET	DERBY	D809 L057
	1852 DENT	DERWENT ST	DERBY	D690 L057
JORDAN HENRY EDWARD	1852 DENT	2 DUKE ST	READING	D788 L020
	1854 DENT	3 FORBURY	READING	D628 L049
JORDAN JOHN	1850 DENT	13 BRAZENNOSE ST	MANCHESTER	D476 L020
	1851 DENT	13 BRAZENNOSE ST	MANCHESTER	D567 L020
	1852 DENT	13 BRAZENNOSE ST	MANCHESTER	D477 L020
JORDAN ROBERT B	1851 SURDENT	SCOTT LANE	DONCASTER	D259 L056
JUDSON B R G	1855 DENT	EGHAM	CHERTSEY	D594 L046
JUNOT FREDERICK CHARLES	1852 SURDENT	CROSS ST	ABERGAVENNY	DA76 L011
KARRAN J	1844 DENT	FINCH RD	DOUGLAS I OF M	DB52 L025
	1848 DENT	19 EDWARD TCE	DOUGLAS I OF M	DB24 L011
	1852 DENT	19 EDWARD TCE	DOUGLAS I OF M	DB73 L079
KARRAN JAMES	1847 DENT	19 EDWARD TCE	DOUGLAS I OF MAN	D505 L025
	1852 DENT	19 EDWARD TCE	DOUGLAS I OF M	DC56 L087
KEATON JOSEPH	1846 DENT	5 ST PETER'S ST	DERBY	D693 L057
KELK EDWIN	1828 DENT	2 SMITH ST	BIRMINGHAM	D025 L006
KELLY THOMAS	1845 DENT	43 CHATHAM ST	MANCHESTER	D474 L020
KELLY THOMAS MOORE	1846 DENT	13 CHATHAM ST	MANCHESTER	D879 L072
	1848 DENT	13 CHATHAM ST	MANCHESTER	D475 L020
	1848 DENT	13 CHATHAM ST	MANCHESTER	D332 L016
	1850 DENT	13 CHATHAM ST	MANCHESTER	D476 L020
	1851 DENT	13 CHATHAM ST	MANCHESTER	D567 L020
	1852 DENT	13 CHATHAM ST	MANCHESTER	D477 L020
	1852 DENT	13 CHAPEL ST	MANCHESTER	D216 L009
	1855 DENT	13 CHATHAM ST	MANCHESTER	D478 L020
KENNEDY R F	1855 SURDENT	33 HIGH ST	COWES I OF W	DA84 L011
KENT FREDERICK CHARLES	1847 DENT	ATHOL ST	DOUGLAS I OF MAN	D505 L025
KERNOTT C M	1839 DENT	GLOSTER HOUSE HIGH ST	COWES	DB43 L078
KING (& HORNER)	1837 DENT	43 CONEY ST	YORK	D257 L010
KING E	1839 DENT	18 MERTON ST	OXFORD	D654 L068
	1847 DENT	121A HIGH ST	OXFORD	D815 L011
	1851 DENT	66 HIGH ST	ROCHESTER	DA77 L011

KING E	1855	DENT	75 ST THOMAS ST	MELCOMBE REGIS	DA84 L011
KING EDWARD	1840	DENT	SHIP ST	BRECON	D143 L020
	1842	DENT	19 HIGH ST	OXFORD	D123 L007
	1844	DENT	WATTON	BRECON	D144 L078
	1846	SURDENT	MAGDALENE ST	OXFORD	D640 L050
	1848	DENT	14 NORTHERNHAY PL	EXETER	DA50 L011
	1849	SURDENT	14 NORTHERNHAY PL	EXETER	D177 L008
	1850	DENT	WATTON	BRECON	DC50 L085
	1850	DENT	MONNOW ST	MONMOUTH	D013 L020
KING EDWARD JOHN	1850	DENT	CATHEDRAL YD	EXETER	D147 L008
KING J H	1843	DENT	22 KING ST	ST HELIER	DC58 L088
KING JOHN HENRY	1839	DENT	22 KING ST	ST HELIER	DB43 L078
KING JOSEPH	1840	DENT	43 CONEY ST	YORK	D734 L063
	1841	DENT	43 CONEY ST	YORK	D241 L009
	1841	DENT	43 CONEY ST	YORK	D331 L016
	1843	SURDENT	43 CONEY ST	YORK (LATE HORNER &	D251 L010
	1845	SURDENT	9 TOWER ST	KING'S LYNN	D650 L011
	1846	DENT	43 CONEY ST	YORK	D258 L010
	1848	DENT	43 CONEY ST	YORK	D332 L016
	1851	SURDENT	43 CONEY ST	YORK	D259 L010
	1855	DENT	43 CONEY ST	YORK	D222 L009
KING JOSEPH (EX HORNER & KING	1840	DENT	43 CONEY ST	YORK	DB88 L006
KING NORMAN	1843	SURDENT	BEDFORD ST	EXETER	D171 L008
	1844	DENT	BEDFORD ST	EXETER	D144 L008
	1844	SURDENT	BEDFORD ST	EXETER	D172 L008
	1845	SURDENT	BEDFORD CLOSE	EXETER	D173 L008
	1846	SURDENT	BEDFORD CLOSE	EXETER	D174 L008
	1847	SURDENT	BEDFORD CLOSE	EXETER	D175 L008
	1848	SURDENT	BEDFORD CIRCUS	EXETER	D176 L008
	1849	SURDENT	BEDFORD CIRCUS	EXETER	D177 L008
	1850	SURDENT	BEDFORD CIRCUS	EXETER	D178 L008
	1850	DENT	7 BEDFORD CIRCUS	EXETER	D147 L008
	1851	SURDENT	BEDFORD CIRCUS	EXETER	D179 L008
	1852	SURDENT	BEDFORD CIRCUS	EXETER	D180 L008
	1852	DENT	7 BEDFORD CIRCUS	EXETER	D788 L020
	1852	DENT	7 BEDFORD CIRCUS	EXETER	D145 L008
	1853	SURDENT	BEDFORD CIRCUS	EXETER	D181 L008
	1853	SURDENT	7 BEDFORD CIRCUS	EXETER	D153 L008
	1854	SURDENT	7 BEDFORD CIRCUS	EXETER	DB71 L025
	1854	SURDENT	BEDFORD CIRCUS	EXETER	D182 L008
	1855	SURDENT	BEDFORD CIRCUS	EXETER	D183 L008
KING NORMAN T	1848	DENT	BEDFORD CIRCUS	EXETER	DA50 L011
KING RICHARD SWIT	1849	SURDENT	MERCERS' ROW	NORTHAMPTON	DA79 L011
KIRK RICHARD SHAW	1848	DENT	BECK LANE	NOTTINGHAM	D506 L023
KIRKBY JAMES	1845	SURDENT	284 ROCKINGHAM ST	SHEFFIELD	D755 L066
	1846	DENT	284 ROCKINGHAM ST	SHEFFIELD	D879 L072
	1848	DENT	284 ROCKINGHAM ST	SHEFFIELD	D332 L016
	1849	SURDENT	284 ROCKINGHAM ST	SHEFFIELD	D756 L066
	1852	DENT	284 ROCKINGHAM ST	SHEFFIELD	D216 L009
	1852	SURDENT	284 ROCKINGHAM ST	SHEFFIELD	D260 L010
	1854	DENT	116 BROOM SPRING LANE	SHEFFIELD	D757 L066
KLOET JACES	1850	DENT	94 WELLINGTON ST SOUTH	STOCKPORT	D709 L034
KLOET JACQUES	1851	DENT	76 WELLINGTON RD	STOCKPORT	D438 L020
KYAN J HOWARD	1855	DENT	7 WESTERN TCE	CHELMSFORD	D594 L046
L'ESTRANGE F	1855	DENT	46 CLAUGHTON RD	BIRKENHEAD	D416 L016
L'ESTRANGE FRANCIS	1849	DENT	88 PRINCE EDWIN ST	LIVERPOOL	D413 L016
	1850	DENT	TRANMERE	BIRKENHEAD	D709 L034

L'ESTRANGE FRANCIS	1851 DENT	88 PRINCE EDWIN ST	LIVERPOOL	D414 L016
	1851 DENT	79 CHESTER ST	BIRKENHEAD	D966 L076
	1853 DENT	85D CHESTER ST	BIRKENHEAD	D415 L016
	1854 DENT	6 CLAUGHTON TCE	BIRKENHEAD	D967 L076
LAING W	1833 DENT	SHERIFF HILL	GATESHEAD	D246 L009
	1836 DENT	FELLING	GATESHEAD	DB34 L011
	1838 DENT	FELLING	GATESHEAD	D239 L009
	1839 DENT	FELLING	GATESHEAD	D240 L009
LAMBERT PETER	1820 JEWELLER DENT	HYDE HILL	BERWICK *	D787 L020
	1828 JEWELLER DENT	HYDE HILL	BERWICK *	D025 L020
	1848 DENT JEWELLER	HIDE HILL	BERWICK *	D332 L016
LAMBERT W	1851 DENT		EAST GRINSTEAD	DA77 L011
	1855 DENT		EAST GRINSTEAD	D594 L046
LAMBERT WILLIAM	1845 DENT		EAST GRINSTEAD	DA66 L011
LANDSDOWNE LAWRENCE	1840 DENT	2 CHAPEL ROW	BATH	D143 L020
LANSDALE R	1854 DENT	QUEEN'S SQ	HIGH WYCOMBE	DA71 L011
LANSDALE RALPH	1853 DENT	QUEEN'S SQ	HIGH WYCOMBE	DA47 L011
LATHAM FRANCIS	1840 DENT	NEW STREET	WORCESTER	D011 L001
LAVENS THOMAS HOWARD	1845 DENT		LEWISHAM	DA66 L011
LAVERS T H	1855 DENT	THE VILLAGE	LEWISHAM	D594 L046
LE BRUN	1843 DENT	5 CAMPBELL PL BATH ST	ST HELIER	DC58 L088
LE BRUN P	1845 DENT	BATH ST	ST HELIER	DA82 L011
	1847 SURDENT	ST MARK'S RD	ST HELIER	D853 L025
	1848 SURDENT	ST MARK'S RD	ST HELIER	DC59 L088
	1849 SURDENT	ST MARK'S RD	ST HELIER	DC60 L088
	1852 DENT	1 EAGLE TCE	ST HELIER	DB72 L025
	1853 SURDENT	BATH ST	ST HELIER	DB75 L080
	1854 SURDENT	VAUXHALL	ST HELIER	DC62 L088
	1855 SURDENT	57 CAMPBELL PL	ST HELIER	DC63 L088
LE DRAY	1845 SURDENT	PARK ST	BRISTOL	D822 L002
	1850 DENT	34 DARLEY ST	BRADFORD	DB35 L078
LE DRAY & CO	1834 DENT	11 COLQUITT ST	LIVERPOOL	D405 L016
	1837 DENT	43 SEEL ST	LIVERPOOL	D407 L016
LE DRAY ANDREW	1837 DENT	48 FAULKNER ST	MANCHESTER	D566 L020
LE DRAY M	1846 SURDENT	PARK ST	BRISTOL	D941 L075
LE DRAY M D & CO	1841 DENT	70 SEEL ST	LIVERPOOL	D409 L016
LE DRAY MARIA & CO	1839 DENT	70 SEEL ST	LIVERPOOL	D408 L016
LE DRAY MONSIEUR	1846 SURDENT	27 PARK ST	BRISTOL	D879 L072
LE GRANTE GEORGE S H	1848 DENT	35 CHURCH ST	MANCHESTER	D332 L016
LEADBETTER E	1850 MECH DENT	22 ST NICHOLAS CHURCHYARD	NEWCASTLE	D214 L009
	1851 SURDENT	23 ST NICHOLAS CHURCHYARD	NEWCASTLE	D215 L009
	1853 DENT	15 ST NICHOLASS CHURCHYARD	NEWCASTLE	D243 L009
	1855 DENT	15 ST NICHOLAS CHURCHYARD	NEWCASTLE	D219 L009
LEADBETTER EDWARD	1847 SURDENT	DEAN CT	NEWCASTLE	D242 L009
	1848 DENT GOLDSM	3 DEAN CT LOW BRIDGE	NEWCASTLE*	D332 L016
	1852 DENT	ST NICHOLAS CHURCHYARD	NEWCASTLE	D216 L009
LEDRAY & LEDRAY	1838 SURDENT	35 BLACKETT ST	NEWCASTLE	D239 L009
LEDRAY (& LEDRAY)	1838 SURDENT	35 BLACKETT ST	NEWCASTLE	D239 L009
LEE	1852 SURDENT	WINDSOR RD	ST HELIER	DC61 L088
LEE J	1852 DENT	2 WINDSOR RD	ST HELIER	DB72 L025
LEGRANTE GEORGE S H	1848 DENT	35 CHURCH ST	MANCHESTER	D475 L020
	1850 DENT	257 ROCHDALE RD	MANCHESTER	D476 L020
LEIGH EDWARD PHILIP	1855 DENT MRCS	3 ADELPHI PL	IPSWICH	D668 L052
LEIGH S G	1851 DENT	99 PORTLAND CRESC	LEEDS	D283 L015
LEIGH SAMUEL GEORGE	1852 DENT	99 PORTLAND CRESC	LEEDS	D216 L009
	1853 SURDENT	96 PORTLAND CRESC	LEEDS	D261 L010
	1855 DENT	99 PORTLAND CRESC	LEEDS	D222 L009

LEVANDER J	1840 DENT	230 HIGH ST	EXETER	D143 L008
	1853 SURDENT	2 CRESCENT ROW	EXETER	D153 L008
	1854 SURDENT	2 CRESCENT ROW	EXETER	DB71 L025
LEVANDER JAMES	1830 DENT	23 SOUTHERNHAY PL	EXETER	D160 L008
	1830 DENT	23 SOUTHERNHAY	EXETER	D119 L008
	1831 DENT	23 SOUTHERNHAY PL	EXETER	D161 L008
	1832 DENT	20 SOUTHERNHAY PL	EXETER	D162 L008
	1833 DENT	20 SOUTHERNHAY PL	EXETER	D163 L008
	1834 DENT	20 SOUTHERNHAY PL	EXETER	D164 L008
	1836 DENT	20 SOUTHERNHAY PL	EXETER	D165 L008
	1837 DENT	20 SOUTHERNHAY PL	EXETER	D166 L008
	1838 DENT	BEDFORD LANE	EXETER	D167 L008
	1840 DENT	BICTON PL	EXMOUTH	D143 L020
	1840 DENT	230 HIGH ST	EXETER	D168 L008
	1841 SURDENT	230 HIGH ST	EXETER	D169 L008
	1842 SURDENT	2 SOUTHERNHAY ST	EXETER	D170 L008
	1843 SURDENT	2 SOUTHERNHAY PL	EXETER	D171 L008
	1844 SURDENT	2 SOUTHERNHAY PL	EXETER	D172 L008
	1844 DENT	2 SOUTHERNHAY PL	EXETER	D144 L008
	1845 SURDENT	2 SOUTHERNHAY ST	EXETER	D173 L008
	1846 SURDENT	2 SOUTHERNHAY ST	EXETER	D174 L008
	1847 SURDENT	2 SOUTHERNHAY ST	EXETER	D175 L008
	1848 SURDENT	2 SOUTHERNHAY	EXETER	D176 L008
	1848 DENT	2 CRESCENT ROW	EXETER	DA50 L011
	1849 SURDENT	2 SOUTHERNHAY PL	EXETER	D177 L008
	1850 DENT	2 CRESC ROW	EXETER	D147 L008
	1850 SURDENT	2 SOUTHERNHAY PL	EXETER	D178 L008
	1851 SURDENT	2 SOUTHERNHAY PL	EXETER	D179 L008
	1852 DENT	2 CRESCENT ROW	EXETER	D788 L020
	1852 DENT	2 CRESCENT ROW SOUTHERNHAY ST	EXETER	D145 L008
	1852 SURDENT	2 SOUTHERNHAY PL	EXETER	D180 L008
	1853 SURDENT	2 SOUTHERNHAY PL	EXETER	D181 L008
	1854 SURDENT	2 SOUTHERNHAY PL	EXETER	D182 L008
	1855 SURDENT	23 SOUTH PL	EXETER	D183 L008
LEVANDER JOHN	1848 DENT	TRIANGLE PL	TEIGNMOUTH	DA50 L011
LEVASON	1832 DENT	UNION PARADE	LEAMINGTON	D315 L014
LEVASON & ALEX & LEVASON	1839 SUR DENT	90 HIGH ST	CHELTENHAM ¢	D654 L068
	1841 SURDENT	98 HIGH ST	CHELTENHAM	D834 L069
LEVASON & DALE	1835 DENT	4 UNION PARADE	LEAMINGTON	D311 L014
	1837 DENT	4 LOWER PARADE	LEAMINGTON	D317 L014
LEVASON (& A)	1840 DENT	90 HIGH ST	CHELTENHAM	D143 L020
LEVASON (& ALEX & LEVASON)	1839 SUR DENT	90 HIGH ST	CHELTENHAM ¢	D654 L068
	1841 SURDENT	98 HIGH ST	CHELTENHAM	D834 L069
LEVASON (& ALEX)	1840 SURDENT	98 HIGH ST	CHELTENHAM	D833 L069
	1842 SURDENT	18 PROMENADE VILLAS	CHELTENHAM	D835 L069
	1842 DENT	18 PROMENADE VILLAS	CHELTENHAM	DB46 L049
	1842 DENT	21 RODNEY TCE	CHELTENHAM	DB46 L049
	1843 SURDENT	18 PROMENADE VILLAS	CHELTENHAM	D836 L069
	1844 SURDENT	18 PROMENADE VILLAS	CHELTENHAM	D837 L069
LEVASON (& DALE)	1838 SURDENT	4 UNION PARADE	LEAMINGTON	D314 L014
	1839 DENT	4 LOW UNION PDE	LEAMINGTON	D301 L002
	1839 DENT	4 LOWER PARADE	LEAMINGTON	D326 L014
	1840 SURDENT	4 LOWER PARADE	LEAMINGTON	D307 L014
	1841 SURDENT	4 LOWER PARADE	LEAMINGTON	D306 L014
LEVASON ALEX & LEVASON	1840 DENT	90 HIGH ST	CHELTENHAM	D143 L020
LEVASON GEORGE	1850 SURDENT	BOURBON ST	AYLESBURY	DA75 L011
	1851 DENT	BOURBON ST	AYLESBURY	DA42 L011

LEVASON JOSEPH	1839 DENT	26 GT GEORGE ST	LIVERPOOL	D408 L016
	1842 DENT	BYE ST	HEREFORD	D123 L020
	1843 SURDENT	21 RODNEY ST	CHELTENHAM	D955 L068
	1847 SURDENT	BRIDGE ST	. HEREFORD	D012 L001
	1850 DENT	BRIDGE ST	HEREFORD	D013 L020
	1852 SURDENT	11 BRIDGE ST	HEREFORD	DB28 L011
LEVASON L	1833 DENT	4 LOWER UNION PARADE	LEAMINGTON	D316 L014
LEVASON LEWIS	1828 DENT	22 WHITEFRIARS	CHESTER	D025 L020
	1833 SURDENT	4 UNION PARADE	LEAMINGTON	D312 L014
	1834 SURDENT	4 UNION PARADE	LEAMINGTON	D313 L014
	1835 DENT	4 LOWER UNION PARADE	LEAMINGTON	D007 L014
	1853 SURDENT	BOURBON ST	AYLESBURY	DA47 L011
	1853 SURDENT	CLAREMONT PL	LONDON	DA47 L011
LEVI J L	1845 DENT	14 DEVONSHIRE PL	BRIGHTON	DA66 L011
LEVISON J L	1828 DENT	21 MASON ST	HULL	D025 L020
	1851 DENT	14 DEVONSHIRE PL	BRIGHTON	DA77 L011
	1854 DENT	14 DEVONSHIRE PL	BRIGHTON	D605 L047
	1855 SURDENT DDS	14 DEVONSHIRE PL	BRIGHTON	D594 L046
LEVISON J.L	1842 DENT	9 COLMORE ROW	BIRMINGHAM	D075 L002
LEVISON JACOB L	1845 DENT	14 DEVONSHIRE PL	BRIGHTON	D606 L047
	1846 DENT	14 DEVONSHIRE PL	BRIGHTON	D601 L047
	1848 DENT	14 DEVONSHIRE PL	BRIGHTON	D602 L047
	1850 DENT	14 DEVONSHIRE PL	BRIGHTON	D603 L047
	1852 DENT	14 DEVONSHIRE PL	BRIGHTON	D604 L047
LEVISON JACOB.LESLIE	1841 DENT	9 COLMORE ROW	BIRMINGHAM	D058 L002
LEWIS	1816 SURDENT	PARIS ST	EXETER	D156 L008
LEWIS GEORGE WHITE	1855 DENT	HIGH ST	HUNTINGDON	DA45 L011
LEWIS J	1822 SURDENT	PARIS ST	EXETER	D157 L008
	1825 SURDENT	MARY'S YD	EXETER	D158 L008
LEWIS JAMES	1823 DENT	PARIS ST	EXETER	D142 L008
	1830 DENT	7 PORTLAND ST	CHELTENHAM	D119 L020
LIDDON GEORGE	1840 DENT	10 WELLINGTON ROW	TEIGNMOUTH	D143 L020
	1848 DENT	10 WELLINGTON ROW	TEIGNMOUTH	DA50 L011
LINDON ANN MARIA	1843 DENT	16 GT BRIDGEWATER ST	MANCHESTER	D473 L020
LINDON BRACEWELL	1836 DENT	59 FALKNER ST	MANCHESTER	D469 L020
	1837 DENT	59 FALKNER ST	MANCHESTER	D566 L020
	1838 DENT	59 FAULKNER ST	MANCHESTER	D470 L020
LINDON JOHN	1824 DENT	64 OLDHAM ST	MANCHESTER	D463 L020
	1828 DENT	26 FALKNER ST	MANCHESTER	D464 L020
LINDON WILLIAM	1828 SURDENT	36 FALKNER ST	MANCHESTER	D025 L020
	1829 SURDENT	36 FALKNER ST	MANCHESTER	D465 L020
	1830 SURDENT	36 FALKNER ST	MANCHESTER	D466 L020
	1832 SURDENT	59 FALKNER ST	MANCHESTER	D467 L020
	1833 SURDENT	59 FALKNER ST	MANCHESTER	D468 L020
	1834 DENT	59 FALKNER ST	MANCHESTER	D236 L009
LITTLE (& HAYMAN)	1850 SURDENT	CUMBERLAND ST	BRISTOL	D946 L075
	1850 DENT	4 CUMBERLAND ST	BRISTOL	D960 L075
	1851 SURDENT	CUMBERLAND ST	BRISTOL	D896 L075
	1852 SURDENT	CUMBERLAND ST	BRISTOL	D897 L075
	1853 DENT	4 CUMBERLAND ST	BRISTOL	D802 L020
	1853 SURDENT	CUMBERLAND ST	BRISTOL	D898 L075
	1853 DENT	4 CUMBERLAND ST	BRISTOL	D951 L075
	1854 SURDENT	CUMBERLAND ST	BRISTOL	D899 L075
	1855 SURDENT	CUMBERLAND ST	BRISTOL	D947 L075
LITTLE H	1830 SURDENT	ST AUBYN ST	DEVONPORT	D491 L022
LITTLE HENRY	1830 DENT	24 GEORGE ST	PLYMOUTH	D119 L008
	1830 SURDENT	GEORGE ST	PLYMOUTH	D491 L022

LITTLE HENRY	1836 DENT	UNION ST	PLYMOUTH	DA44 L011
	1840 DENT	3 GEORGE TCE	PLYMOUTH	D143 L00B
	1844 DENT	3 GEORGE TCE	PLYMOUTH	D492 L022
	1844 DENT	3 GEORGE'S TCE	PLYMOUTH	D144 L00B
	1847 DENT	3 GEORGE ST	PLYMOUTH	D152 L008
LITTLE W H	1840 SURDENT	29 BARRACK ST	DEVONPORT	D143 L020
LITTLEFIELD JAMES	1839 DENT	HIGH ST	RYDE I OF W	DB43 L078
LLOYD & SON	1843 DENT	96 BOLD ST	LIVERPOOL	D410 L016
	1843 DENT	96 BOLD ST	LIVERPOOL	D434 L019
	1845 DENT	96 BOLD ST	LIVERPOOL	D411 L016
	1846 DENT	96 BOLD ST	LIVERPOOL	D879 L072
	1847 DENT	96 BOLD ST	LIVERPOOL	D412 L016
	1848 DENT	96 BOLD ST	LIVERPOOL	D332 L016
LLOYD (& BLAIR)	1818 DENT	42 BOLD ST	LIVERPOOL	D432 L016
	1818 DENT	41 BOLD ST	LIVERPOOL	D302 L002
	1819 DENT	41 BOLD ST	LIVERPOOL	D735 L064
	1821 DENT	51 BOLD ST	LIVERPOOL	D399 L016
	1823 DENT	51 BOLD ST	LIVERPOOL	D400 L016
LLOYD (& FATH)	1843 DENT	96 BOLD ST	LIVERPOOL	D434 L019
	1843 DENT	96 BOLD ST	LIVERPOOL	D410 L016
	1845 DENT	96 BOLD ST	LIVERPOOL	D411 L016
	1846 DENT	96 BOLD ST	LIVERPOOL	D879 L072
	1847 DENT	96 BOLD ST	LIVERPOOL	D412 L016
	1848 DENT	96 BOLD ST	LIVERPOOL	D332 L016
LLOYD E	1848 DENT	GEORGE ST	RICHMOND	DB45 L011
	1851 DENT	26 ABOVE BAR	SOUTHAMPTON	D342 L017
	1852 DENT	6 SUSSEX PL SHIRLEY	SOUTHAMPTON	DB72 L025
	1852 DENT	26 ABOVE BAR	SOUTHAMPTON	DB72 L025
	1853 DENT	30 ABOVE BAR	SOUTHAMPTON	D343 L017
	1855 SURDENT	30 ABOVE BAR	SOUTHAMPTON	DA84 L011
	1855 DENT	50 UNION ST	RYDE I OF W	DA84 L011
	1855 DENT	GEORGE ST	RICHMOND	D594 L046
LLOYD E (SAVORY & MOORE)	1851 CHEM DENT	POST OFFICE	RICHMOND +	DA83 L011
LLOYD EDWARD	1852 DENT	26 ABOVE BAR	SOUTHAMPTON	D788 L020
	1852 DENT	26 ABOVE BAR	SOUTHAMPTON	D346 L017
LLOYD EDWIN	1855 DENT	31 ABOVE BAR	SOUTHAMPTON	D344 L017
LLOYD G F	1855 DENT	12 GRANBY ST	LEICESTER	D511 L023
LLOYD GEORGE FIELDHOUSE	1854 DENT	GRANBY ST	LEICESTER	D660 L024
LLOYD RICHARD	1841 DENT	96 BOLD ST	LIVERPOOL	D409 L016
	1849 DENT	96 BOLD ST	LIVERPOOL	D413 L016
	1851 DENT	96 BOLD ST	LIVERPOOL	D414 L016
	1851 DENT	96 BOLD ST	LIVERPOOL	D438 L020
	1852 DENT	96 BOLD ST	LIVERPOOL	D216 L009
	1853 DENT	96 BOLD ST	LIVERPOOL	D415 L016
	1855 DENT	96 BOLD ST	LIVERPOOL	D416 L016
LLOYD THOMAS	1828 DENT	59 BOLD ST	LIVERPOOL	D025 L020
	1835 DENT	67 BOLD ST	LIVERPOOL	D406 L016
LLOYD THOMAS BRIDGE	1834 DENT	45 PRINCESS ST	MANCHESTER	D236 L009
	1836 DENT	40 MOSLEY ST	MANCHESTER	D469 L020
	1837 DENT	40 MOSLEY ST	MANCHESTER	D566 L020
	1838 DENT	40 MOSELY ST	MANCHESTER	D470 L020
	1840 DENT	40 MOSLEY ST	MANCHESTER	D471 L020
	1841 DENT	40 MOSLEY ST	MANCHESTER	D331 L016
	1841 DENT	40 MOSELY ST	MANCHESTER	D472 L020
	1843 DENT	40 MOSLEY ST	MANCHESTER	D473 L020
	1845 DENT	40 MOSLEY ST	MANCHESTER	D474 L020
	1846 DENT	40 MOSLEY ST	MANCHESTER	D879 L072

LLOYD THOMAS W	1824 DENT	59 BOLD ST	LIVERPOOL	D401 L016
	1827 DENT	59 BOLD ST	LIVERPOOL	D402 L016
	1829 DENT	59 BOLD ST	LIVERPOOL	D404 L016
	1832 DENT	67 BOLD ST	LIVERPOOL	D445 L016
	1834 DENT	70 BOLD ST	LIVERPOOL	D405 L016
LLOYD THOMAS WHITFIELD	1825 DENT	59 BOLD ST	LIVERPOOL	D444 L016
	1834 DENT	67 BOLD ST	LIVERPOOL	D236 L009
	1837 DENT	67 BOLD ST	LIVERPOOL	D566 L020
	1837 DENT	73 BOLD ST	LIVERPOOL	D407 L016
	1839 DENT	96 BOLD ST	LIVERPOOL	D408 L016
LOGAN D	1848 DENT	TRINITY TCE	CHELTENHAM	D954 L069
	1849 DENT	3 ORIEL VILLAS	CHELTENHAM	DB81 L082
LOGAN DAVID	1847 DENT	2 TRINITY TCE	CHELTENHAM	D890 L068
	1851 DENT	3 ORIEL VILLAS	CHELTENHAM	D953 L069
	1852 DENT	3 ORIEL VILLAS	CHELTENHAM	D952 L069
	1853 SURDENT	3 ORIEL VILLAS	CHELTENHAM	D956 L068
LOGAN DR	1846 SURDENT	21 RODNEY TCE	CHELTENHAM	D839 L069
	1847 SURDENT	21 RODNEY TCE	CHELTENHAM	D840 L069
	1848 SURDENT	3 ORIEL VILLAS	CHELTENHAM	D841 L069
	1849 SURDENT	3 ORIEL VILLAS	CHELTENHAM	D842 L069
LOMAX JAMES	1846 DENT	3 OXFORD ST	MANCHESTER	D879 L072
	1848 DENT	3 OXFORD ST	MANCHESTER	D475 L020
	1848 DENT	YORKSHIRE ST	ROCHDALE	D332 L016
	1848 DENT	3 OXFORD ST	MANCHESTER	D332 L016
LOMAX JAMES WOOD	1850 DENT	79 MOSLEY ST	MANCHESTER	D476 L020
	1851 DENT	79 MOSELY ST	MANCHESTER	D567 L020
	1852 DENT	79 MOSLEY ST	MANCHESTER	D216 L009
	1852 DENT	79 MOSLEY ST	MANCHESTER	D477 L020
	1855 DENT	79 MOSLEY ST	MANCHESTER	D478 L020
LOUDE L C	1839 DENT	CHURCH ST	WOLVERHAMPTON	D301 L002
	1839 DENT	CHURCH ST	WOLVERHAMPTON	D697 L058
LOWE E	1848 DENT	6 PIER ST	RYDE I OF W	D357 L017
LOWE EDWIN	1839 DENT	PIER ST	RYDE I OF W	DB43 L078
	1844 DENT	6 PIER ST	RYDE I OF W	D144 L068
LOWS ANDREW	1847 DENT	55 CASTLE ST	CARLISLE	D443 L019
	1848 DENT	55 CASTLE ST	CARLISLE	D332 L016
	1852 DENT	55 CASTLE ST	CARLISLE	D216 L009
	1855 DENT	MIDDLEGATE	PENRITH	D222 L020
	1855 DENT	4 DEVONSHIRE ST	CARLISLE	D222 L020
LUKYN	1845 SURDENT	18 LOWER PARADE	LEAMINGTON	D309 L014
	1848 SURDENT	24 LOWER PARADE	LEAMINGTON	D308 L014
	1849 SURDENT	24 LOWER PARADE	LEAMINGTON	D310 L014
LUKYN & SPURR	1850 DENT	7 BROAD ST	NOTTINGHAM	D013 L020
LUKYN C	1845 DENT	HERTFORD ST	COVENTRY	D077 L006
LUKYN CHRISTOPHER	1850 DENT	HERTFORD ST	COVENTRY	D013 L002
	1850 SURDENT	HERTFORD ST	COVENTRY	D063 L002
	1850 SURDENT	HERTFORD ST	COVENTRY	D714 L002
LUKYN EDWARD	1850 SURDENT	114 WARWICK ST	LEAMINGTON	D063 L002
LUKYN J	1848 DENT	BROAD ST	NOTTINGHAM	D800 L020
LUKYN JOHN	1844 DENT	BROAD ST	NOTTINGHAM	D509 L023
	1847 DENT	7 BROAD ST	NOTTINGHAM	D505 L023
	1848 DENT	BROAD ST	NOTTINGHAM	D506 L023
LUKYN W	1845 DENT		LEAMINGTON	D077 L006
	1846 DENT	24 LOWER PARADE	LEAMINGTON	D303 L014
	1855 DENT	36 BROAD ST	NOTTINGHAM	D511 L023
LUKYN WILLIAM	1830 DENT	LONDON PL	OXFORD	D119 L007
	1850 DENT	24 LOWER PARADE	LEAMINGTON	D013 L002

LUKYN WILLIAM	1853 SURDENT	36 BROAD ST	NOTTINGHAM	D507 L023
	1854 DENT	26 BROAD ST	NOTTINGHAM	D510 L023
LYON H	1853 DENT	22 PETTY CURY	CAMBRIDGE	D655 L051
LYON HENRY	1850 DENT	22 PETTY CURY	CAMBRIDGE	DA91 L011
	1855 SURDENT	HOBSON ST	CAMBRIDGE	DA45 L011
LYON LEMUEL	1855 DENT	MUSEUM ST	IPSWICH	D668 L052
LYON WILLIAM	1855 SURDENT	BRIDGE ST	CAMBRIDGE	DA45 L011
LYONS LEO	1798 DENT	THUNDERBOLT ST	BRISTOL	D900 L075
LYONS MAURICE	1850 DENT	143 SUFFOLK ST	BHAM	D013 L002
LYONS MORRIS	1845 DENT	20 ANN STREET	BIRMINGHAM	D077 L002
	1849 SURDENT	143 SUFFOLK STREET	BIRMINGHAM	D062 L002
	1850 SURDENT	143 SUFFOLK STREET	BIRMINGHAM	D063 L002
	1852 DENT	143 SUFFOLK STREET	BIRMINGHAM	D078 L002
	1854 DENT	143 SUFFOLK STREET	BIRMINGHAM	D069 L002
LYONS MORRIS (MAURICE)	1855 SURDENT	143 SUFFOLK STREET	BIRMINGHAM	D064 L002
LYONS MOSES	1839 DENT	HOWARD ST	YARMOUTH	D654 L068
MACGREGOR RICHARD	1839 DENT	PORTLAND ST	SOUTHAMPTON	D337 L017
MACKENZIE	1839 DENT	CAMPBELL HOUSE BELMONT RD	ST HELIER	DB43 L078
	1843 DENT	2 DAVID PL	ST HELIER	DC58 L088
MACKLESTON FREDERICK	1790 DENT	COVENTRY ST	LONDON	D274 L011
MACKLIN THOMAS	1852 DENT	ST MARY ST	WEYMOUTH	D788 L020
MACLEAN	1840 DENT	ESPLANADE	WEYMOUTH	D143 L020
MACLEAN ALEXANDER	1842 DENT	5 FREDERICK PL	WEYMOUTH	DB46 L049
MADDEN J W	1853 SURDENT	2 QUEEN ST	EXETER	D153 L008
	1854 SURDENT	3 CASTLE ST	EXETER	DB71 L025
MADDEN W J	1852 SURDENT	QUEEN ST	EXETER	D180 L008
	1853 SURDENT	QUEEN ST	EXETER	D181 L008
	1854 SURDENT	3 CASTLE ST	EXETER	D182 L008
	1855 SURDENT	4 HIGH ST	EXETER	D183 L008
MADDEN WILLIAM JOHN	1852 DENT	QUEEN ST	EXETER	D145 L008
	1852 DENT	QUEEN ST	EXETER	D788 L020
MAGENCE CHARLES	1842 DENT	65 ST MARY ST	WEYMOUTH	DB46 L049
MAGENEE C	1840 DENT	65 ST MARY ST	WEYMOUTH	D143 L020
MAGOR	1847 SURDENT	LEMON ST	TRURO	DC64 L067
MAGOR MARTIN	1847 SURDENT	CHAPEL ST	PENZANCE	DC64 L067
	1852 SURDENT	CHAPEL ST	PENZANCE	D788 L020
MAISH E B	1854 SURDENT	ST MICHAEL'S CRESC	BRISTOL	D899 L075
	1855 SURDENT	ST MICHAEL'S CRESC	BRISTOL	D947 L075
MALLAN & CO	1842 DENT	30 PARK ST	BRISTOL	DB46 L049
MALLAN (& FATH M & BRO 1)	1834 DENT	BOLD ST	LIVERPOOL	D405 L016
MALLAN (& FATH M & BRO 2)	1834 DENT	BOLD ST	LIVERPOOL	D405 L016
MALLAN JAMES & M & S	1841 DENT	29 BOLD ST	LIVERPOOL	D409 L016
MALLAN M S	1834 DENT	46 BOLD ST	LIVERPOOL	D236 L009
	1837 DENT	46 BOLD ST	LIVERPOOL	D566 L020
MALLAN MESSRS	1840 SURDENT	30 PARK ST	BRISTOL	D945 L075
	1841 SURDENT	30 PARK ST	BRISTOL	D937 L075
	1842 SURDENT	30 PARK ST	BRISTOL	D938 L075
	1843 SURDENT	30 PARK ST	BRISTOL	D939 L075
MALLAN MICHAEL & SONS	1834 DENT	BOLD ST	LIVERPOOL	D405 L016
MALLAN MICHAEL (& J & S)	1841 DENT	29 BOLD ST	LIVERPOOL	D409 L016
MALLAN SIMON (& J & M)	1841 DENT	29 BOLD ST	LIVERPOOL	D409 L016
MALLAN T	1850 DENT	6 GAOL GATE ST	STAFFORD	D099 L006
MALLAN T H	1854 DENT	LIVERPOOL RD	STOKE ON TRENT	D015 L001
MALLORY T T	1823 DENT	21 BUTCHER ST	PORTSEA	D142 L017
	1839 DENT	21 BUTCHER ST	PORTSEA	DB43 L078
	1852 DENT	BUTCHER ST	PORTSEA	D346 L017
MANN G A	1821 DENT	NORFOLK ST	SHEFFIELD	D748 L066

MANN G A	1822 DENT	NORFOLK ST	SHEFFIELD	D005 L020
MANN GEORGE	1799 DENT	CHAPEL BAR	NOTTINGHAM	D499 L023
	1822 DENT	MOUNT ST	NOTTINGHAM	D005 L020
	1828 DENT	HORTON LANE	NEWARK	D025 L020
MANNE ELIZABETH	1851 DENT	8 ETHERINGTON PL	HULL	D379 L018
	1851 SURDENT	8 ETHERINGTON PL	HULL	D259 L010
MANNE G A	1824 SURDENT	11 ST JAMES'S BARTON	BRISTOL	D923 L075
	1825 SURDENT	11 ST JAMES'S BARTON	BRISTOL	D924 L075
	1826 SURDENT	11 ST JAMES'S BARTON	BRISTOL	D925 L075
	1827 SURDENT	11 ST JAMES'S BARTON	BRISTOL	D926 L075
	1835 SURDENT		BEVERLEY (SAT)	D365 L018
	1835 SURDENT	11 SAVILE ST	HULL	D365 L018
	1838 DENT	22 WHITEFRIARGATE	HULL	D375 L018
	1839 DENT	22 WHITEFRIARGATE	HULL	D376 L018
	1841 DENT	22 WHITEFRIARGATE	HULL	D241 L009
	1842 DENT	22 WHITEFRIARGATE	HULL	D377 L018
	1848 DENT	8 ETHERINGTON PL	HULL	D378 L018
MANNE GEORGE	1798 DENT		NOTTINGHAM	D279 L011
	1831 DENT	HAWTON LANE	NEWARK	D501 L057
MANNE GEORGE A	1837 SURDENT	22 WHITEFRIARGATE	HULL	D257 L010
	1840 SURDENT	22 WHITEFRIARGATE	HULL	D888 L006
MANNE GEORGE ALRED	1828 DENT	WHEELER GATE	NOTTINGHAM	D025 L020
	1831 DENT	WHEELER GATE	NOTTINGHAM	D501 L024
MANNE GEORGE ARTHUR	1834 DENT	11 SAVILE ST	HULL	D236 L009
	1837 DENT	11 SAVILE ST	HULL	D566 L020
	1841 DENT	22 WHITEFRIARGATE	HULL	D331 L016
	1846 SURDENT	22 WHITEFRIARGATE	HULL	D258 L010
	1848 DENT	8 ETHERINGTON PL	HULL	D332 L016
	1849 DENT		HULL	D333 L016
	1849 DENT	MISS WAITE'S EASTGATE	LOUTH (WED)	D333 L016
	1850 DENT		HULL	D013 L020
	1850 DENT	MISS WAITE'S EASTGATE	LOUTH (WED)	D013 L020
MARDEN J W	1855 DENT	BROAD ST	LYME REGIS	DA84 L011
MARGETSON WILLIAM	1853 DENT	BOND ST	WAKEFIELD	D261 L010
MARKHAM H	1853 DENT	3 INGHAM PL	S SHIELDS	D243 L009
MARKHAM HENRY	1848 DENT	44 CARLIOL ST	NEWCASTLE	D332 L016
	1851 SURDENT	3 INGRAM ST	S SHIELDS	D292 L013
MARKHAM J	1855 DENT	MARKET PL	REIGATE	D594 L046
MARKLAND E	1846 SURDENT	MARKET PL	YARMOUTH	DA85 L011
MARKLAND EDWIN	1850 DENT	MARKET PL	YARMOUTH	DA91 L011
	1853 DENT	MARKET PL	YARMOUTH	D655 L051
MARKS ROBERT	1855 DENT	8 ETHERINGTON PL	HULL	D222 L009
MARLEY J	1855 DENT	21 GRAINGER ST	NEWCASTLE	D223 L009
MARSH ROBERT.J	1852 DENT CHEM	42 CHEAPSIDE	BIRMINGHAM *	D078 L002
MARSHALL JOHN	1840 DENT	FORE ST	TAUNTON	D676 L055
	1840 DENT	FORE ST	TAUNTON	D143 L020
MARTIN (& WALLER)	1845 DENT	68 HIGH ST	GUILDFORD	DA66 L011
MARTIN J	1848 DENT	148 HIGH ST	PORTSMOUTH	D357 L017
	1852 DENT	HIGH ST	PORTSMOUTH	DB72 L025
MARTIN JOHN	1839 DENT	148 HIGH ST	PORTSMOUTH	DB43 L078
	1844 DENT	148 HIGH ST	PORTSMOUTH	D144 L068
	1852 DENT	133 HIGH ST	PORTSMOUTH	D346 L017
	1852 DENT	132 HIGH ST	PORTSMOUTH	D788 L020
	1855 SURDENT	HIGH ST	PORTSMOUTH	DA84 L011
MARTIN STABLES	1852 DENT	17 ST THOMAS ST	PORTSMOUTH	D346 L017
MASEY WILLIAM	1811 DENT	REDCLIFF HILL	BRISTOL	D284 L011
MASON JAMES	1855 DENT	29 BOARDMAN ST	MANCHESTER	D478 L020

MASON W	1853 DENT	EASTHILL	YARMOUTH	D655 L051
MASON WILLIAM	1850 DENT	EAST HILL	YARMOUTH	DA91 L011
	1852 DENT	1 CATHEDRAL YD	EXETER	D788 L020
	1852 DENT	1 CATHEDRAL YD	EXETER	D145 L008
	1853 SURDENT	CATHEDRAL YD	EXETER	D181 L008
	1853 SURDENT	1 DEANERY PL	EXETER	D153 L008
	1854 SURDENT	CATHEDRAL YD	EXETER	D182 L008
	1854 SURDENT	CATHEDRAL YD	EXETER	DB71 L025
	1855 SURDENT	7 QUEEN ST	EXETER	D183 L008
MASSEY J	1850 DENT	ALBION ST	SHELTON	D099 L006
MASSEY JOHN	1835 DENT	HIGH ST	HANLEY	D007 L001
	1841 SURDENT	HIGH ST	HANLEY	D028 L002
	1846 SURDENT	ALBION ST	SHELTON	D713 L061
	1850 DENT	ALBION ST	SHELTON	D013 L001
	1851 SURDENT	ALBION ST	HANLEY	D104 L006
MASSEY WILLIAM	1855 DENT	HEMER TCE LINACRE MARSH	LIVERPOOL	D416 L016
MATTHEWS ALFRED	1847 DENT	NORTH PDE	BRADFORD	D276 L015
	1853 SURDENT	8 NORTH PDE	BRADFORD	D261 L010
MATTHEWS ALFRED M	1848 DENT	NORTH PDE	BRADFORD	D332 L016
	1850 DENT	6 NORTH PDE	BRADFORD	DB35 L078
	1855 DENT	NORTH PDE	BRADFORD	D222 L009
MATTHEWS DAVID	1839 DENT	SUN ST	CANTERBURY	D584 L011
MAUDUIT A	1852 DENT	48 DON ST	ST HELIER	DB72 L025
	1853 SURDENT	DON ST	ST HELIER	DB75 L080
	1854 SURDENT	BROAD ST	ST HELIER	DC62 L088
	1855 SURDENT	BROAD ST	ST HELIER	DC63 L088
MAURE ELIZABETH .	1852 DENT	8 ETHERINGTON PL	HULL	D216 L009
MAVIUS	1852 SURDENT	ST MARK'S TCE	ST HELIER	DC61 L088
	1853 SURDENT	ST MARK'S TCE	ST HELIER	DB75 L080
	1854 SURDENT	ST MARK'S TCE	ST HELIER	DC62 L088
	1855 SURDENT	ST MARK'S TCE	ST HELIER	DC63 L088
MCADAM GEORGE	1840 DENT	KING ST	HEREFORD	D143 L020
	1842 DENT	ST OWEN ST	HEREFORD	D123 L020
	1847 SURDENT	KING ST	HEREFORD	D012 L001
	1852 SURDENT	KING ST	HEREFORD	DB28 L011
MCADAM GEORGE C	1850 DENT	KING ST	HEREFORD	D013 L020
MCGREGOR R H G	1850 DENT	LONDON RD & 63 BROAD ST	WORCESTER	D099 L011
MCGREGOR R.H.G	1847 DENT	50 FOREGATE STREET	WORCESTER	D012 L001
	1851 SURDENT	CATHERINE HILL HSE LOUDON RD	WORC	D014 L001
	1851 SURDENT	63 BROAD STREET	WORCESTER	D014 L001
	1855 SURDENT	63 BROAD STREET	WORCESTER	D016 L001
MCGREGOR RICHARD.H.G	1850 DENT	50 FOREGATE STREET	WORCESTER	D013 L001
	1853 DENT	63 BROAD STREET	WORCESTER	D031 L004
	1854 DENT	63 BROAD STREET	WORCESTER	D015 L001
MCKENZIE	1845 DENT	2 DAVID PL	ST HELIER	DA82 L011
	1847 SURDENT	NORFOLK VILLA ROUGE BOUILLON	ST HELIER	DB53 L025
	1848.SURDENT	NORFOLK VILLA ROUGE BOUILLON	ST HELIER	DC59 L088
MCKENZIE D	1849 SURDENT	NORFOLK VILLA ROUGE BOUILLON	ST HELIER	DC60 L088
MCKIERNAN THOMAS	1832 DENT	37 SIR THOMAS BDGS	LIVERPOOL	D445 L016
MCKIERNAN THOMAS EDWARD	1834 DENT	5 OLD HALL ST	LIVERPOOL	D236 L009
	1834 DENT	39 ST THOMAS BDGS	LIVERPOOL	D236 L009
	1837 DENT	39 SIR THOMAS' BDGS	LIVERPOOL	D566 L020
	1837 DENT	5 OLDHALL ST	LIVERPOOL	D566 L020
MCOWEN W H	1844 SURDENT	10 PITTVILLE ST	CHELTENHAM	D837 L069
	1848 DENT	84 WINCHCOMB ST	CHELTENHAM	D954 L069
	1849 DENT	2 GROSVENOR ST	CHELTENHAM	DB81 L082
	1850 SURDENT	2 GROSVENOR ST	CHELTENHAM	D843 L069

MCOWEN W H	1850 DENT	2 GROSVENOR ST	CHELTENHAM	DA74 L011
	1851 DENT	2 GROSVENOR ST	CHELTENHAM	D953 L069
	1852 DENT	2 GROSVENOR ST	CHELTENHAM	D952 L069
MCOWEN WILLIAM	1843 DENT	27 HENRIETTA ST	CHELTENHAM	D955 L068
MCOWEN WILLIAM HENRY	1842 DENT	27 HENRIETTA ST	CHELTENHAM	DB46 L049
	1847 DENT	6 PITTVILLE ST	CHELTENHAM	D890 L068
	1852 DENT	2 GROSVENOR ST	CHELTENHAM	D788 L020
	1853 SURDENT	2 GROSVENOR ST	CHELTENHAM	D956 L068
MCPHERSON JOHN	1828 DENT	WOODEN BRIDGE	NORTH SHIELDS	D025 L020
MEACHAM J	1854 DENT	PARK LANE ROUND HILL	BIRMINGHAM	D069 L002
MEACHAM JAMES	1839 DENT	QUEEN ST	WOLVERHAMPTON	D301 L002
	1839 DENT	QUEEN ST	WOLVERHAMPTON	D697 L058
	1839 DENT	113 SNOW HILL	BIRMINGHAM	D083 L002
	1839 DENT	113 SNOWHILL	BHAM	D301 L002
	1841 DENT	113 SNOW HILL	BIRMINGHAM	D058 L002
	1842 DENT	113 SNOW HILL	BIRMINGHAM	D075 L002
	1845 DENT	119 SNOW HILL	BIRMINGHAM	D077 L002
	1846 DENT	119 SNOW HILL	BIRMINGHAM	D879 L072
	1847 DENT	119 SNOW HILL	BIRMINGHAM	D061 L002
	1849 SURDENT	119 SNOW HILL	BIRMINGHAM	D062 L002
	1850 SURDENT	119 SNOW HILL	BIRMINGHAM	D063 L002
	1850 DENT	119 SNOWHILL	BHAM	D013 L002
	1852 DENT	20 NEW STREET	BIRMINGHAM	D078 L002
	1855 SURDENT	20 NEW STREET	BIRMINGHAM	D064 L002
	1855 SURDENT	HOME LEE COTTAGE ASTON	BIRMINGHAM	D064 L002
MEADOWS J	1855 DENT	HOTEL ST	LEICESTER	D511 L023
	1855 DENT	38 HIGH ST	ROCHESTER	D594 L046
MEDD JOSEPH	1853 DENT	56 WESTGATE ST	GLOUCESTER	D951 L075
MEDWIN A	1851 DENT	4 BLACKHEATH RD	GREENWICH	DA77 L011
MEDWIN AARON	1845 DENT	3 BLACKHEATH RD	LONDON	DA66 L011
	1849 DENT CHEM DRUGGIST	4 BLACKHEATH RD	GREENWICH *	D587 L011
MEEARS J W	1855 DENT	115 & 90 HIGH ST	CROYDON	D594 L046
MELLOR EBENEZER	1848 DENT	96 BROAD LANE	SHEFFIELD	D332 L016
	1852 DENT	96 BROAD LANE	SHEFFIELD	D216 L009
	1854 DENT	96 BROAD LANE	SHEFFIELD	D757 L066
	1855 DENT	96 BROAD ST	SHEFFIELD	D222 L009
MENS T	1855 DENT	EAST HILL	COLCHESTER	D594 L046
MENS THOMAS GILES	1848 SURDENT	121 HIGH ST	COLCHESTER	DA53 L011
MEREDITH JOSEPH	1833 SURDENT	17 COLMORE ROW	BIRMINGHAM	D079 L002
	1835 DENT	17 COLMORE ROW	BIRMINGHAM	D057 L002
	1852 DENT	HOME LEE CRESCENT	BIRMINGHAM	D078 L002
	1852 DENT	17 COLMORE ROW	BIRMINGHAM	D078 L002
	1854 DENT	17 COLMORE ROW	BIRMINGHAM	D069 L002
	1855 SURDENT	HOME 47 LEE CRESCENT	BIRMINGHAM	D064 L002
	1855 SURDENT	17 COLMORE ROW	BIRMINGHAM	D064 L002
MERRICK T	1848 DENT	10 GEORGE ST	HULL	D378 L018
MERRICK THOMAS	1846 SURDENT	14 NORTH CHURCH ST	HULL	D258 L010
	1848 DENT	10 GEORGE ST	HULL	D332 L016
	1851 SURDENT	10 GEORGE ST	HULL	D259 L010
	1851 DENT	10	HULL	D379 L018
	1852 DENT	10 GEORGE ST	HULL	D216 L009
	1855 DENT	10 GEORGE ST	HULL	D222 L009
MERRYWEATHER J	1844 DENT	10 BLACKETT ST	NEWCASTLE	D213 L009
MESSENGER WILLIAM	1839 DENT	30 STEELHOUSE LANE	BIRMINGHAM	D083 L002
MICHEL	1812 DENT	YORK ST	BATH	D114 L007
	1826 SURDENT	16 YORK ST	BATH	D117 L007
	1829 SURDENT	16 YORK ST	BATH	D118 L007

MICHEL P	1819	SURDENT	16 YORK ST	BATH	D115 L007
	1824	SURDENT	16 YORK ST	BATH	D116 L007
	1846	SURDENT	1 ALFRED ST	BATH	D124 L007
MICHEL P (MONSIEUR)	1833	SURDENT	10 BLADUDS BUILDINGS	BATH	D120 L007
MICHEL PETER	1840	DENT	1 ALFRED ST	BATH	D143 L020
	1841	SURDENT	1 ALFRED ST	BATH	D122 L007
	1848	SURDENT	6 CHAPEL ROW QUEENS SQ	BATH	D125 L007
	1849	SURDENT	6 CHAPEL ROW	BATH	D126 L007
	1852	SURDENT	6 CHAPEL ROW	BATH	D788 L020
MICHEL PIERRE	1830	SURDENT	16 YORK ST	BATH	D119 L007
	1837	SURDENT	10 BLADUD BDGS	BATH	D121 L007
	1850	SURDENT	6 CHAPEL ROW	BATH	D127 L007
MICHELL PETER	1822	SURDENT	16 YORK ST	BATH	D005 L020
MIDDLETON CHARLES	1828	DENT	1 TEMPLAR ST	LEEDS	D025 L020
	1851	DENT	98 WAVERLEY ST	HULL	D379 L018
MIDDLETON T PATCHETT	1851	DENT	71 PICCADILLY	MANCHESTER	D567 L020
	1852	DENT	71 PICCADILLY	MANCHESTER	D477 L020
MIDDLETON THOMAS	1852	DENT	22 ST ANN'S SQ	MANCHESTER	D216 L009
MIDDLETON THOMAS P	1851	DENT	OPENSHAW	DENTON	D438 L020
MIDDLETON THOMAS PATCHETT	1845	DENT	71 PICCADILLY	MANCHESTER	D474 L020
	1846	DENT	71 PICCADILLY	MANCHESTER	D879 L072
	1848	DENT	71 PICCADILLY	MANCHESTER	D475 L020
	1848	DENT	71 PICCADILLY	MANCHESTER	D332 L016
	1850	DENT	71 PICCADILLY	MANCHESTER	D476 L020
MILL	1849	SURDENT	27 HARMER ST	GRAVESEND	DC16 L084
MILL T	1851	DENT	UPPER BRIXTON PL BRIXTON	LONDON	DA77 L011
MILLER CHARLES	1811	TOOTHDRAWER BARBER		ROMSEY *	D284 L011
MILLIDGE W H	1855	DENT	50 HIGH ST	NEWPORT I OF W	DA84 L011
MILLIDGE WILLIAM HENRY	1852	DENT	50 HIGH ST	NEWPORT I OF W	D346 L017
MILLS J	1850	SURDENT	27 HARMER ST	GRAVESEND	DA75 L011
MILNER JAMES	1855	DENT	10 ST JAMES ST	HULL	D222 L009
MITCHELL J W	1852	DENT	8 PAVILION PDE	BRIGHTON	D604 L047
	1854	DENT	8 PAVILION PDE	BRIGHTON	D605 L047
	1855	SURDENT	20 WIGMORE ST	LONDON	D594 L046
	1855	SURDENT	8 PAVILION PDE	BRIGHTON	D594 L046
MITCHELL JOHN	1853	DENT	115 KIRKGATE	WAKEFIELD	D261 L010
MITCHELL PETER	1852	DENT	14 CAMDEN COTTAGES GAYS HILL	BATH	D128 L007
MOLINEUX HENRY	1839	DENT	60 SHIP ST	BRIGHTON	D584 L011
	1839	DENT CUPPER	3 MARKET ST	BRIGHTON *	D607 L047
	1843	SURDENT	3 MARKET ST	BRIGHTON	D600 L047
	1845	DENT	3 MARKET ST	BRIGHTON	DA66 L011
	1846	DENT	MARKET ST	BRIGHTON	D601 L047
	1848	DENT	3 MARKET ST	BRIGHTON	D602 L047
	1850	DENT	12 GRENVILLE PL	BRIGHTON	D603 L047
MONTAGUE ALEXANDER	1841	DENT	14 BRIDGE STREET	WORCESTER	D028 L002
MOORE EDWARD	1839	DENT	11 HATTON GDNS	LIVERPOOL	D408 L016
	1841	DENT	11 HATTON GDNS	LIVERPOOL	D409 L016
	1843	DENT	11 HATTON GDNS	LIVERPOOL	D410 L016
	1843	DENT	11 HATTON GDNS	LIVERPOOL	D434 L019
	1852	DENT	DUNSTANVILLE TCE	FALMOUTH	D788 L020
	1852	DENT	RIVER ST	TRURO	D788 L020
MOORE H	1847	DENT	PILGRIM PL	WINDSOR	D815 L011
	1853	DENT	19 THAMES ST	WINDSOR	D627 L049
MOORE HENRY	1832	DENT	HIGH ST	UXBRIDGE	D819 L002
	1842	DENT	4 PILGRIM PL	WINDSOR	DB46 L049
	1844	DENT	4 PILGRIM PL	WINDSOR	D626 L049
	1846	DENT	4 PILGRIM PL PEASCOD ST	WINDSOR	DB79 L082

MOORE HENRY	1847 DENT	4 PILGRIM PL	WINDSOR	DB84 L049
	1851 DENT	4 PILGRIM PL PEASCOD ST	WINDSOR	DA83 L011
	1852 DENT	4 PILGRIM PL	WINDSOR	D788 L020
	1853 SURDENT	18 THAMES ST	WINDSOR	DA47 L011
	1854 DENT	18 THAMES ST	WINDSOR	D628 L049
MOORE WILLIAM VANDERKEMP	1852 DENT	BRUNSWICK PL	TEIGNMOUTH	D788 L020
MORES (& BIRD)	1829 SURDENT	113 GREENGATE	SALFORD	D465 L020
MORGAN (& DALE)	1854 DENT	107 WARWICK ST	LEAMINGTON	D015 L001
MORGAN WILLIAM	1850 DENT	MONNOW ST	MONMOUTH	D013 L020
	1852 DENT	MONNOW ST	MONMOUTH	DA76 L011
MORLEY H	1855 DENT	6 LONDON ST	DERBY	D511 L023
MORLEY HENRY	1850 DENT	36 ST HELEN'S ST	DERBY	D013 L020
	1852 DENT	36 ST HELEN'S ST	DERBY	D690 L057
	1854 SURDENT	LONDON ST	DERBY	D660 L057
MORTIMER HENRY THOMAS	1841 DENT	NEW LENTON	NOTTINGHAM	D331 L016
	1046 DENT	REDCROSS GT	LEICESTER	D658 L024
MORTON LEWIS	1833 DENT	39 BLACKETT ST	NEWCASTLE	D246 L009
	1834 DENT	39 BLACKETT ST	NEWCASTLE	D236 L009
MOSELEY	1851 SURDENT	13 NORTHERNHAY PL	EXETER	D179 L008
MOSELEY & DRAKE	1855 SURDENT	HIGH ST	WOLVERHAMPTON	D098 L006
MOSELEY A	1847 SURDENT	30 PARK ST	BRISTOL	D942 L075
	1850 SURDENT	33 PARK ST	BRISTOL	D946 L075
	1851 SURDENT	33 PARK ST	BRISTOL	D896 L075
	1852 SURDENT	33 PARK ST	BRISTOL	D897 L075
	1853 SURDENT	33 PARK ST	BRISTOL	D898 L075
	1854 SURDENT	33 PARK ST	BRISTOL	D899 L075
	1855 SURDENT	33 PARK ST	BRISTOL	D947 L075
	1855 DENT	MARKET PL	DEVIZES	DA84 L011
MOSELEY ABRAHAM	1846 SURDENT	30 PARK ST	BRISTOL	D879 L072
	1852 DENT	33 PARK ST	BRISTOL	D788 L020
MOSELEY B	1850 SURDENT	29 LOWER PARADE	LEAMINGTON	D063 L002
MOSELEY BEDFORD	1850 SURDENT	29 LOWER PARADE	LEAMINGTON	D013 L002
MOSELEY C	1849 DENT	FISH MARKET	KENDAL (ALT WKS)	D441 L019
	1851 DENT	FISH MARKET	KENDAL (ALT WKS)	D437 L019
MOSELEY CHARLES	1848 DENT	4 BACK LANE	BLACKBURN	D332 L016
	1851 DENT	3 FISHERGATE HILL	PRESTON	D727 L020
	1851 DENT	29 DUKE ST	LONDON	D727 L020
	1851 DENT	FISHERGATE HILL	PRESTON	D438 L020
	1855 DENT	29 DUKE ST	LONDON	D732 L064
	1855 DENT	3 FISHERGATE HILL	PRESTON	D732 L064
	1855 DENT	NETHEREND	PENRITH	D222 L020
MOSELEY GILLAM	1854 DENT	MARKET PL	CHESTERFIELD	D660 L057
	1854 DENT		SHEFFIELD	D660 L057
	1854 DENT	BATH BDGS 205 GLOSSOP RD	SHEFFIELD	D757 L066
	1855 DENT	205 GLOSSOP RD	SHEFFIELD	D222 L009
MOSELEY L	1850 SURDENT	10 STRAND	TORQUAY	D147 L008
	1852 SURDENT	13 NORTHERNHAY PL	EXETER	D180 L008
MOSELEY LAWRENCE	1841 DENT	50 GEORGE ST	HULL	D241 L009
MOSELEY MESSRS	1851 SURDENT	29 DUKE ST	LONDON	D259 L010
	1851 SURDENT	15 WHITEFRIARGATE	HULL	D259 L010
MOSELEY SIMEON	1851 SURDENT	DUDLEY ST	WOLVERHAMPTON	D699 L059
	1855 DENT	3 ST NICHOLAS ST	SCARBORO	D550 L031
	1855 DENT	3 ST NICHOLAS ST	SCARBORO	D262 L010
MOSELY & DRAKE	1854 DENT	48 HIGH ST	NEWCASTLE UNDER LYME	D015 L001
	1854 DENT		WOLVERHAMPTON	D015 L001
	1855 SURDENT	HIGH ST	WOLVERHAMPTON	D064 L011
MOSELY & MOSELY	1851 SURDENT	34 GRAINGER ST	NEWCASTLE	D215 L009

MOSELY (& CO)	1852 DENT	34 GRAINGER ST	NEWCASTLE	D216 L009
MOSELY (& FATHER E)	1853 DENT	34 GRAINGER ST	NEWCASTLE	D243 L009
	1854 DENT	10 ELDON SQ	NEWCASTLE	D218 L009
	1855 DENT	10 ELDON SQ	NEWCASTLE	D219 L009
	1855 DENT	219 HIGH ST	SUNDERLAND	D223 L009
	1855 DENT	10 ELDON SQ	NEWCASTLE	D223 L009
	1855 DENT	61 GROSVENOR ST	LONDON	D223 L009
	1855 DENT	HIGH ST	STOCKTON	D223 L009
MOSELY (& MOSELY)	1851 SURDENT	34 GRAINGER ST	NEWCASTLE	D215 L009
MOSELY A	1848 SURDENT	30 PARK ST	BRISTOL	D943 L075
	1849 SURDENT	33 PARK ST	BRISTOL	D944 L075
MOSELY ABRAHAM	1848 DENT	30 PARK ST	BRISTOL	DA50 L011
	1848 DENT	30 PARK ST	BRISTOL	D125 L075
	1849 DENT	30 PARK ST	BRISTOL	D891 L068
	1850 DENT	33 PARK ST	BRISTOL	D960 L075
	1853 DENT	33 PARK ST	BRISTOL	D802 L020
	1853 DENT	33 PARK ST	BRISTOL	D951 L075
MOSELY B	1854 DENT	23 GAY ST	BATH	D129 L007
MOSELY CHARLES	1851 DENT	3 FISHERGATE HILL	PRESTON	D437 L019
	1851 DENT	29 DUKE ST	LONDON	D437 L019
	1852 DENT	66 CASTLE ST	CARLISLE	D216 L009
	1854 DENT	29 DUKE ST	LONDON	D439 L019
	1854 DENT	3 FISHERGATE HILL	PRESTON	D439 L019
MOSELY CHARLES & L	1855 DENT	92 BOLD ST	LIVERPOOL	D416 L016
MOSELY CHARLES L	1854 DENT	21 KING ST	BLACKBURN	D439 L019
	1855 DENT	21 KING ST	BLACKBURN	D732 L064
MOSELY E	1842 DENT	9 WHITEFRIARGATE	HULL	D377 L018
	1853 DENT	82 NEW ELVET	DURHAM	D243 L009
	1853 SURDENT	219 HIGH ST	SUNDERLAND	D243 L009
	1854 DENT	22 GAY ST	BATH	D129 L007
	1854 DENT	HIGH ST	DUNSTABLE	DA71 L011
MOSELY E & S	1850 DENT	34 GRAINGER ST	NEWCASTLE	D214 L009
MOSELY E & SON	1853 DENT	34 GRAINGER ST	NEWCASTLE	D243 L009
	1855 DENT	10 ELDON SQ	NEWCASTLE	D219 L009
	1855 DENT	HIGH ST	STOCKTON	D223 L009
	1855 DENT	61 GROSVENOR ST	LONDON	D223 L009
	1855 DENT	10 ELDON SQ	NEWCASTLE	D223 L009
	1855 DENT	219 HIGH ST	SUNDERLAND	D223 L009
MOSELY E (& S)	1848 DENT	15 WHITEFRIARGATE	HULL	D378 L018
MOSELY EPHRAIM	1851 SURDENT	PRISSICK ST	HARTLEPOOL	D292 L013
	1851 SURDENT	13 KEPPEL ST	S SHIELDS	D292 L013
	1851 SURDENT	NORTHGATE	DARLINGTON	D292 L013
	1851 SURDENT	61 GROSVENOR ST GROSVENOR SQ	LONDON	D292 L013
	1851 SURDENT	HIGH ST	STOCKTON ON TEES	D292 L013
	1852 SURDENT	82 NEW ELVET	DURHAM	D287 L013
	1853 SURDENT	82 NEW ELVET	DURHAM	D286 L013
	1855 DENT	NORTHGATE	DARLINGTON	D222 L009
	1855 DENT	319 HIGH ST	SUNDERLAND	D222 L009
	1855 DENT	81 NEW ELVET	DURHAM	D222 L009
	1855 DENT	10 ELDON SQ	NEWCASTLE	D222 L009
MOSELY EPHRAIM & S	1848 DENT	15 WHITEFRIARGATE	HULL	D332 L016
	1852 DENT	15 WHITEFRIARGATE	HULL	D216 L009
MOSELY EPHRAIM & SON	1854 DENT	10 ELDON SQ	NEWCASTLE	D218 L009
MOSELY H	1855 DENT	36 SILVER ST	LINCOLN	D682 L056
MOSELY H B	1837 SURDENT	25 BROCK ST	BATH	D121 L007
MOSELY J L	1842 DENT	11 LONDON ST	READING	D625 L049
	1847 DENT	11 LONDON ST	READING	DB84 L049

MOSELY L	1843 SURDENT	2 UPPER SOUTHERNHAY	EXETER	D171 L008
	1844 SURDENT	5 UPPER SOUTHERNHAY	EXETER	D172 L008
	1844 DENT	ADJ CHEQUERS INN SPEENHAMLAND	NEWBURY (THURS)	D626 L049
	1844 DENT	11 LONDON ST	READING (FRI SAT)	D626 L049
	1844 DENT	12 BERNERS ST	LONDON	D626 L049
	1855 DENT	CARDIFF ARMS INN	CARDIFF (DCC)	DC47 L085
MOSELY LEWIN	1844 DENT	5 UPPER SOUTHERNHAY PL	EXETER	D144 L008
MOSELY LEWIN (& C)	1855 DENT	92 BOLD ST	LIVERPOOL	D416 L016
MOSELY S	1851 DENT	29 DUKE ST	LONDON	D379 L018
	1851 DENT	15 WHITEFRIARGATE	HULL	D379 L018
MOSELY S & E	1848 DENT	15 WHITEFRIARGATE	HULL	D378 L018
MOSELY S (& E)	1850 DENT	34 GRAINGER ST	NEWCASTLE	D214 L009
MOSELY SIMEON (& E)	1848 DENT	15 WHITEFRIARGATE	HULL	D332 L016
	1852 DENT	15 WHITEFRIARGATE	HULL	D216 L009
MOSLEY	1851 DENT	3 FISHERGATE HILL	PRESTON	D673 L053
	1853 DENT	3 FISHERGATE HILL	PRESTON	D533 L028
	1855 SURDENT	HIGH ST	BANBURY	DB01 L011
MOSLEY A	1844 SURDENT	30 PARK ST	BRISTOL	D940 L075
	1845 SURDENT	30 PARK ST	BRISTOL	D822 L002
	1846 SURDENT	30 PARK ST	BRISTOL	D941 L075
MOSLEY CHARLES	1848 DENT	66 CASTLE ST	CARLISLE	D332 L016
	1855 DENT	21 LOWTHER ST	CARLISLE	D222 L020
MOSLEY EPHRAIM	1854 SURDENT	82 NEW ELVET	DURHAM	D289 L013
	1855 DENT	15 WHITEFRIARGATE	HULL	D222 L009
	1855 SURDENT	82 NEW ELVET	DURHAM	DB76 L081
MOSLEY L	1853 SURDENT	46 DARLEY ST	BRADFORD	D261 L010
MOSLEY LAWRENCE LANSDOWNE	1841 DENT	50 GEORGE ST	HULL	D331 L016
MOSLEY MESSRS	1846 SURDENT	15 WHITEFRIARGATE	HULL	D258 L010
	1855 DENT		READING	DA90 L011
MOSLEY SIMEON	1845 SURDENT	TUESDAY MARKET PL	KING'S LYNN	D650 L011
	1855 DENT	3 ST NICHOLAS ST	SCARBORO	D222 L009
MOSS BARNETT	1836 DENT	22 GARTSIDE	MANCHESTER	D469 L020
	1837 DENT	22 GARTSIDE ST	MANCHESTER	D566 L020
	1838 DENT	22 GARTSIDE ST	MANCHESTER	D470 L020
	1841 DENT	91 PICCADILLY	MANCHESTER	D331 L016
	1843 DENT	91 PICCADILLY	MANCHESTER	D473 L020
	1845 DENT	91 PICCADILLY	MANCHESTER	D474 L020
	1846 DENT	91 PICCADILLY	MANCHESTER	D879 L072
MOSS EMANUEL	1828 SURDENT	49 FALKNER ST	MANCHESTER	D025 L020
	1829 SURDENT	49 FAULKNER ST	MANCHESTER	D565 L020
MOSS ISAAC	1831 SURDENT	27 COLLEGE ST	BRISTOL	D929 L075
MOULD THOMAS	1840 SURDENT	62 ST AUBYN ST	DEVONPORT	D143 L020
	1844 DENT	38 ST AUBYN ST	DEVONPORT	D492 L022
	1844 DENT	38 ST AUBYN ST	DEVONPORT	D144 L008
	1850 SURDENT	21 ST AUBYN ST	DEVONPORT	D147 L008
	1852 DENT	21 ST AUBYN ST	DEVONPORT	D788 L020
	1852 DENT	21 ST AUBYN ST	DEVONPORT	D145 L008
	1852 DENT	21 ST AUBYN ST	DEVONPORT	D493 L022
MUMMERY J R	1855 SURDENT	26 CASTLE ST	DOVER	D594 L046
MUMMERY JOHN	1845 DENT	25 CASTLE ST	DOVER	DA66 L011
MUMMERY JOHN R	1847 DENT	25 CASTLE ST	DOVER	D586 L044
MUMMERY JOHN RIGDEN (JUN)	1849 SURDENT	25 CASTLE ST	DOVER	D587 L011
MURPHY	1829 DENT		DERBY	D774 L066
	1833 DENT	GREAT CHARLES STREET	BIRMINGHAM	D079 L002
	1851 DENT	6 INFIRMARY ST	LEEDS	D283 L015
MURPHY & SHERWIN	1830 DENT	73 NORFOLK ST	SHEFFIELD	D751 L066
MURPHY EDWARD	1828 DENT	33 EXETER ST	DERBY	D025 L020

MURPHY EDWARD	1831 DENT	GEORGE ST	DERBY	D501 L057
MURPHY G B	1847 DENT	15 VICTORIA ST	DERBY	D505 L025
MURPHY J	1817 DENT	PARK SQ	LEEDS	D038 L015
MURPHY J B	1831 DENT	5 GEORGE ST	DERBY	D501 L057
	1850 DENT	32 VICTORIA ST	DERBY	D013 L020
	1852 DENT	32 VICTORIA ST	DERBY	D690 L057
MURPHY J K	1842 DENT	7 GRINSTON ST	HULL	D377 L018
MURPHY J L	1839 DENT	44 CHERRY ST	BHAM	D301 L002
	1850 DENT	22 ANN ST	BIRMINGHAM	D099 L011
MURPHY J.L	1839 DENT	44 CHERRY STREET	BIRMINGHAM	D083 L002
	1842 DENT	33 PARADISE STREET	BIRMINGHAM	D075 L002
MURPHY JAMES	1840 SURDENT	46 GEORGE ST	HULL	D888 L006
	1854 DENT	ANGEL ROW	NOTTINGHAM	D510 L023
MURPHY JAMES B	1835 DENT	LONDON RD	DERBY	D007 L014
	1840 DENT	ST PETER'S VICARAGE HOUSE	DERBY	D734 L063
	1843 DENT	ST PETER'S ST	DERBY	D694 L057
	1849 SURDENT	VICTORIA ST	DERBY	D803 L057
	1849 SURDENT		QUORNDON (DERB)	D803 L057
	1850 SURDENT	VICTORIA ST	DERBY	D809 L057
	1850 SURDENT		QUORNDON (DERB)	D809 L057
MURPHY JAMES BRABAZON	1846 DENT	15 VICTORIA ST	DERBY	D693 L057
	1855 DENT	32 VICTORIA ST	DERBY	D511 L023
	1855 DENT	37 TRINITY TCE (RES)	DERBY	D511 L023
MURPHY JEREMIAH.L	1845 DENT	33 PARADISE STREET	BIRMINGHAM	D077 L002
MURPHY JOHN	1847 DENT	33 PARADISE STREET	BIRMINGHAM	D061 L002
	1849 SURDENT	22 ANN STREET	BIRMINGHAM	D062 L002
	1850 SURDENT	22 ANN STREET	BIRMINGHAM	D063 L002
MURPHY JOHN L	1837 DENT	44 CHERRY ST	BIRMINGHAM	D566 L020
	1846 DENT	33 PARADISE ST	BIRMINGHAM	D879 L072
MURPHY JOHN.L	1835 DENT	42 UPPER TEMPLE STREET	BIRMINGHAM	D057 L002
MURPHY JOHN.LOTHER	1841 DENT	44 CHERRY STREET	BIRMINGHAM	D058 L002
MURPHY JOSEPH	1809 SURDENT	COMMERCIAL ST	LEEDS	D285 L015
	1814 SURDENT	COMMERCIAL ST	LEEDS	D330 L016
	1816 DENT	COMMERCIAL ST	LEEDS	D049 L016
	1818 SUR DENT	COMMERCIAL ST	LEEDS *	D302 L002
	1819 SUR DENT	COMMERCIAL ST	LEEDS *	D735 L064
	1822 SURDENT	PARK SQ	LEEDS	D255 L010
	1822 SURDENT	PARK SQ	LEEDS	D005 L030
	1826 SURDENT	33 PARK SQ	LEEDS	D040 L015
	1828 DENT	29 PARK SQ	LEEDS	D025 L020
	1833 SURDENT	PARK SQ	LEEDS	D778 L066
	1848 DENT	4 OXFORD ROW	LEEDS	D332 L016
MURPHY JOSEPH C	1837 DENT	ALBION ST	LEEDS	D257 L010
MURPHY JOSEPH KINNAIRD	1849 SURDENT	206 WEST ST	SHEFFIELD	D756 L066
MURRAY WILLIAM	1852 DENT	CHURCH ST	LISKEARD	D788 L020

NAILER WILLIAM	1770	BLEEDER TOOTHDRAWER	84 DUDLEY STREET	BIRMINGHAM +	D033 L002
	1774	TOOTHDRAWER	84 DUDLEY STREET	BIRMINGHAM	D034 L002
	1775	TOOTHDRAWER	84 DUDLEY STREET	BIRMINGHAM	D035 L002
NATHAN WOLFF	1835	DENT	32 PARK LANE	LIVERPOOL	D406 L016
	1837	DENT	32 PARK LANE	LIVERPOOL	D407 L016
NEEDHAM JOHN	1854	DENT	34 REGENT ST	SHEFFIELD	D757 L066
	1855	DENT	34 REGENT ST	SHEFFIELD	D222 L009
NEEP	1839	DENT	ST ANDREW'S HILL	NORWICH	D654 L011
NEEP EDWARD	1836	DENT	64 BETHEL ST	NORWICH	D649 L051
NEEP W E J	1853	DENT	5 POST OFFICE ST	NORWICH	D655 L051
NEEP WILLIAM EDWARD	1845	DENT	POST OFFICE ST	NORWICH	D650 L051
	1850	DENT	POST OFFICE ST	NORWICH	D652 L051
	1854	DENT	POST OFFICE ST	NORWICH	D651 L051
NEEP WILLIAM EDWARD JOHN	1850	DENT	5 POST OFFICE ST	NORWICH	D491 L011
	1852	SURDENT	5 POST OFFICE ST	NORWICH	D653 L051
NELSON & JONES	1846	DENT	13 MT PLEASANT	LIVERPOOL	D303 L014
NELSON DANIEL	1851	DENT	13 MT PLEASANT	LIVERPOOL	D438 L020
	1852	DENT	13 MT PLEASANT	LIVERPOOL	D216 L009
NELSON GEORGE	1854	DENT	CROSS ST	PRESTON	D439 L019
	1855	DENT	CROSS ST	PRESTON	D732 L064
NELSON NATHAN	1841	DENT	16 NEWINGTON	LIVERPOOL	D409 L016
	1846	DENT	9 UPPER DUKE ST	LIVERPOOL	D879 L072
NELSON NATHANIEL	1839	DENT	16 NEWINGTON	LIVERPOOL	D408 L016
	1843	DENT	16 NEWINGTON	LIVERPOOL	D410 L016
	1845	DENT	16 NEWINGTON	LIVERPOOL	D411 L016
	1846	DENT	NEWINGTON	LIVERPOOL	D303 L014
	1847	DENT	13 MT PLEASANT	LIVERPOOL	D412 L016
	1848	DENT	13 MT PLEASANT	LIVERPOOL	D332 L016
	1849	DENT	13 MT PLEASANT	LIVERPOOL	D413 L016
	1851	DENT	13 MT PLEASANT	LIVERPOOL	D414 L016
	1853	DENT	13 MT PLEASANT	LIVERPOOL	D415 L016
	1855	DENT	28 SEYMOUR ST	LIVERPOOL	D416 L016
NELSON NATHANIEL & W	1843	DENT	16 NEWINGTON	LIVERPOOL	D434 L019
NELSON W (& N)	1843	DENT	16 NEWINGTON	LIVERPOOL	D434 L019
NEWLAND JAMES	1826	DENT	HIGH ST	STAMFORD	D864 L070
	1828	DENT	HIGH ST	STAMFORD	D025 L020
NEWMAN WILLIAM JOHN	1855	DENT	99 BOLD ST	LIVERPOOL	D416 L016
NICHOLSON JOSEPH	1855	SURDENT	48 SADLER ST	DURHAM	DB76 L081
	1855	SURDENT	10 MARKET PL	DURHAM	DB76 L081
NIGHTINGALE & SONS	1853	DENT	7 NEW BRIDGE ST	NEWCASTLE	D243 L009
	1855	DENT	7 NEW BRIDGE ST	NEWCASTLE	D219 L009
	1855	DENT	223 HIGH ST	SUNDERLAND	D223 L009
NIGHTINGALE (& FATH & BRO 1)	1853	DENT	7 NEW BRIDGE ST	NEWCASTLE	D243 L009
	1855	DENT	223 HIGH ST	SUNDERLAND	D223 L009
	1855	DENT	7 NEW BRIDGE ST	NEWCASTLE	D219 L009
NIGHTINGALE (& FATH & BRO 2)	1853	DENT	7 NEW BRIDGE ST	NEWCASTLE	D243 L009
	1855	DENT	7 NEW BRIDGE ST	NEWCASTLE	D219 L009
	1855	DENT	223 HIGH ST	SUNDERLAND	D223 L009
NIGHTINGALE C	1855	DENT	EAST PERCY ST	N SHIELDS	D223 L009
NIGHTINGALE D	1833	DENT	NEW BRIDGE ST	NEWCASTLE	D246 L009
	1836	DENT	NEW BRIDGE ST	NEWCASTLE	DB34 L011
	1838	SURDENT	NEW BRIDGE ST	NEWCASTLE	D239 L009
	1850	DENT	7 NEW BRIDGE ST	NEWCASTLE	D214 L009
	1851	SURDENT	7 NEW BRIDGE ST	NEWCASTLE	D215 L009
	1855	DENT	10 NEW BRIDGE ST	NEWCASTLE	D223 L009
NIGHTINGALE DANIEL	1827	SURDENT	WELLINGTON PL PILGRIM ST	NEWCASTLE	D211 L009
	1827	DENT	10 NEWGATE ST	NEWCASTLE	D211 L009

NIGHTINGALE DANIEL	1828 DENT	26 MOSLEY ST	NEWCASTLE	D025 L020
	1829 DENT	26 MOSLEY ST	NEWCASTLE	D212 L009
	1834 DENT	1 NEW BRIDGE ST	NEWCASTLE	D236 L009
	1837 DENT	1 NEW BRIDGE ST	NEWCASTLE	D566 L020
	1839 SURDENT	NEW BRIDGE ST	NEWCASTLE	D240 L009
	1841 DENT	7 NEW BRIDGE ST	NEWCASTLE	D241 L009
	1847 SURDENT	7 NEW BRIDGE ST	NEWCASTLE	D242 L009
	1848 DENT	7 NEW BRIDGE ST	NEWCASTLE	D332 L016
	1852 DENT	7 NEW BRIDGE ST	NEWCASTLE	D216 L009
NIGHTINGALE DANIEL & T	1855 DENT	7 NEW BRIDGE ST	NEWCASTLE	D222 L009
NIGHTINGALE THOMAS (& D)	1855 DENT	7 NEW BRIDGE ST	NEWCASTLE	D222 L009
NIGHTINGALE WILLIAM	1844 DENT	NEW BRIDGE ST	NEWCASTLE	D213 L009
NORMAN R R B	1853 DENT	ST GEORGE'S RD	YARMOUTH	D655 L051
NORMAN RICHARD	1850 DENT	ST GEORGE'S RD	YARMOUTH	DA91 L011
NORTHEN JOHN	1828 DENT	ST JOHN'S LANE	HALIFAX	D025 L020
NORTHERN JOHN	1809 SURDENT	WOODHOUSE LANE	LEEDS	D285 L015
	1816 DENT	AKED'S RD	HALIFAX	D049 L002
	1816 DENT	AKED'S RD	HALIFAX	D049 L016
	1818 SUR DENT	AKED'S RD	HALIFAX *	D302 L002
	1819 SUR DENT	AKED'S ST	HALIFAX *	D735 L064
	1822 DENT	ST JOHN'S LANE	HALIFAX	D005 L030
	1830 SURDENT	3 ST JOHN'S LANE	HALIFAX	D256 L010
NOWELL CHARLES	1855 DENT	36 SILVESTER ST	HULL	D222 L009
OLIVER MICHAEL	1794 DENT	4 MURRAY ST	LIVERPOOL	D282 L011
ORMROD JOHN	1794 DENT	6 SUGAR LANE	MANCHESTER	D282 L011
	1797 DENT	6 SUGAR LANE	MANCHESTER	D452 L020
	1800 DENT	6 SUGAR LANE	MANCHESTER	D453 L020
	1802 DENT	6 SUGAR LANE	MANCHESTER	D454 L020
ORMROD MARY	1804 DENT	5 SUGAR LANE	MANCHESTER	D455 L020
	1808 DENT	5 SUGAR LANE	MANCHESTER	D456 L020
ORROCK JAMES	1853 SURDENT	29 PELHAM ST	NOTTINGHAM	D507 L023
	1854 DENT	PELHAM ST	NOTTINGHAM	D510 L023
ORVISS R	1853 DENT	23 NORFOLK ST	KING'S LYNN	D655 L051
ORVISS R W	1845 SURDENT	13 NEW CONDUIT ST	KING'S LYNN	D650 L011
	1846 DENT	23 NORFOLK ST	KING'S LYNN	DA85 L011
	1854 DENT (SUR & MECH)	23 NORFOLK ST	KING'S LYNN	D651 L051
OSBORNE C	1851 SURDENT	12 BLACKETT ST	NEWCASTLE	D215 L009
OWEN HENRY	1852 DENT	103 MEDLOCK ST HULME	MANCHESTER	D216 L009
	1855 DENT	100 OXFORD ST	CHORLTON	D478 L020
OWEN RICHARD	1855 SURDENT	COCK ST	WOLVERHAMPTON	D064 L011
	1855 SURDENT	COCK ST	WOLVERHAMPTON	D098 L006
OXLEY LOUIS	1840 DENT	43 ALBION ST	LEEDS	D734 L063
	1841 DENT	42 ALBION ST	LEEDS	D331 L016
	1841 DENT	43 ALBION ST	LEEDS	D241 L009
	1842 SURDENT	20 PARK SQ	LEEDS	D060 L015
	1845 SURDENT	20 PARK ROW	LEEDS	D275 L015
	1846 DENT	20 PARK SQ	LEEDS	D879 L072
	1846 SURDENT	20 PARK ROW	LEEDS	D713 L061
	1848 DENT	20 PARK SQ	LEEDS	D332 L016
	1851 DENT	20 PARK SQ	LEEDS	D283 L015
	1852 DENT	20 PARK SQ	LEEDS	D216 L009
	1853 SURDENT	20 PARK SQ	LEEDS	D261 L010
OXLEY THOMAS LOUIS	1847 SURDENT	20 PARK SQ	LEEDS	D276 L015
	1855 DENT	20 MARKET SQ	LEEDS	D222 L009
PALK E	1849 DENT	38 HIGH ST	SOUTHAMPTON	D345 L017
PALMER G	1854 DENT	PALMER PLACE LODGE ROAD	BIRMINGHAM	D069 L002
PALMER J	1849 DENT	ST GEORGE'S SQ	STAMFORD	D681 L056

PALMER J E	1855 DENT	ST MARY'S ST	STAMFORD	D682 L056
	1855 DENT	EASTGATE	SLEAFORD	D682 L056
PALMER J G	1839 DENT	34 TEMPLE ROW	BHAM	D301 L002
PALMER J.G	1833 DENT (SURGICAL AND M34 TEMPLE ROW		BHAM	D079 L002
	1842 DENT	34 TEMPLE ROW	BIRMINGHAM	D075 L002
PALMER JOSEPH GUNN	1837 DENT	34 TEMPLE ROW	BIRMINGHAM	D566 L020
	1846 DENT	34 TEMPLE ROW	BIRMINGHAM	D879 L072
PALMER JOSEPH.G	1845 DENT	34 TEMPLE ROW	BIRMINGHAM	D077 L002
PALMER JOSEPH.GUNN	1835 DENT	34 TEMPLE ROW	BIRMINGHAM	D057 L002
	1841 DENT	34 TEMPLE ROW	BIRMINGHAM	D058 L002
PALMER ROBERT	1800 DRUGGIST DENT	13 LADY MEAD	BATH *	D111 L007
PALMER T G	1839 SURDENT	24 REGENT ST	CHELTENHAM	D832 L069
	1839 SURDENT	BATH ST	CHELTENHAM	D654 L068
	1839 SURDENT	PROMENADE VILLAS	CHELTENHAM	D957 L068
	1840 DENT	BATH ST	CHELTENHAM	D143 L020
	1840 SURDENT	SOUTH CAMBRAY HOUSE	CHELTENHAM	D833 L069
	1841 SURDENT	SOUTH CAMBRAY HOUSE	CHELTENHAM	D834 L069
	1842 SURDENT	1 BATH ST	CHELTENHAM	D835 L069
	1843 SURDENT	1 BATH ST	CHELTENHAM	D836 L069
	1844 SURDENT	1 BATH ST	CHELTENHAM	D837 L069
	1845 SURDENT	1 ROYAL CRESC	CHELTENHAM	D838 L069
	1846 SURDENT	1 ROYAL CRESC	CHELTENHAM	D839 L069
	1847 SURDENT	1 ROYAL CRESC	CHELTENHAM	D840 L069
	1848 SURDENT	1 ROYAL CRESC	CHELTENHAM	D841 L069
	1849 SURDENT	1 ROYAL CRESC	CHELTENHAM	D842 L069
	1851 SURDENT	1 ROYAL CRESC	CHELTENHAM	D844 L069
	1852 SURDENT	1 ROYAL CRESC	CHELTENHAM	D845 L069
	1853 SURDENT	1 ROYAL CRESC	CHELTENHAM	D847 L069
	1853 SURDENT	1 ROYAL CRESC	CHELTENHAM	D846 L069
PALMER T GILL	1848 DENT	1 ROYAL CRESC	CHELTENHAM	D954 L069
	1849 DENT	1 ROYAL CRESC	CHELTENHAM	D881 L082
PALMER THOMAS G	1844 SURDENT	1 BATH ST	CHELTENHAM	D959 L069
PALMER THOMAS GILL	1842 DENT	1 BATH ST	CHELTENHAM	D846 L049
	1847 DENT	1 ROYAL CRESC	CHELTENHAM	D890 L068
	1850 DENT	1 ROYAL CRESC	CHELTENHAM	DA74 L011
	1851 DENT	1 ROYAL CRESC	CHELTENHAM	D953 L069
	1852 DENT	1 ROYAL CRESC	CHELTENHAM	D952 L069
	1852 DENT	1 ROYAL CRESC	CHELTENHAM	D788 L020
	1853 SURDENT	1 ROYAL CRESC	CHELTENHAM	D956 L068
PAM ALBERT	1831 SURDENT	BURDETT PL	HASTINGS	D582 L044
	1833 SURDENT	DISPENSARY HIGH ST	HASTINGS	D583 L044
	1839 DENT	HIGH ST	HASTINGS	D584 L011
	1840 SURDENT	DISPENSARY HIGH ST	HASTINGS	D585 L044
PARDOE CHARLES CAYGILL	1838 DENT	13 OXFORD ST	MANCHESTER	D470 L020
	1840 DENT	112 OXFORD ST	CHORLTON	D471 L020
	1841 DENT	112 OXFORD ST	CHORLTON	D472 L020
	1841 DENT	112 OXFORD ST CHORLTON	MANCHESTER	D331 L016
	1845 DENT	53 PETER ST	MANCHESTER	D474 L020
	1846 DENT	53 PETER ST	MANCHESTER	D879 L072
	1848 DENT	10 DICKINSON ST	MANCHESTER	D332 L016
	1848 DENT	10 DICKINSON ST	MANCHESTER	D475 L020
PARKINSON	1839 SUR DENT	12 PARK ST	BRISTOL *	D654 L068
	1840 DENT	12 PARK ST	BRISTOL	D143 L020
	1845 DENT	10 OLD STEINE	BRIGHTON	DB70 L025
PARKINSON E	1851 DENT	10 OLD STEINE	BRIGHTON	DA77 L011
	1855 DENT	10 OLD STEYNE	BRIGHTON	D594 L046
PARKINSON EDWARD	1839 DENT	10 OLD STEYNE	BRIGHTON	D584 L011

PARKINSON EDWARD	1839 DENT	10 OLD STEINE	BRIGHTON	D607 L047
	1843 SURDENT	10 OLD STEYNE	BRIGHTON	D600 L047
	1845 DENT	10 OLD STEINE	BRIGHTON	DA66 L011
	1845 DENT	10 OLD STEINE	BRIGHTON	D606 L047
	1846 DENT	10 OLD STEINE	BRIGHTON	D601 L047
	1848 DENT	10 OLD STEINE	BRIGHTON	D602 L047
	1850 DENT	10 OLD STEINE	BRIGHTON	D603 L047
	1852 DENT	10 OLD STEINE	BRIGHTON	D604 L047
	1854 DENT	10 OLD STEINE	BRIGHTON	D605 L047
PARKINSON F	1833 SURDENT	6 PARAGON BDGS	BATH	D120 L007
	1838 SURDENT	12 PARK ST	BRISTOL	D935 L075
	1839 SURDENT	12 PARK ST	BRISTOL	D936 L075
	1840 DENT	3 PRINCESS BDGS	BATH	D143 L020
	1840 SURDENT	12 PARK ST	BRISTOL	D945 L075
	1841 SURDENT	12 PARK ST	BRISTOL	D937 L075
	1846 SURDENT	3 PRINCES BDGS	BATH	D124 L007
PARKINSON FELIX	1829 SURDENT	6 PARAGON BUILDINGS	BATH	D118 L007
	1830 SURDENT	6 PARAGON BUILDINGS	BATH	D119 L007
	1837 SURDENT	3 PRINCESS BDGS	BATH	D121 L007
	1841 SURDENT	3 PRINCES BDGS	BATH	D122 L007
	1842 SURDENT	6 PARAGON BDGS	BATH	D123 L007
	1848 SURDENT	3 PRINCES BDGS	BATH	D125 L007
	1849 SURDENT	3 PRINCES BDGS	BATH	D126 L007
PARKINSON G	1850 SURDENT	3 PRINCES BDGS	BATH	D127 L007
	1852 DENT	3 PRINCES BDGS	BATH	D128 L007
PARKINSON GEORGE	1852 SURDENT	3 PRINCES BDGS	BATH	D788 L020
	1854 DENT	3 PRINCES BDGS	BATH	D129 L007
PARKINSON JAMES	1852 DENT	3 ST PETER'S SQ	MANCHESTER	D216 L009
	1855 DENT	3 ST PETER'S SQ	MANCHESTER	D478 L020
PARKINSON JOHN	1784 DENT	CHURCH LANE WHITECHAPEL	LONDON	D273 L011
PARKINSON SAMUEL M	1855 DENT	120 BOLD ST	LIVERPOOL	D416 L016
PARKINSON SOLOMON	1853 DENT	18A ISLINGTON	LIVERPOOL	D415 L016
PARKINSON WALTER	1848 DENT	27 GT GEORGE ST	LIVERPOOL	D332 L016
PARROTT THOMAS	1850 DENT	16 BUCKWELL ST	PLYMOUTH	D147 L008
PARSLEY JAMES	1787 SURDENT	BROAD ST	BRISTOL	D110 L075
	1792 BARBERSURGEON	20 BROAD ST	BRISTOL	D892 L075
PARSON C T	1850 SURDENT	17 ORCHARD ST	BRISTOL	D946 L075
	1851 SURDENT	17 ORCHARD ST	BRISTOL	D896 L075
	1852 SURDENT	17 ORCHARD ST	BRISTOL	D897 L075
	1853 SURDENT	17 ORCHARD ST	BRISTOL	D898 L075
	1854 SURDENT	17 ORCHARD ST	BRISTOL	D899 L075
	1855 SURDENT	17 ORCHARD ST	BRISTOL	D947 L075
PARSON JOSEPH H	1839 DENT	94 BOLD ST	LIVERPOOL	D408 L016
	1841 DENT	16 PARKER ST	LIVERPOOL	D409 L016
	1846 DENT	30 BOLD ST	LIVERPOOL	D303 L014
PARSON T C	1845 DENT	66 PARK ST	BRISTOL	D822 L002
	1846 SURDENT	66 PARK ST	BRISTOL	D941 L075
	1847 SURDENT	17 ORCHARD ST	BRISTOL	D942 L075
	1848 SURDENT	17 ORCHARD ST	BRISTOL	D943 L075
	1849 SURDENT	17 ORCHARD ST	BRISTOL	D944 L075
PARSON THOMAS C	1846 SURDENT	66 PARK ST	BRISTOL	D879 L072
	1848 DENT	17 ORCHARD ST	BRISTOL	D125 L075
	1848 DENT	17 ORCHARD ST	BRISTOL	DA50 L011
	1849 DENT	17 ORCHARD ST	BRISTOL	D891 L068
	1850 DENT	17 ORCHARD ST	BRISTOL	D960 L075
	1852 DENT	17 ORCHARD ST	BRISTOL	D788 L020
	1853 DENT	17 ORCHARD ST	BRISTOL	D802 L020

PARSON THOMAS C	1853 DENT	17 ORCHARD ST	BRISTOL	D951 L075
PARSONE JOSEPH HENRY	1853 SURDENT	4 WARD'S END	HALIFAX (LATE GREAVED261 L010
PARSONS J H	1850 DENT	MRS PATTINSON MANN'HAM LANE	BRADFORD (THURS)	DB35 L078
PARSONS JOSEPH H	1843 DENT	16 PARKER ST	LIVERPOOL	D410 L016
	1843 DENT	16 PARKER ST	LIVERPOOL	D434 L019
	1845 DENT	16 PARKER ST	LIVERPOOL	D411 L016
	1846 DENT	30 BOLD ST	LIVERPOOL	D879 L072
	1847 DENT	30A BOLD ST	LIVERPOOL	D412 L016
PARSONS JOSEPH HENRY	1848 DENT	CLARE HALL RD	HALIFAX	D332 L016
	1848 DENT	30 BOLD ST	LIVERPOOL	D332 L016
	1850 SURDENT	WARD'S END	HALIFAX	D571 L041
	1855 DENT	CLARE HALL RD	HALIFAX	D222 L009
PARSONS ROBERT	1837 DENT	27 CONEY ST	YORK	D257 L010
	1840 DENT	27 CONEY ST	YORK	D734 L063
	1840 DENT	27 CONEY ST	YORK	D888 L006
	1841 DENT	35 CONEY ST	YORK	D331 L016
	1841 DENT	27 CONEY ST	YORK	D241 L009
	1843 SURDENT	33 CONEY ST	YORK	D251 L010
	1846 DENT	33 CONEY ST	YORK	D258 L010
	1848 DENT	10 HIGH OUSEGATE	YORK	D332 L016
	1851 SURDENT	33 CONEY ST	YORK	D259 L010
PARSONS THOMAS	1855 DENT	33 CONEY ST	YORK	D222 L009
PATRICK & SON	1836 DENT	BRIDGE ST	LITTLE BOLTON	D469 L020
PATRICK (& FATH)	1836 DENT	BRIDGE ST	LITTLE BOLTON	D469 L020
PATRICK HUGH	1943 DENT	14 BOUNDARY ST	CHORLTON	D473 L020
PATRICK ROBERT	1843 DENT	WOOD ST	BOLTON	D473 L020
	1844 DENT	WOOD ST	BOLTON	D436 L019
	1845 DENT	WOOD ST	BOLTON	D786 L020
	1848 DENT	2 WOOD ST	BOLTON	DA86 L011
	1848 DENT	WOOD ST	BOLTON	D332 L016
	1851 DENT	2 WOOD ST	BOLTON	D438 L020
	1854 DENT	2 WOOD ST	BOLTON	D439 L019
	1855 DENT	2 WOOD ST	BOLTON	B732 L064
PATTERSON CHARLES	1841 DENT	3 NORMAN COURT	HULL	D241 L009
	1841 DENT	NORMAN CT	HULL	D331 L016
PAYNE T	1852 DENT	9 PORTLAND ST	SOUTHAMPTON	DB72 L025
PAYNE T P	1849 DENT	8 BECKFORD TCE	SOUTHAMPTON	D341 L017
	1851 DENT	9 PORTLAND ST	SOUTHAMPTON	D342 L017
	1855 SURDENT	9 PORTLAND ST	SOUTHAMPTON	DA84 L011
PAYNE THOMAS	1847 DENT	8 BECKFORD TCE	SOUTHAMPTON	D340 L017
	1849 DENT	8 BECKFORD TCE	SOUTHAMPTON	D345 L017
	1855 DENT	9 PORTLAND ST	SOUTHAMPTON	D344 L017
PAYNE THOMAS P	1852 DENT	9 PORTLAND ST	SOUTHAMPTON	D788 L020
	1852 DENT	9 PORTLAND ST	SOUTHAMPTON	D346 L017
	1853 DENT	9 PORTLAND ST	SOUTHAMPTON	D343 L017
PAYNE THOMAS PIBBLE	1845 SURDENT	4 NEW RD	SOUTHAMPTON	D339 L017
PEACOCK JAMES	1794 SUR DENT	31 UNION ST	LIVERPOOL *	D282 L011
PEAL JOSEPH	1855 DENT	11 PRINCESS ST	NEWCASTLE	D222 L009
PEARSALL & PENNY	1849 SURDENT	17 RODNEY TCE	CHELTENHAM	D842 L069
	1849 DENT	17 RODNEY TCE	CHELTENHAM	DB81 L082
PEARSALL R	1839 SURDENT	17 RODNEY TCE	CHELTENHAM	D832 L069
	1839 SURDENT	17 RODNEY TCE	CHELTENHAM	D654 L068
	1840 SURDENT	17 RODNEY TCE	CHELTENHAM	D833 L069
	1840 DENT	17 RODNEY TCE	CHELTENHAM	D143 L020
	1843 SURDENT	17 RODNEY TCE	CHELTENHAM	D836 L069
	1844 SURDENT	17 RODNEY TCE	CHELTENHAM	D837 L069
	1845 SURDENT	17 RODNEY TCE	CHELTENHAM	D838 L069

PEARSALL R	1846 SURDENT	17 RODNEY TCE	CHELTENHAM	D839 L069
	1847 SURDENT	17 RODNEY TCE	CHELTENHAM	D840 L069
	1848 DENT	17 RODNEY TCE	CHELTENHAM	D954 L069
	1848 SURDENT	17 RODNEY TCE	CHELTENHAM	D841 L069
PEARSALL ROBERT	1830 DENT	17 RODNEY TCE	CHELTENHAM	D119 L020
	1839 SURDENT	RODNEY TCE	CHELTENHAM	D957 L068
	1842 DENT	17 RODNEY TCE	CHELLTENHAM	DB46 L049
	1844 SURDENT	17 RODNEY TCE	CHELTENHAM	D959 L069
	1847 DENT	17 RODNEY TCE	CHELTENHAM	D890 L068
PEATSON HENRY ROBERT	1855 DENT	102 BROUGHTON ST	MANCHESTER	D478 L020
PECK LEONARD W	1850 SURDENT	302 HIGH ST	CHATHAM	DA75 L011
PECK W	1851 DENT	312 HIGH ST	CHATHAM	DA77 L011
PECK WILLIAM	1838 SUR DENT CUPP CHEM	123 HIGH ST	CHATHAM *	DA73 L011
	1845 DENT	312 HIGH ST	CHATHAM	DA66 L011
PENNY (& PEARSALL)	1849 DENT	17 RODNEY TCE	CHELTENHAM	DB81 L082
	1849 SURDENT	17 RODNEY TCE	CHELTENHAM	D842 L069
PENNY G S	1850 SURDENT	17 RODNEY TCE	CHELTENHAM	D843 L069
	1851 SURDENT	17 RODNEY TCE	CHELTENHAM	D844 L069
	1852 SURDENT	17 RODNEY TCE	CHELTENHAM	D845 L069
	1853 SURDENT	14 RODNEY TCE	CHELTENHAM	D847 L069
	1853 SURDENT	2 RODNEY TCE	CHELTENHAM	D846 L069
PENNY G T	1850 DENT	17 RODNEY TCE	CHELTENHAM	DA74 L011
	1851 DENT	17 RODNEY TCE	CHELTENHAM	D953 L069
	1852 DENT	17 RODNEY TCE	CHELTENHAM	D952 L069
PENNY GEORGE S	1853 SURDENT	14 RODNEY TCE	CHELTENHAM	D956 L068
PENNY GEORGE STOTHART	1852 DENT	17 RODNEY TCE	CHELTENHAM	D788 L020
PENNY GEORGE STOTHERT	1848 DENT	15 OXFORD ST	MANCHESTER	D475 L020
	1848 DENT	15 OXFORD ST	MANCHESTER	D332 L016
PERFECT G	1855 DENT	HYDE PARK RD	SOUTHSEA	DA84 L011
PERRY T A	1839 DENT CUPPER	ATHOLL ST	DOUGLAS I OF M *	DB25 L011
	1845 DENT		STRATFORD	D077 L006
PERRY WILLIAM	1794 SUR DENT	9 KING ST	LIVERPOOL *	D282 L011
	1800 SUR DENT	41 SEEL ST	LIVERPOOL *	D389 L016
	1803 SUR DENT	41 SEEL ST	LIVERPOOL *	D390 L016
	1804 SUR DENT	41 SEEL ST	LIVERPOOL *	D391 L016
	1805 SUR DENT	41 SEEL ST	LIVERPOOL *	D393 L016
	1807 SUR DENT	47 SEEL ST	LIVERPOOL *	D394 L016
	1810 SUR DENT	47 SEEL ST	LIVERPOOL *	D395 L016
	1811 SUR DENT	44 SEEL ST	LIVERPOOL *	D396 L016
	1811 SUR DENT	47 SEEL ST	LIVERPOOL *	D284 L011
	1813 SUR DENT	47 SEEL ST	LIVERPOOL *	D397 L016
	1814 SURDENT	47 SEEL ST	LIVERPOOL	D330 L016
	1814 SUR DENT	47 SEEL ST	LIVERPOOL *	D398 L016
	1816 DENT	47 SEEL ST	LIVERPOOL	D049 L016
	1816 SUR DENT	46 SEEL ST (SURGERY)	LIVERPOOL *	D431 L016
	1816 SUR DENT	6 HIGHER LANE EVERTON	LIVERPOOL *	D431 L016
	1818 DENT	47 SEEL ST	LIVERPOOL	D302 L002
	1818 SUR DENT	9 CHURCH ST EVERTON	LIVERPOOL *	D432 L016
	1819 SUR DENT	47 SEEL ST	LIVERPOOL *	D735 L064
	1822 SUR DENT	55 SEEL ST	LIVERPOOL *	D005 L020
	1823 DENT	55 SEEL ST	LIVERPOOL	D400 L016
	1824 DENT	55 SEEL ST	LIVERPOOL	D401 L016
	1825 DENT	55 SEEL ST	LIVERPOOL	D444 L016
	1827 DENT	55 SEEL ST	LIVERPOOL	D402 L016
	1829 DENT	55 SEEL ST	LIVERPOOL	D404 L016
	1834 DENT	55 SEEL ST	LIVERPOOL	D236 L009
	1837 DENT PHYS	55 SEEL ST	LIVERPOOL *	D566 L020

PERRY WILLIAM (JUN)	1821 SURDENT MD	55 SEEL ST	LIVERPOOL	D399 L016
	1821 SURDENT MD	9 CHURCH ST EVERTON	LIVERPOOL	D399 L016
	1823 DENT	55 SEEL ST	LIVERPOOL	D400 L016
	1825 DENT MD	55 SEEL ST	LIVERPOOL	D444 L016
PERRY WILLIAM (SEN)	1821 SURDENT	55 SEEL ST	LIVERPOOL	D399 L016
	1821 SURDENT	9 CHURCH ST EVERTON	LIVERPOOL	D399 L016
PERRY WILLIAM D	1835 DENT	55 SEEL ST	LIVERPOOL	D406 L016
	1837 DENT	61 SEEL ST	LIVERPOOL	D407 L016
	1839 DENT	49 SEEL ST	LIVERPOOL	D408 L016
PERRY WILLIAM DUNCAN	1832 DENT	55 SEEL ST	LIVERPOOL	D445 L016
	1834 DENT	55 SEEL ST	LIVERPOOL	D405 L016
PHILLIPS (& STOKES)	1851 SURDENT	51 BLACKETT ST	NEWCASTLE	D215 L009
	1855 DENT	51 BLACKETT ST	NEWCASTLE	D222 L009
PHILLIPS G & H	1851 DENT	HIGH ST	TUNBRIDGE WELLS	DA77 L011
PHILLIPS GEORGE	1845 DENT		DENMARK HILL	DA66 L011
PHILLIPS H (& C)	1851 DENT	HIGH ST	TUNBRIDGE WELLS	DA77 L011
PHILLIPS SAUL	1846 DENT	120 ST JAMES'S ST	BRIGHTON	D601 L047
PHILLIPS THOMAS	1854 DENT	45 SMALLBROOK STREET	BIRMINGHAM	D069 L002
	1855 SURDENT	45 SMALLBROOK STREET	BIRMINGHAM	D064 L002
PHILLIPS W	1848 DENT	BONFIRE CORNER	PORTSEA	D357 L017
	1852 DENT	BONFIRE CORNER	PORTSEA	DB72 L025
PHILLIPS WILLIAM	1852 DENT	CROSS ST	PORTSEA	D346 L017
PICNOT (& DIXON)	1846 DENT	13 WELLINGTON ST	LEEDS	D879 L072
	1847 SURDENT	13 WELLINGTON ST	LEEDS	D276 L015
	1848 DENT	13 WELLINGTON ST	LEEDS	D332 L016
	1849 DENT	13 WELLINGTON ST	LEEDS	D277 L015
	1851 DENT	13 WELLINGTON ST	LEEDS	D283 L015
	1852 DENT	13 WELLINGTON ST	LEEDS	D216 L009
	1855 DENT	13 WELLINGTON ST	LEEDS	D222 L009
PICNOT THEODORE	1853 SURDENT	13 WELLINGTON ST	LEEDS	D261 L010
PIERPOINT (& FAULKNER)	1840 DENT	18 OLDHAM ST	MANCHESTER	D471 L020
	1841 DENT	18 OLDHAM ST	MANCHESTER	D331 L016
	1841 DENT	18 OLDHAM ST	MANCHESTER	D472 L020
PIERREPOINT (& FAULKNER)	1843 DENT	18 OLDHAM ST	MANCHESTER	D473 L020
PIERREPOINT JOHN	1845 DENT	18 OLDHAM ST	MANCHESTER	D474 L020
	1848 DENT	18 OLDHAM ST	MANCHESTER	D475 L020
	1848 DENT	18 OLDHAM ST	MANCHESTER	D332 L016
	1850 DENT	18 OLDHAM ST	MANCHESTER	D476 L020
	1852 DENT	18 OLDHAM ST	MANCHESTER	D477 L020
	1852 DENT	18 OLDHAM ST	MANCHESTER	D216 L009
	1855 DENT	18 OLDHAM ST	MANCHESTER	D478 L020
PIERREPONT JOHN	1846 DENT	18 OLDHAM ST	MANCHESTER	DB79 L072
	1851 DENT	18 GIDHAM ST	MANCHESTER	D567 L020
PILLING EDMUND	1843 DENT SURINSTR MAKER	RICHMOND TCE	BLACKBURN ⁑	D473 L020
	1848 DENT SURGINSTRMAKER	2 HIGH ST	BLACKBURN ⁑	D332 L016
	1851 DENT SURINSTRMAK	UNION ST	BLACKBURN⁑	D438 L020
	1852 DENT SURINSTRMAK	UNION ST	BLACKBURN ⁑	D001 L020
	1854 DENT	5 UNION ST	BLACKBURN	D439 L019
	1855 DENT	5 UNION ST	BLACKBURN	D732 L064
PILLING JAMES	1851 DENT	11 ASTLEY GATE	BLACKBURN	D438 L020
	1852 DENT	11 ASTLEY GATE	BLACKBURN	D801 L020
	1854 DENT	11 ASTLEY GATE	BLACKBURN	D439 L019
	1855 DENT	11 ASTLEY GATE	BLACKBURN	D732 L064
PINNOCK JOHN	1792 DENT PERFUMER	ST JAMES CHURCHYARD	BRISTOL ⁑	D892 L075
PLATTIN H	1853 DENT	BRIDGE ST	FAKENHAM	D655 L051
PLATTIN HOWARD	1850 DENT	SWAN ST	FAKENHAM	DA91 L011
PLUMBLY J W	1839 DENT	HIGH ST	COWES	DB43 L078

POINTING JOHN	1852 DENT CUPPER	26 PARK ST	BRISTOL *	D788 L020
PONSFORD	1845 DENT	BROAD ST	ST HELIER	DA82 L011
POTTS W DURANT	1853 SURDENT	22 PITTVILLE ST	CHELTENHAM	D956 L068
POULTON S	1854 DENT	2 LONDON ST	READING	DA71 L011
POUNDALL W	1848 DENT	ST MARY'S GATE	DERBY	D800 L020
POUNDALL W L	1855 DENT	20 VICTORIA ST	DERBY	D511 L023
POUNDALL WILLIAM	1852 DENT	CARRINGTON ST	DERBY	D690 L057
	1854 DENT	PARK ST	DERBY	D660 L057
POUNDALL WILLIAM LLOYD	1849 SURDENT	CORN MARKET	DERBY	D803 L057
	1850 DENT	10 CORN MKT	DERBY	D013 L020
	1850 SURDENT	CORN MARKET	DERBY	D809 L057
PRATT & SON	1839 DENT CUPPER	EAST ST	CHICHESTER *	D584 L011
PRATT (& FATH)	1839 DENT CUPPER	EAST ST	CHICHESTER *	D584 L011
PRATT R	1855 DENT	7 SOUTH ST	GREENWICH	D594 L046
PREBBLE JAMES	1849 DENT	159 HIGH ST	MARGATE	D587 L044
PRESTWICH WRIGHT	1850 DENT	8 HENRY ST	BURY	D728 L020
PREW	1824 SURDENT	2 CHARLES ST	BATH	D116 L007
	1826 SURDENT	5 CHARLES ST	BATH	D117 L007
	1829 SURDENT (LATE ASSIST8 EDGAR BUILDINGS		BATH	D118 L007
PREW J	1833 SURDENT	58 PARK ST	BRISTOL	D931 L075
	1834 SURDENT	58 PARK ST	BRISTOL	D932 L075
	1835 SURDENT	58 PARK ST	BRISTOL	D820 L002
	1836 SURDENT	58 PARK ST	BRISTOL	D933 L075
	1838 SURDENT	58 PARK ST	BRISTOL	D935 L075
	1839 SURDENT	58 PARK ST	BRISTOL	D936 L075
	1840 SURDENT	58 PARK ST	BRISTOL	D945 L075
	1841 SURDENT	58 PARK ST	BRISTOL	D937 L075
	1842 SURDENT	58 PARK ST	BRISTOL	D938 L075
	1843 SURDENT	58 PARK ST	BRISTOL	D939 L075
	1844 SURDENT	58 PARK ST	BRISTOL	D940 L075
	1845 SURDENT	58 PARK ST	BRISTOL	D822 L002
	1846 SURDENT	58 PARK ST	BRISTOL	D941 L075
	1846 SURDENT	8 EDGAR BDGS	BATH	D124 L007
PREW JAMES	1830 SURDENT	8 EDGAR BUILDINGS	BATH	D119 L007
	1831 SURDENT	58 PARK ST	BRISTOL	D929 L075
	1832 SURDENT	58 PARK ST	BRISTOL	D930 L075
	1833 SURDENT	8 EDGAR BDGS	BATH	D120 L007
	1837 SURDENT	8 EDGAR BDGS	BATH	D121 L007
	1839 SUR DENT	57 PARK ST	BRISTOL *	D654 L068
	1840 DENT	8 EDGAR BDGS	BATH	D143 L020
	1840 DENT	57 PARK ST	BRISTOL	D143 L020
	1841 SURDENT	8 EDGAR BDGS	BATH	D122 L007
	1842 SURDENT	8 EDGAR BDGS	BATH	D123 L007
	1842 DENT	57 PARK ST	BRISTOL	DB46 L049
	1846 SURDENT	37 PARK ST	BRISTOL	D879 L072
PRICHARD AUGUSTIN	1852 DENT	PARK ROW	BRISTOL	D788 L020
PRIDEAUX FRANCIS	1852 DENT	FORE ST	TAUNTON	D788 L020
PRIDEAUX T S	1845 SURDENT	4 PORTLAND ST	SOUTHAMPTON	D339 L017
	1847 DENT	4 PORTLAND ST	SOUTHAMPTON	D340 L017
	1848 DENT	4 PORTLAND ST	SOUTHAMPTON	D357 L017
	1849 DENT	4 PORTLAND ST	SOUTHAMPTON	D345 L017
	1849 DENT	4 PORTLAND ST	SOUTHAMPTON	D341 L017
PRIDEAUX THOMAS	1843 SURDENT	4 PORTLAND ST	SOUTHAMPTON	D338 L017
	1844 DENT	UNION ST	RYDE I OF W	D144 L068
PRIDEAUX THOMAS SIMS	1844 DENT	4 PORTLAND ST	SOUTHAMPTON	D144 L068
PRYNN C T R	1855 DENT	16 SAVILLE ROW	NEWCASTLE	D223 L009
PULFORD WILLIAM	1850 DENT	22 SHADWELL ST	BHAM	D013 L002

QUINTIN A & A T	1849 DENT	2 NORFOLK TCE	GLOUCESTER	D891 L068
QUINTIN A T (& A)	1849 DENT	2 NORFOLK TCE	GLOUCESTER	D891 L068
QUINTIN A V	1852 SURDENT	4 BEDFORD BDGS	CHELTENHAM	D845 L069
	1853 SURDENT	4 BEDFORD BDGS	CHELTENHAM	D847 L069
	1853 SURDENT	4 BEDFORD BDGS	CHELTENHAM	D846 L069
QUINTIN ADOLPHUS	1847 DENT	ALTON ST	ROSS	D012 L001
QUINTIN ADOLPHUS & A	1852 DENT	NORFOLK TCE	GLOUCESTER	D788 L020
QUINTIN ADOLPHUS U (& LC & AT	1853 DENT	1 NORFOLK TCE	GLOUCESTER	D951 L075
QUINTIN ADOLPHUS URIAH	1853 SURDENT	4 BEDFORD BDGS	CHELTENHAM	D956 L068
QUINTIN ADOLPHUS W	1850 DENT	7 GROSVENOR PL	CHELTENHAM	DA74 L011
	1851 DENT	CRESCENT PL	CHELTENHAM	D953 L069
	1852 DENT	4 BEDFORD BDGS	CHELTENHAM	D952 L069
QUINTIN AUG-US TH (& L C A V)	1847 DENT	2 NORFOLK TCE	GLOUCESTER	D012 L001
QUINTIN AUGUSTUS (& A)	1852 DENT	NORFOLK TCE	GLOUCESTER	D788 L020
QUINTIN AUGUSTUS TH (&LC &AU)	1853 DENT	1 NORFOLK TCE	GLOUCESTER	D951 L075
QUINTIN LOUIS CHARLES	1842 DENT	BRIDGE ST	HEREFORD	D123 L020
QUINTIN LOUIS CHAS & A U & A	1853 DENT	1 NORFOLK TCE	GLOUCESTER	D951 L075
QUINTIN LS CHAS ADOL-US V & A	1847 DENT	2 NORFOLK TCE	GLOUCESTER	D012 L001
RAMSDEN GEORGE	1841 DENT	ALBION CT KIRKGATE	BRADFORD	D331 L016
RAMSDEN HARRY	1848 DENT	17 ST JOHN ST	LEEDS (TUES SAT)	D332 L016
RAMSDEN HENRY	1845 SURDENT	9 ALBION CT	BRADFORD	D569 L041
	1847 DENT	9 ALBION ST	LEEDS	D276 L015
	1848 DENT	9 ALBION ST	BRADFORD	D332 L016
	1850 DENT	29 DARLEY ST	BRADFORD	DB35 L078
	1853 SUR DENT	28 DARLEY ST	BRADFORD	D261 L010*
	1853 SUR DENT		SHIPLEY	D261 L010*
	1855 DENT	28 DARLEY ST	BRADFORD	D222 L009
	1855 DENT	SKINNER LANE	SHIPLEY	D222 L009
RANSOM R	1855 SURDENT	3 VERULAM PL	HASTINGS	D594 L046
RANSOM ROBERT	1852 SURDENT	3 VERULAM PL	HASTINGS	DA54 L011
RANSOM WILLIAM	1855 DENT	4 STAFFORD ST	LIVERPOOL	D416 L016
RANSON WILLIAM	1852 DENT	BENACRE STREET	BIRMINGHAM	D078 L002
RAYMENT THOMAS	1798 DENT		STAMFORD	D279 L011
READ MESSRS	1854 DENT	65 GRAND PDE	BRIGHTON	D605 L047
READ T & W	1855 SURDENT	65 GRAND PDE	BRIGHTON	D594 L046
	1855 SURDENT	8 HOLLES ST	LONDON	D594 L046
READ W (& T)	1855 SURDENT	8 HOLLES ST	LONDON	D594 L046
	1855 SURDENT	65 GRAND PDE	BRIGHTON	D594 L046
REDWARD E	1855 DENT	64 UNION ST	RYDE I OF W	DA84 L011
REDWARD W	1848 DENT	59 UNION ST	PORTSEA	D357 L017
	1852 DENT	UNION ST	PORTSEA	DB72 L025
REDWARD W C	1852 DENT	25 UNION ST	PORTSEA	D346 L017
	1855 SURDENT	25 UNION ST	PORTSEA	DA84 L011
REDWARD WILLIAM	1839 DENT	UNION ST	PORTSEA	DB43 L078
REILLY MAURICE.S	1855 SURDENT	87 HENEAGE STREET	BIRMINGHAM	D064 L002
RESTIEUX	1783 DENT	19 LOWER CLOSE SQ	NORWICH	D878 L072
RESTUE ANDREW	1792 DENT	NORTH ST DOCK	HULL	D371 L018
RICHARDSON FRANK	1853 SURDENT	PARK ST	NOTTINGHAM	D507 L023
RICHARDSON GEORGE	1853 DENT	SILVER STREET	WORCESTER	D031 L004
	1855 SURDENT	SILVER STREET	WORCESTER	D016 L001
RICHARDSON J	1834 DENT CUPPER	17 ABOVE BAR	SOUTHAMPTON *	D335 L017
	1838 DENT	13 SAVILE ST	HULL	D375 L018
	1839 DENT	13 SAVILE ST	HULL	D376 L018
	1842 DENT	13 SAVILE ST	HULL	D377 L018
	1848 DENT	13 SAVILE ST	HULL	D378 L018
RICHARDSON JOHN	1831 SURDENT	4 WORSHIP ST	HULL	D380 L018
	1834 DENT	4 WORSHIP ST	HULL	D236 L009

RICHARDSON JOHN	1835	SURDENT CHEM/DR	7 WORSHIP ST	HULL *	D365	L018
	1837	SURDENT	7 WORSHIP ST	HULL	D257	L010
	1837	DENT	4 WORSHIP ST	HULL	D566	L020
	1840	SURDENT	13 SAVILE ST	HULL	D888	L006
	1841	DENT	13 SAVILE ST	HULL	D241	L009
	1841	DENT	13 SAVILE ST	HULL	D331	L016
	1846	SURDENT	13 SAVILE ST	HULL	D258	L010
	1848	DENT	13 SAVILE ST	HULL	D332	L016
	1851	SURDENT	13 SAVILE ST	HULL	D259	L010
	1851	DENT	13 SAVILE ST	HULL	D379	L018
	1852	DENT	13 SAVILE ST	HULL	D216	L009
	1855	DENT	13 SAVILE ST	HULL	D222	L009
RICHERAUD FERDINAND	1846	DENT	173 OXFORD ST CHORLTON	MANCHESTER	D879	L072
RICHERAUD MORRIS	1845	DENT	6 HARDY ST	LIVERPOOL	D411	L016
RIDLEY A	1850	SURDENT	WHITBURN ST	SUNDERLAND	D214	L009
RISSIEUX	1784	DENT (DAINTIST)	LOWER CLOSE SQ	NORWICH	D273	L011
RITSON JOSEPH	1855	DENT	BACK ST	BRAMPTON	D222	L020
ROBARTS GEORGE	1844	DENT	WEST ST	TAVISTOCK	D144	L068
	1852	DENT	15 DEVONSHIRE TCE	PLYMOUTH	D493	L022
ROBB (& DAVENPORT)	1855	DENT	27 WHITEFRIARGATE	HULL	D222	L009
ROBERTS	1855	DENT	HIGH ST	CANTERBURY	D594	L046
ROBERTS BENJAMIN	1845	SURDENT	15 NORTH PDE	BRADFORD	D569	L041
	1848	DENT	21 DARLEY ST	BRADFORD	D332	L016
	1850	DENT	42 DARLEY ST	BRADFORD	DB35	L078
ROBERTS CHARLES	1839	CUPPER DENT	96 WINCHESTER ST	CHELTENHAM *	D654	L068
	1840	DENT	96 WINCHESTER ST	CHELTENHAM	D143	L020
ROBERTS GEORGE	1852	DENT	15 DEVONSHIRE TCE	PLYMOUTH	D788	L020
	1852	DENT	15 DEVONSHIRE TCE	PLYMOUTH	D145	L008
ROBERTS J B	1849	DENT	NORTH ST	BOURN	D681	L056
ROBERTSON H B	1850	DENT	GLEBE ST	STOKE ON TRENT	D099	L006
ROBERTSON HENRY BLAIR	1850	DENT SUR	GLEBE ST	STOKE ON TRENT *	D013	L001
ROBERTSON J	1850	DENT	47 FOREGATE ST	WORCESTER	D099	L011
	1852	DENT	8 EDGAR BDGS	BATH	D128	L007
ROBERTSON JAMES	1839	DENT	109 NORFOLK ST	SHEFFIELD	D301	L002
	1840	DENT	109 NORFOLK ST	SHEFFIELD	D734	L063
	1847	DENT	47 FOREGATE STREET	WORCESTER	D012	L001
	1848	SURDENT	8 EDGARS BDGS	BATH	D125	L007
	1849	SURDENT	8 EDGAR BDGS	BATH	D126	L007
	1850	DENT	47 FOREGATE STREET	WORCESTER	D013	L001
	1850	SURDENT	8 EDGARS BDGS	BATH	D127	L007
	1851	SURDENT	47 FOREGATE STREET	WORCESTER	D014	L001
	1852	SURDENT	8 EDGAR BDGS	BATH	D788	L020
	1853	DENT	47 FOREGATE STREET	WORCESTER	D031	L004
	1854	DENT	8 EDGARS BDGS	BATH	D129	L007
	1854	DENT	47 FOREGATE STREET	WORCESTER	D015	L001
	1855	SURDENT	48 FOREGATE STREET	WORCESTER	D016	L001
ROBERTSON WILLIAM	1823	SUR DENT	11 SQUARE	BIRMINGHAM *	D052	L002
	1824	DENT		BHAM (TUES AT LEAMIND	D319	L014
	1825	SURDENT	11 SQUARE	BIRMINGHAM	D053	L002
	1828	DENT	11 OLD SQ	BIRMINGHAM	D025	L006
	1828	DENT	17 SQUARE	BIRMINGHAM	D054	L002
	1829	DENT	17 SQUARE	BIRMINGHAM	D055	L002
	1830	DENT	17 SQUARE	BIRMINGHAM	D056	L002
	1833	SURDENT	SQUARE	BIRMINGHAM	D079	L002
	1835	DENT	SQUARE	BIRMINGHAM	D057	L002
	1837	DENT	SQUARE	BIRMINGHAM	D566	L020
	1839	SURDENT	8 OLD SQUARE	BIRMINGHAM	D083	L002

ROBERTSON WILLIAM	1841 DENT	8 OLD SQUARE	BIRMINGHAM	D058 L002
	1842 DENT	OLD SQUARE	BIRMINGHAM	D075 L002
	1845 DENT	8 SQUARE	BIRMINGHAM	D077 L002
	1846 DENT	8 OLD SQ	BIRMINGHAM	D879 L072
	1847 SURDENT	8 OLD SQUARE	BIRMINGHAM	D061 L002
	1849 SURDENT	8 OLD SQUARE	BIRMINGHAM	D062 L002
	1850 SURDENT	8 OLD SQUARE	BIRMINGHAM	D063 L002
	1850 DENT	8 OLD SQ	BHAM	D013 L002
	1852 DENT	8 OLD SQUARE	BIRMINGHAM	D078 L002
	1854 DENT	8 OLD SQUARE	BIRMINGHAM	D069 L002
	1855 SURDENT	8 OLD SQUARE	BIRMINGHAM	D064 L002
ROBINSON GEORGE MOORE	1849 DENT	WIDE BARGATE	BOSTON	D870 L056
ROBINSON JOHN	1815 SURDENT TDR	55 GT BRIDGEWATER ST	MANCHESTER *	D459 L020
	1817 SURDENT TDRAWER	92 DEANSGATE	MANCHESTER *	D460 L020
	1819 SURDENT	ST JOHN'S ST	MANCHESTER	D461 L020
	1821 SURDENT	ST JOHN'S ST	MANCHESTER	D462 L020
	1822 DENT	ST JOHN'S ST	MANCHESTER	D005 L020
	1824 SURDENT	21 ST JOHN'S ST	MANCHESTER	D463 L020
	1824 SURDENT	21 ST JOHN ST	MANCHESTER	D401 L019
	1829 SURDENT	21 ST JOHN'S ST	MANCHESTER	D465 L020
	1830 SURDENT	21 ST JOHN'S ST	MANCHESTER	D466 L020
ROBINSON S R	1855 SURDENT	JEWRY ST	WINCHESTER	DA84 L011
RODGERS	1842 DENT	GALLOWTREEGATE	LEICESTER	D662 L024
	1843 DENT	GALLOWTREEGATE	LEICESTER	D664 L024
RODWAY H B	1850 DENT	3 PARK CRESC	TORQUAY	D147 L008
RODWAY HENRY BARON	1848 DENT	3 PARK CRESC	TORQUAY	DA50 L011
RODWAY HENRY BARRON	1852 DENT	3 PARK CRESC	TORQUAY	D788 L020
	1852 DENT	3 PARK CRESC	TORQUAY	D145 L008
ROGERS	1845 SURDENT	LAURA PL LEEDS RD	BRADFORD	D569 L041
	1845 SURDENT	4 CLARE HALL RD	HALIFAX	D570 L041
ROGERS (& ST CROIX)	1843 DENT	29 DICKINSON ST	MANCHESTER	D473 L020
ROGERS C D	1854 DENT	OLD RECTORY HOUSE	NEWBURY	DA71 L011
ROGERS D	1845 DENT	MARKET HILL HIGH ST	WOOLWICH	DA66 L011
ROGERS J	1850 DENT	44 BROAD ST	WORCESTER	D099 L011
ROGERS JOSEPH	1847 DENT	44 BROAD STREET	WORCESTER	D012 L001
	1850 DENT	44 BROAD STREET	WORCESTER	D013 L001
	1851 SURDENT	44 BROAD STREET	WORCESTER	D014 L001
	1853 DENT	44 BROAD STREET	WORCESTER	D031 L004
	1854 DENT	BROAD STREET	WORCESTER	D015 L001
	1855 SURDENT	44 BROAD STREET	WORCESTER	D016 L001
ROGERS NATHAN C	1851 SURDENT	28 BRIDGE ST	SUNDERLAND	D292 L013
ROGERS THOMAS	1846 DENT	24 GALLOWTREEGATE	LEICESTER	D658 L024
	1847 DENT	MANNINGHAM LANE	BRADFORD	D276 L015
	1848 DENT	16 PARK SQ	LEEDS	D332 L016
	1848 DENT	NORTH PDE	BRADFORD	D332 L016
	1849 DENT	16 PARK SQ	LEEDS	D277 L015
	1851 DENT	3 HANOVER BDGS	SOUTHAMPTON	D342 L017
	1851 DENT	24 PARK ROW	LEEDS	D283 L015
	1851 DENTSUR	WOOD ST	WAKEFIELD (FRI)	DB54 L025
	1852 DENT	16 PARK SQ	LEEDS	D216 L009
	1853 SURDENT	24 PARK ROW	LEEDS	D261 L010
	1855 DENT	24 PARK ROW	LEEDS	D222 L009
ROSE & SIMPSON	1834 DENT	26 DUKE ST	LIVERPOOL	D405 L016
	1835 DENT	126 DUKE ST	LIVERPOOL	D406 L016
ROSE (& BROOKS)	1834 DENT	126 DUKE ST	LIVERPOOL	D236 L009
ROSE D (& R)	1837 DENT	41 MT PLEASANT	LIVERPOOL	D566 L020
	1841 DENT	7 CHADDOCK ST	PRESTON	D472 L020

ROSE DANIEL	1835 DENT		41 MT PLEASANT	LIVERPOOL	D406 L016
ROSE DONALD	1832 DENT		41 MT PLEASANT	LIVERPOOL	D445 L016
	1834 DENT		41 MT PLEASANT	LIVERPOOL	D236 L009
	1841 DENT		69 MT PLEASANT	LIVERPOOL	D409 L016
	1843 DENT		69 MT PLEASANT	LIVERPOOL	D410 L016
	1843 DENT		69 MT PLEASANT	LIVERPOOL	D434 L019
	1845 DENT		69 MT PLEASANT	LIVERPOOL	D411 L016
ROSE DONALD (& R)	1837 DENT		41 MT PLEASANT	LIVERPOOL	D407 L016
	1839 DENT		79 MT PLEASANT	LIVERPOOL	D408 L016
ROSE ELIZABETH	1832 DENT		127 DUKE ST	LIVERPOOL	D445 L016
	1834 DENT		126 DUKE ST	LIVERPOOL	D236 L009
ROSE JAMES	1823 DENT		130 DUKE ST	LIVERPOOL	D400 L016
	1824 DENT		130 DUKE ST	LIVERPOOL	D401 L016
	1825 DENT		130 DUKE ST	LIVERPOOL	D444 L016
	1827 DENT		13 DUKE ST	LIVERPOOL	D402 L016
	1828 DENT		130 DUKE ST	LIVERPOOL	D025 L020
	1829 DENT		139 DUKE ST	LIVERPOOL	D404 L016
	1829 DENT		BRECK LANE EVERTON	LIVERPOOL	D404 L016
	1845 DENT		155 DUKE ST	LIVERPOOL	D411 L016
ROSE JAMES EDWARD	1845 DENT		BARK ST	BOLTON	D786 L020
	1846 DENT		69 MT PLEASANT	LIVERPOOL	D303 L014
	1846 DENT		69 MT PLEASANT	LIVERPOOL	DB79 L072
	1847 DENT		69 MT PLEASANT	LIVERPOOL	D412 L016
	1848 DENT		69 MT PLEASANT	LIVERPOOL	D332 L016
	1849 DENT		69 MT PLEASANT	LIVERPOOL	D413 L016
	1851 DENT		69 MT PLEASANT	LIVERPOOL	D414 L016
	1853 DENT		69 MT PLEASANT	LIVERPOOL	D415 L016
	1855 DENT		52 MT PLEASANT	LIVERPOOL	D416 L016
ROSE JOHN FREDERICK	1851 DENT		46 LUNE ST	PRESTON	D727 L020
	1851 DENT		46 LUNE ST	PRESTON	D438 L020
	1851 DENT		46 LUNE ST	PRESTON	D437 L019
	1851 DENT		46 LUNE ST	PRESTON	D673 L053
	1853 DENT		46 LUNE ST	PRESTON	D533 L028
	1854 DENT		FISHERGATE	PRESTON	D439 L019
	1855 DENT		FISHERGATE	PRESTON	D732 L064
ROSE R & D	1837 DENT		41 MT PLEASANT	LIVERPOOL	D566 L020
	1841 DENT		7 CHADDOCK ST	PRESTON	D472 L020
ROSE ROBERT	1837 DENT		5 CHADDOCK ST	PRESTON	DB68 L078
	1841 DENT		5 CHADDOCK ST	PRESTON	D534 L028
	1843 DENT		46 LUNE ST	PRESTON	D473 L020
	1844 DENT		46 LUNE ST	PRESTON	D436 L019
	1846 DENT		46 LUNE ST	PRESTON	D713 L072
	1848 DENT		46 LUNE ST	PRESTON	D332 L016
ROSE ROBERT & D	1837 DENT		41 MT PLEASANT	LIVERPOOL	D407 L016
	1839 DENT		79 MT PLEASANT	LIVERPOOL	D408 L016
ROTHWELL JAMES	1841 DENT	DENTINSTR MAKER	WALLGATE	WIGAN *	D472 L020
	1843 DENT	DENT INSTR MAN	WALLGATE	WIGAN *	D434 L019
	1846 DENT	DENTINSTRMAK	WALLGATE	WIGAN*	D713 L061
	1851 DENT	DENTINSTRMAK	WALLGATE	WIGAN *	D438 L020
	1852 DENT		WALLGATE	WIGAN	D537 L029
	1854 DENT		WALLGATE	WIGAN	D439 L019
	1855 DENT		WALLGATE	WIGAN	D732 L064
ROWE C	1848 DENT		GEORGE'S ROW	LANDPORT	D357 L017
	1848 DENT			WIMBORNE	D357 L011
	1852 DENT		GEORGE'S ROW	LANDPORT	DB72 L025
	1855 DENT		HIGH ST	WIMBORNE	DA84 L011
ROWE C A	1855 SURDENT		GEORGE'S ST	LANDPORT	DA84 L011

ROWLAND (& FATH S)	1829 DENT	ST JAMES ST	LIVERPOOL	D404 L016
	1829 DENT	47 TITHEBARN ST	LIVERPOOL	D404 L016
	1832 DENT	VINCENT ST	LIVERPOOL	D445 L016
	1832 DENT	26 ST JAMES ST	LIVERPOOL	D445 L016
	1832 DENT	99 TITHEBARN ST	LIVERPOOL	D445 L016
	1834 DENT	71 ST JAMES ST	LIVERPOOL	D405 L016
	1835 DENT	68 ST JAMES ST	LIVERPOOL	D406 L016
	1835 DENT	98 TITHEBARN ST	LIVERPOOL	D406 L016
	1837 DENT PERF	125 TITHEBARN ST	LIVERPOOL *	D566 L020
	1837 DENT	97 TITHEBARN ST	LIVERPOOL	D407 L016
	1837 DENT	69 ST JAMES ST	LIVERPOOL	D407 L016
	1837 DENT PERF	64 ST JAMES ST	LIVERPOOL *	D566 L020
ROWLAND CHARLES	1841 DENT	6 TITHEBARN ST	LIVERPOOL	D409 L016
ROWLAND CHARLES S	1839 DENT	6 TITHEBARN ST	LIVERPOOL	D408 L016
ROWLAND S	1839 DENT	137 ST JAMES ST	LIVERPOOL	D408 L016
	1841 DENT	137 ST JAMES ST	LIVERPOOL	D409 L016
ROWLAND S & SON	1829 DENT	47 TITHEBARN ST	LIVERPOOL	D404 L016
	1829 DENT	ST JAMES ST	LIVERPOOL	D404 L016
	1832 DENT	99 TITHEBARN ST	LIVERPOOL	D445 L016
	1832 DENT	26 ST JAMES ST	LIVERPOOL	D445 L016
	1832 DENT	VINCENT ST	LIVERPOOL	D445 L016
	1834 DENT	71 ST JAMES ST	LIVERPOOL	D405 L016
	1835 DENT	68 ST JAMES ST 98 TITHEBARN ST	LIVERPOOL	D406 L016
	1837 DENT	69 ST JAMES ST 97 TITHEBARN ST	LIVERPOOL	D407 L016
ROWLAND SMITH	1843 DENT	1 JORDAN ST	LIVERPOOL	D434 L019
	1843 DENT	164 MILL ST	LIVERPOOL	D434 L019
	1845 DENT	202 MILL ST	LIVERPOOL	D411 L016
	1845 DENT	3 HILL ST	LIVERPOOL	D411 L016
	1846 DENT	3 HILL ST & MILL ST	LIVERPOOL	D879 L072
	1847 DENT	226 MILL ST	LIVERPOOL	D412 L016
	1847 DENT	3 HILL ST	LIVERPOOL	D412 L016
ROWLAND SMITH & SON	1837 DENT PERF	64 ST JAMES ST	LIVERPOOL *	D566 L020
	1837 DENT PERF	125 TITHEBARN ST	LIVERPOOL *	D566 L020
ROWNE A	1855 DENT	62 CUMBERLAND ST	PORTSEA	DA84 L011
ROWNEY (& DAVENPORT)	1855 DENT	27 WHITEFRIARS' GATE	HULL	D682 L056
	1855 DENT	CHEQUERGATE	LOUTH	D682 L056
ROWNEY THOMAS R	1854 DENT	NORFOLK ST	KING'S LYNN	D651 L051
ROWNTREE M	1848 DENT	ST JAMES ST	NOTTINGHAM	D800 L020
	1855 DENT	FRYER LANE	NOTTINGHAM	D511 L023
ROWNTREE MATTHEW	1841 DENT	CASTLE GATE	NOTTINGHAM	D331 L016
	1844 DENT	BROAD ST	NOTTINGHAM	D509 L023
	1847 DENT	ST JAMES ST	NOTTINGHAM	D505 L023
	1848 DENT	ST JAMES'S ST	NOTTINGHAM	D506 L023
	1850 DENT	FRIAR LANE	NOTTINGHAM	D013 L020
	1853 SURDENT	FRIAR LANE	NOTTINGHAM	D507 L023
	1854 DENT	FRIAR LANE	NOTTINGHAM	D510 L023
RUMBLE G	1855 DENT	174 HIGH ST	LINCOLN	D682 L056
RUSHFORTH JOHN	1828 DENT BONE SETTER	SPEDING'S YD	BARNSLEY *	D025 L020
	1840 DENT	PEAS HILL NOOK	BARNSLEY	D734 L063
	1841 DENT	PEASHILL NOOK	BARNSLEY	D241 L009
RUSHWORTH JOHN	1841 DENT	CHEAPSIDE	BARNSLEY	D331 L016
RUSPINI	1793 SURDENT	6 KINGSTON BDGS	BATH	DB21 L011
	1794 SURDENT	6 NR THE PUMP ROOM	BATH	DB22 L011
	1796 SURDENT	4 KINGSTON BDGS	BATH	DB23 L011
RUSPINI BARTHOLOMEW	1784 SURDENT	12 PALL MALL	LONDON	D273 L011
RUST J A	1853 DENT	YORK ROW	WISBEACH	D655 L051
RUST JEREMIAH A	1851 SURDENT	HIGH ST	WISBEACH	DA48 L011

Name	Year	Type	Address	Town	Ref 1	Ref 2
RUST JEREMIAH ANDERSON	1850	DENT	MARKET ST	WISBEACH	DA91	L011
RUTTER J	1853	SURDENT	136 BRIGGATE	LEEDS	D261	L010
RUTTER JOHN	1852	DENT	33 NEWSOME'S YD	LEEDS	D216	L009
	1855	DENT	33 NEWSOME'S YD	LEEDS	D222	L009
RYMER SAMUEL LEE	1853	DENT	26 GEORGE ST	CROYDON	D612	L048
	1855	DENT	52 NORTH END	CROYDON	D613	L048
SAFFORD I T	1793	DENT	QUEEN SQ	BRISTOL	D893	L075
SAFFORD T I	1795	DENT	49 QUEEN SQ	BRISTOL	D894	L075
	1797	DENT	40 QUEEN SQ	BRISTOL	D895	L075
	1798	DENT	40 QUEEN SQ	BRISTOL	D900	L075
	1799	DENT	40 QUEEN SQ	BRISTOL	D901	L075
	1801	DENT	40 QUEEN SQ	BRISTOL	D902	L075
	1803	DENT	49 QUEEN SQ	BRISTOL	D903	L075
	1805	DENT	49 QUEEN SQ	BRISTOL	D904	L075
	1806	SURDENT	49 QUEEN SQ	BRISTOL	D905	L075
	1807	SURDENT	49 QUEEN SQ	BRISTOL	D906	L075
SAFFORD T S	1787	DENT WATCHMAKER	QUEEN SQ	BRISTOL *	D110	L011
SAFFORD THOMAS J	1811	SURDENT	49 QUEEN SQ	BRISTOL	D910	L075
SAFFORD THOMAS JEFFREY	1792	DENT	49 QUEEN SQ	BRISTOL	D892	L075
SANDBROOK BENJAMIN	1835	DENT	27 SUFFOLK STREET	BIRMINGHAM	D057	L002
SAUNDERS JOSIAH	1846	DENT	3 JESUS LANE	CAMBRIDGE	DA85	L011
SAYLES CHARLES LEWIS	1841	DENT	71 FARGATE	SHEFFIELD	D331	L016
	1846	DENT	1 FARGATE	SHEFFIELD	D879	L072
SAYLES F A	1849	DENT	140 HIGH ST	LINCOLN	D681	L056
	1850	SURDENT	MR HAWKSLEY'S CHURCHGATE	RETFORD (APR OCT)	D013	L001
	1855	DENT	GUILDHALL ST	LINCOLN	D682	L056
	1855	DENT	HIGH ST	LINCOLN	D682	L056
SAYLES FRANCIS ALBAN	1849	DENT	140 HIGH ST	LINCOLN	D333	L016
SAYLES FREDERICK A	1826	DENT	SILVER ST	LINCOLN	D864	L070
SAYLES FREDERICK ALBAN	1842	DENT	38 SILVER ST	LINCOLN	D865	L070
	1843	SURDENT	38 SILVER ST	LINCOLN	D685	L070
	1849	SURDENT	140 HIGH ST	LINCOLN	D870	L056
	1850	DENT	140 HIGH ST	LINCOLN	D013	L020
	1851	SURDENT	140 HIGH ST	LINCOLN	DB54	L025
SAYLES L C	1822	DENT	29 FARGATE	SHEFFIELD	D255	L010
	1825	DENT SUR	10 NORFOLK ST	SHEFFIELD *	D749	L066
	1828	DENT	FARGATE	SHEFFIELD	D025	L011
	1828	SURGICAL DENT	FARGATE	SHEFFIELD	D025	L020
	1828	DENT SUR	FARGATE	SHEFFIELD *	D750	L066
	1830	DENT	82 FARGATE	SHEFFIELD	D751	L066
	1833	DENT	SURREY ST	SHEFFIELD	D752	L066
	1834	DENT	SURREY ST	SHEFFIELD	D236	L009
	1839	DENT	71 FARGATE	SHEFFIELD	D301	L002
	1840	DENT	71 FARGATE	SHEFFIELD	D734	L063
	1841	DENT	71 FARGATE	SHEFFIELD	D241	L009
SAYLES LEWIS CHARLES	1837	DENT	29 FARGATE	SHEFFIELD	D257	L010
	1837	DENT	FARGATE	SHEFFIELD	D566	L020
	1841	DENT	71 FARGATE	SHEFFIELD	D754	L066
	1841	DENT	71 FARGATE	SHEFFIELD	D753	L066
	1845	SURDENT	71 FARGATE	SHEFFIELD	D755	L066
	1848	DENT	71 FARGATE	SHEFFIELD	D332	L016
	1849	SURDENT	71 FARGATE	SHEFFIELD	D756	L066
	1852	SURDENT	71 FARGATE	SHEFFIELD	D260	L010
	1852	DENT	71 FARGATE	SHEFFIELD	D216	L009
	1854	DENT	71 FARGATE	SHEFFIELD	D757	L066
SCHOFIELD WILLIAM	1850	DENT	22 SANDY LANE	HEATON NORRIS	D709	L034
SCHOLEFIELD JAMES	1850	DENT	SOUTH ST	HUDDERSFIELD	D539	L030

SCHOLEFIELD JAMES	1853 SURDENT	11 SOUTH ST	HUDDERSFIELD	D261 L010
	1855 DENT	SOUTH ST	HUDDERSFIELD	D222 L009
SCOTT	1843 DENT	20 COLOMBERIE	ST HELIER	DC58 L088
	1855 SURDENT	2 NORTHGATE ST	BURY ST EDMUNDS	D668 L011
SCOTT SARAH ANN	1828 DENT	63 DALE END	BIRMINGHAM	D025 L006
SCOTT SARAH.A	1829 DENT	122 GREAT CHARLES STREET	BIRMINGHAM	D055 L002
	1830 DENT	122 GREAT CHARLES STREET	BIRMINGHAM	D056 L002
SCOTT SARAH.ANN	1828 DENT	122 GREAT CHARLES STREET	BIRMINGHAM	D054 L002
SCRIVENER P	1846 DENT	MARKET PL	STOWMARKET	DA85 L011
SEDMOND JOSEPH	1822 SURDENT	FRANKFORT ST	PLYMOUTH	DB77 L022
	1823 SURDENT	FRANKFORT ST	PLYMOUTH	DB51 L025
	1830 SURDENT	FRANKFORT ST	PLYMOUTH	D491 L022
	1830 DENT	42 FRANKFORT ST	PLYMOUTH	D119 L008
	1836 DENT	FRANKFORT ST	PLYMOUTH	DA44 L011
	1840 DENT	32 FRANKFORT ST	PLYMOUTH	D143 L008
	1844 DENT	12 UNION PL	PLYMOUTH	D144 L008
	1844 DENT	12 UNION PL	PLYMOUTH	D492 L022
SEDMOND MR & MRS	1797 DENT	PRINCES ST	BRISTOL	D895 L075
	1798 DENT	PRINCES ST	BRISTOL	D900 L075
SEDMOND MRS (& MR)	1797 DENT	PRINCES ST	BRISTOL	D895 L075
	1798 DENT	PRINCES ST	BRISTOL	D900 L075
SEDMOND RICHARD	1847 DENT	FRANKFORT ST	PLYMOUTH	D152 L008
	1850 DENT	14 PRINCESS ST	PLYMOUTH	D147 L008
	1852 DENT	4 COURTENAY ST	PLYMOUTH	D493 L022
SELVEY J	1850 DENT	109 GT CHARLES ST	BIRMINGHAM	D099 L011
SELVEY JOSEPH	1847 DENT	11 BRITTLE STREET	BIRMINGHAM	D061 L002
	1849 SURDENT	109 GREAT CHARLES STREET	BIRMINGHAM	D062 L002
	1850 SURDENT	109 GREAT CHARLES STREET	BIRMINGHAM	D063 L002
	1850 DENT	119 GT CHARLES ST	BHAM	D013 L002
	1852 DENT	109 GREAT CHARLES STREET	BIRMINGHAM	D078 L002
	1854 DENT	109 GREAT CHARLES STREET	BIRMINGHAM	D069 L002
	1855 SURDENT	109 GREAT CHARLES STREET	BIRMINGHAM	D064 L002
SHALE T WADSON	1852 DENT	24 DAVID ST	MANCHESTER	D477 L020
SHALE T WATSON	1851 DENT	21 DAVID ST	MANCHESTER	D567 L020
SHALE THEODORE WADSON	1848 DENT	24 DAVID ST	MANCHESTER	D332 L016
SHALE THOMAS WADSON	1848 DENT	24 DAVID ST	MANCHESTER	D475 L020
	1850 DENT	24 DAVID ST	MANCHESTER	D476 L020
	1852 DENT	24 DAVID ST	MANCHESTER	D216 L009
	1855 DENT	24 DAVID ST	MANCHESTER	D478 L020
SHAW JAMES	1830 DENT	BETHEL ST	NORWICH	D119 L020
SHAW JOHN	1855 DENT	7 HOUGHTON ST	NOTTINGHAM	D511 L023
SHEFFIELD & SON	1852 DENT	24 ABBEY ST	CARLISLE	D216 L009
SHEFFIELD (& FATH T)	1829 DENT	ABBEY ST	CARLISLE	D440 L019
SHEFFIELD (& FATH)	1852 DENT	24 ABBEY ST	CARLISLE	D216 L009
SHEFFIELD JOHN	1855 DENT	24 ABBEY ST	CARLISLE	D222 L020
SHEFFIELD THOMAS	1828 DENT	ABBEY ST	CARLISLE	D025 L008
	1831 SURDENT	255 HIGH ST	EXETER	D161 L008
	1832 SURDENT	MARY'S YD	EXETER	D162 L008
	1833 DENT	PALACE GATE	EXETER	D163 L008
	1834 SURDENT	PALACE GATE	EXETER	D164 L008
	1836 SURDENT	PALACE GATE	EXETER	D165 L008
	1837 DENT	24 ABBEY ST	CARLISLE	DA49 L011
	1837 SURDENT	PALACE GATE	EXETER	D166 L008
	1838 SURDENT	PALACE GATE	EXETER	D167 L008
	1839 SURDENT	PALACE GATE	EXETER	D151 L008
	1840 SURDENT	PALACE GATE	EXETER	D168 L008
	1840 DENT	ABBEY ST	CARLISLE	DA70 L011

SHEFFIELD THOMAS	1840 DENT	PALACE ST	EXETER	D143 L008
	1841 SURDENT	PALACE GATE	EXETER	D169 L008
	1842 SURDENT	PALACE GATE	EXETER	D170 L008
	1843 SURDENT	PALACE GATE	EXETER	D171 L008
	1844 DENT	PALACE ST	EXETER	D144 L008
	1844 SURDENT	PALACE GATE	EXETER	D172 L008
	1845 SURDENT	PALACE GATE	EXETER	D173 L008
	1846 SURDENT	PALACE GATE	EXETER	D174 L008
	1847 DENT	24 ABBEY ST	CARLISLE	D443 L019
	1847 SURDENT	PALACE GATE	EXETER	D175 L008
	1848 SURDENT	PALACE GATE	EXETER	D176 L008
	1848 DENT	24 ABBEY ST	CARLISLE	D332 L016
	1848 DENT	PALACE ST	EXETER	DA50 L011
	1849 SURDENT	PALACE GATE	EXETER	D177 L008
	1850 SURDENT	PALACE GATE	EXETER	D178 L008
	1850 DENT	PALACE GATE	EXETER	D147 L008
	1851 SURDENT	PALACE GATE	EXETER	D179 L008
	1852 SURDENT	PALACE GATE	EXETER	D180 L008
	1852 DENT	PALACE ST	EXETER	D788 L020
	1852 DENT	PALACE ST	EXETER	D145 L008
	1853 SURDENT	PALACE ST	EXETER	D153 L008
	1853 SURDENT	PALACE GATE	EXETER	D181 L008
	1854 SURDENT	PALACE GATE	EXETER	D182 L008
	1854 SURDENT	PALACE ST	EXETER	DB71 L025
	1855 SURDENT	PALACE GATE	EXETER	D183 L008
SHEFFIELD THOMAS & SON	1829 DENT	ABBEY ST	CARLISLE	D440 L019
SHEPHERD H	1852 DENT	NORFOLK ST	SOUTHSEA	D872 L025
SHEPHERD HENRY	1852 DENT	13 ST PAUL'S SQ	SOUTHSEA	D346 L017
	1855 DENT	SOMERSET LODGE GREEN RD	SOUTHSEA	DA84 L011
SHERWIN (& MURPHY)	1830 DENT	73 NORFOLK ST	SHEFFIELD	D751 L066
SHERWIN JAMES	1833 DENT	65 NORFOLK ST	SHEFFIELD	D752 L066
	1834 DENT	65 NORFOLK ST	SHEFFIELD	D236 L009
	1837 DENT	65 NORFOLK ST	SHEFFIELD	D566 L020
	1837 DENT	65 NORFOLK ST	SHEFFIELD	D257 L010
	1841 DENT	14 SURREY ST	SHEFFIELD	D754 L066
	1841 DENT	14 SURREY ST	SHEFFIELD	D753 L066
	1841 DENT	14 SURREY ST	SHEFFIELD	D331 L016
	1845 SURDENT	14 SURREY ST	SHEFFIELD	D755 L066
	1846 DENT	14 SURREY ST	SHEFFIELD	D879 L072
	1848 DENT	14 SURREY ST	SHEFFIELD	D332 L016
	1849 SURDENT	14 SURREY ST	SHEFFIELD	D756 L066
	1852 SURDENT	14 SURREY ST	SHEFFIELD	D260 L010
	1852 DENT	14 SURREY ST	SHEFFIELD	D216 L009
	1854 DENT	14 SURREY ST	SHEFFIELD	D757 L066
	1855 DENT	14 SURREY ST	SHEFFIELD	D222 L009
SHEW	1796 SURDENT	4 FOUNTAIN BDGS	BATH	DB23 L011
	1801 SURDENT	12 BELMONT ROW	BATH	D849 L025
	1812 SURDENT	1 BLADUDS BUILDINGS	BATH	D114 L007
	1836 SURDENT	51 PARK ST	BRISTOL	D933 L075
	1838 SURDENT	51 PARK ST	BRISTOL	D935 L075
	1839 SURDENT	51 PARK ST	BRISTOL	D936 L075
	1840 SURDENT	51 PARK ST	BRISTOL	D945 L075
	1841 SURDENT	51 PARK ST	BRISTOL	D937 L075
	1842 SURDENT	51 PARK ST	BRISTOL	D938 L075
	1843 SURDENT	51 PARK ST	BRISTOL	D939 L075
	1844 SURDENT	51 PARK ST	BRISTOL	D940 L075
	1845 SURDENT	51 PARK ST	BRISTOL	D822 L002

SHEW	1846 SURDENT	51 PARK ST	BRISTOL	D941 L075
	1847 SURDENT	51 PARK ST	BRISTOL	D942 L075
	1848 SURDENT	51 PARK ST	BRISTOL	D943 L075
	1849 SURDENT	51 PARK ST	BRISTOL	D944 L075
	1850 SURDENT	51 PARK ST	BRISTOL	D946 L075
	1851 SURDENT	51 PARK ST	BRISTOL	D896 L075
	1852 SURDENT	51 PARK ST	BRISTOL	D897 L075
	1853 SURDENT	51 PARK ST	BRISTOL	D898 L075
SHEW & SHEW	1805 SURDENT	12 BELMONT	BATH	D112 L007
	1809 SURDENT	12 BELMONT	BATH	D113 L007
	1830 SURDENT	1 BLADUDS BUILDINGS	BATH	D119 L007
	1833 SURDENT	1 BLADUDS BDGS	BATH	D120 L007
SHEW & SON	1809 SURDENT	12 BELMONT	BATH	D046 L011
	1830 SURDENT	51 PARK ST	BRISTOL	D119 L020
	1832 SURDENT	51 PARK ST	BRISTOL	D930 L075
	1833 SURDENT	51 PARK ST	BRISTOL	D931 L075
	1834 SURDENT	51 PARK ST	BRISTOL	D932 L075
	1835 SURDENT	51 PARK ST	BRISTOL	D820 L002
SHEW (& FATH H)	1828 SURDENT	51 PARK ST	BRISTOL	D927 L075
	1829 SURDENT	51 PARK ST	BRISTOL	D821 L002
	1830 SURDENT	51 PARK ST	BRISTOL	D928 L075
	1831 SURDENT	PARK ST	BRISTOL	D929 L075
SHEW (& FATH)	1809 SURDENT	12 BELMONT	BATH	D046 L011
	1830 SURDENT	51 PARK ST	BRISTOL	D119 L020
	1832 SURDENT	51 PARK ST	BRISTOL	D930 L075
	1833 SURDENT	51 PARK ST	BRISTOL	D931 L075
	1834 SURDENT	51 PARK ST	BRISTOL	D932 L075
	1835 SURDENT	51 PARK ST	BRISTOL	D820 L002
SHEW (& FATHER R)	1837 SURDENT	BLADUD BDGS	BATH	D121 L007
	1841 SURDENT	BLADUD BDGS	BATH	D122 L007
SHEW (& SHEW)	1805 SURDENT	12 BELMONT	BATH	D112 L007
	1809 SURDENT	12 BELMONT	BATH	D113 L007
	1830 SURDENT	1 BLADUDS BUILDINGS	BATH	D119 L007
	1833 SURDENT	1 BLADUDS BDGS	BATH	D120 L007
SHEW C	1839 SUR DENT	51 PARK ST	BRISTOL *	D654 L068
	1840 DENT	51 PARK ST	BRISTOL	D143 L020
	1854 SURDENT	51 PARK ST	BRISTOL	D899 L075
	1855 SURDENT	51 PARK ST	BRISTOL	D947 L075
SHEW CHARLES	1848 DENT	51 PARK ST	BRISTOL	D125 L075
	1848 DENT	51 PARK ST	BRISTOL	DA50 L011
	1849 DENT	51 PARK ST	BRISTOL	D891 L068
	1850 DENT	51 PARK ST	BRISTOL	D960 L075
	1852 DENT	51 PARK ST	BRISTOL	D788 L020
	1853 DENT	51 PARK ST	BRISTOL	D802 L020
	1853 DENT	51 PARK ST	BRISTOL	D951 L075
SHEW CHARLES WEARE	1846 SURDENT	51 PARK ST	BRISTOL	D879 L072
SHEW G	1839 SURDENT	15 RODNEY TCE	CHELTENHAM	D654 L068
	1839 SURDENT	RODNEY TCE	CHELTENHAM	D957 L068
	1839 SURDENT	15 RODNEY TCE	CHELTENHAM	D832 L069
	1840 DENT	15 RODNEY TCE	CHELTENHAM	D143 L020
	1840 SURDENT	15 RODNEY TCE	CHELTENHAM	D833 L069
	1841 SURDENT	15 RODNEY TCE	CHELTENHAM	D834 L069
	1842 SURDENT	15 RODNEY TCE	CHELTENHAM	D835 L069
	1843 SURDENT	15 RODNEY TCE	CHELTENHAM	D836 L069
	1844 SURDENT	15 RODNEY TCE	CHELTENHAM	D837 L069
	1845 SURDENT	15 RODNEY TCE	CHELTENHAM	D838 L069
	1846 SURDENT	15 RODNEY TCE	CHELTENHAM	D839 L069

SHEW G	1847 SURDENT	15 RODNEY TCE		CHELTENHAM	D840 L069
	1848 DENT	15 RODNEY TCE		CHELTENHAM	D954 L069
	1848 SURDENT	15 RODNEY TCE		CHELTENHAM	D841 L069
	1849 DENT	15 RODNEY TCE		CHELTENHAM	D881 L082
	1849 SURDENT	15 RODNEY TCE		CHELTENHAM	D842 L069
SHEW GEORGE	1800 SURDENT	12 BELMONT		BATH	D111 L007
	1830 DENT	86 HIGH ST		CHELTENHAM	D119 L020
	1842 DENT	15 RODNEY TCE		CHELTENHAM	D846 L049
	1843 DENT	15 RODNEY TCE		CHELTENHAM	D955 L068
SHEW HENRY	1847 DENT	15 RODNEY TCE		CHELTENHAM	D890 L068
	1803 SURDENT	HANMER'S BDG PARK ST		BRISTOL	D903 L075
	1805 SURDENT	HANMER'S BDG PARK ST		BRISTOL	D904 L075
	1806 SURDENT	HANMER'S BDG PARK ST		BRISTOL	D905 L075
	1807 SURDENT	HANMER'S BDG PARK ST		BRISTOL	D906 L075
	1808 SURDENT	HANMER'S BDG PARK ST		BRISTOL	D907 L075
	1809 SURDENT	51 PARK ST		BRISTOL	D908 L075
	1810 SURDENT	51 PARK ST		BRISTOL	D909 L075
	1811 SURDENT	51 PARK ST		BRISTOL	D910 L075
	1812 SURDENT	51 PARK ST		BRISTOL	D911 L075
	1813 SURDENT	51 PARK ST		BRISTOL	D912 L075
	1814 SURDENT	51 PARK ST		BRISTOL	D913 L075
	1815 SURDENT	51 PARK ST		BRISTOL	D914 L075
	1816 SURDENT	51 PARK ST		BRISTOL	D915 L075
	1816 DENT	51 PARK ST		BRISTOL	D948 L075
	1817 SURDENT	51 PARK ST		BRISTOL	D916 L075
	1817 DENT	51 PARK ST		BRISTOL	D949 L075
	1818 SURDENT	51 PARK ST		BRISTOL	D917 L075
	1818 DENT	51 PARK ST		BRISTOL	D950 L075
	1819 SURDENT	51 PARK ST		BRISTOL	D918 L075
	1820 SURDENT	51 PARK ST		BRISTOL	D919 L075
	1821 SURDENT	51 PARK ST		BRISTOL	D920 L075
	1822 SURDENT	51 PARK ST		BRISTOL	D005 L020
	1822 SURDENT	51 PARK ST		BRISTOL	D921 L075
	1823 SURDENT	51 PARK ST		BRISTOL	D922 L075
	1824 SURDENT	51 PARK ST		BRISTOL	D923 L075
	1825 SURDENT	51 PARK ST		BRISTOL	D924 L075
	1826 SURDENT	51 PARK ST		BRISTOL	D925 L075
	1827 SURDENT	51 PARK ST		BRISTOL	D926 L075
SHEW HENRY & SON	1828 SURDENT	51 PARK ST		BRISTOL	D927 L075
	1829 SURDENT	51 PARK ST		BRISTOL	D821 L002
	1830 SURDENT	51 PARK ST		BRISTOL	D928 L075
	1831 SURDENT	PARK ST		BRISTOL	D929 L075
SHEW HENRY (SHOE)	1801 SURDENT	3 HANMER'S BDG PARK ST		BRISTOL	D902 L075
SHEW HENRY W	1842 DENT	51 PARK ST		BRISTOL	D846 L049
SHEW R	1819 SURDENT	1 BLADUDS BUILDINGS		BATH	D115 L007
	1824 SURDENT	1 BLADUDS BUILDINGS		BATH	D116 L007
	1826 SURDENT	1 BLADUDS BUILDINGS		BATH	D117 L007
	1829 SURDENT	1 BLADUDS BUILDINGS		BATH	D118 L007
	1846 SURDENT	10 BLADUD BDGS		BATH	D124 L007
SHEW ROBERT	1800 DENT	COLMORE ROW		BHAM	D300 L002
	1808 SURDENT	23 COLMORE ROW		BIRMINGHAM	D045 L002
	1809 SURDENT	23 COLMORE ROW		BIRMINGHAM	D046 L002
	1812 SURDENT	COLMORE ROW		BIRMINGHAM	D047 L002
	1815 SURDENT	COLMORE ROW		BIRMINGHAM	D048 L002
	1816 SURDENT	25 COLMORE ROW		BIRMINGHAM	D049 L016
	1816 DENT SUR	25 COLMORE ROW		BIRMINGHAM +	D049 L002
	1822 SURDENT	1 BLADUD BDGS		BATH	D005 L020

SHEW ROBERT	1840 DENT	1 BLADUD'S BDGS	BATH	D143 L020
	1842 SURDENT	1 BLADUDS BDGS	BATH	D123 L007
	1848 SURDENT	10 BLADUD BDGS	BATH	D125 L007
	1849 SURDENT	10 BLADUD BDGS	BATH	D126 L007
	1850 SURDENT	10 BLADUDS BDGS	BATH	D127 L007
	1852 SURDENT	10 BLADUD BDGS	BATH	D788 L020
	1852 DENT	10 BLADUD BDGS	BATH	D128 L007
	1854 DENT	10 BLADUDS BDGS	BATH	D129 L007
SHEW ROBERT & SON	1837 SURDENT	BLADUD BDGS	BATH	D121 L007
	1841 SURDENT	BLADUD BDGS	BATH	D122 L007
SHILLOCK J B	1851 DENT	HIGH ST	BROMLEY	DA77 L011
SIEMINS ADOLPHUS	1849 DENT	HIGH ST	LINCOLN	D333 L016
	1850 DENT	HIGH ST	LINCOLN	D013 L020
SIEMMS ADOLPH	1855 SURDENT	16 BELLBARN ROAD	BIRMINGHAM	D064 L002
SIGMOND	1796 SURDENT	35 MILSOM ST	BATH	DB23 L011
	1800 SURDENT	2 EDGAR BUILDINGS	BATH	D111 L007
	1801 SURDENT	2 EDGAR BDGS	BATH	DB49 L025
	1805 SURDENT	1 EDGARS BUILDINGS	BATH	D112 L007
	1809 SURDENT	1 EDGAR BDGS	BATH	D046 L011
	1809 SURDENT	6 YORK BUILDINGS	BATH	D113 L007
	1812 SURDENT	8 EDGARS BUILDINGS	BATH	D114 L007
	1819 SURDENT	8 EDGAR BUILDINGS	BATH	D115 L007
	1824 SURDENT	8 EDGAR BUILDINGS	BATH	D116 L007
SIGMOND I	1794 DENT	CHURCH YD	EXETER	D282 L011
SIGMOND JOSEPH	1822 SURDENT	8 EDGAR BDGS	BATH	D005 L020
SILVESTER G.I	1840 DENT	57 HIGH STREET	WORCESTER	D011 L001
SIME PETER	1844 DENT	3 GEORGE ST	DEVONPORT	D144 L008
	1844 DENT	3 GEORGE ST	DEVONPORT	D492 L022
SIMMONS ISAAC	1813 DENT CORN EXTRACTOR	57 HART ST	MANCHESTER *	D458 L020
SIMMS ADOLPH	1851 SURDENT	15 WORSHIP ST	HULL	D259 L010
SIMPSON (& ROSE)	1834 DENT	26 DUKE ST	LIVERPOOL	D405 L016
	1835 DENT	126 DUKE ST	LIVERPOOL	D406 L016
SIMPSON J	1855 DENT	CLARENDON PL	MAIDSTONE	D594 L046
SIMPSON JAMES	1846 DENT	66 GEORGE ST	MANCHESTER	D879 L072
	1850 DENT CUPPER	KING ST	MAIDSTONE *	D592 L045
	1854 DENT	CLARENDON PL	MAIDSTONE	DB82 L082
SIMPSON JOHN	1837 DENT	23 HARFORD ST	LIVERPOOL	D566 L020
	1837 DENT	23 HARFORD ST	LIVERPOOL	D407 L016
	1838 DENT	29 PICCADILLY	MANCHESTER	D470 L020
	1840 DENT	29 PICCADILLY	MANCHESTER	D471 L020
	1841 DENT	29 PICCADILLY	MANCHESTER	D331 L016
	1841 DENT	29 PICCADILLY	MANCHESTER	D472 L020
SIMS ROBERT	1833 DENT	ALBION STREET	BIRMINGHAM	D079 L002
	1842 DENT	51 CURZON PLACE	BIRMINGHAM	D075 L002
	1842 DENT	UNION PASSAGE	BIRMINGHAM	D075 L002
	1845 DENT	51 UNION PASSAGE	BIRMINGHAM	D077 L002
	1846 DENT	51 UNION PASSAGE	BIRMINGHAM	D879 L072
	1847 SURDENT	51 UNION PASSAGE	BIRMINGHAM	D061 L002
	1849 SURDENT	51 UNION PASSAGE	BIRMINGHAM	D062 L002
	1849 SURDENT	HOME DIXONS LANE	BIRMINGHAM	D062 L002
	1850 DENT	51 UNION PASSAGE	BHAM	D013 L002
	1850 SURDENT	HOME DIXONS LANE	BIRMINGHAM	D063 L002
	1850 SURDENT	51 UNION PASSAGE	BIRMINGHAM	D063 L002
	1852 DENT	51 UNION PASSAGE	BIRMINGHAM	D078 L002
	1852 DENT	HOME SKIRT LANE	BIRMINGHAM	D078 L002
	1854 DENT	SKIRTS LANE	BIRMINGHAM	D069 L002
	1854 DENT	51 UNION PASSAGE	BIRMINGHAM	D069 L002

Name	Year/Type	Address	City	Ref
SIMS ROBERT	1855 SURDENT	HOME SKIRTS LANE	BIRMINGHAM	D064 L002
	1855 SURDENT	51 UNION PASSAGE	BIRMINGHAM	D064 L002
SINCLAIR	1845 DENT	WEST ST	BRIGHTON	DB70 L025
SINCLAIR & BEW	1832 DENT	116 ST JAMES ST	BRIGHTON	DB19 L011
	1833 DENT	116 ST JAMES ST	BRIGHTON	D583 L044
	1840 DENT	116 ST JAMES ST	BRIGHTON	D585 L044
SINCLAIR A	1851 DENT	22 WEST ST	BRIGHTON	DA77 L011
	1855 DENT	22 WEST ST	BRIGHTON	D594 L046
SINCLAIR ARCHIBALD	1839 DENT	57 OLD STEINE	BRIGHTON	D607 L047
	1839 DENT	57 OLD STEYNE	BRIGHTON	D584 L011
	1843 SURDENT	22 WEST ST	BRIGHTON	D600 L047
	1845 DENT	22 WEST ST	BRIGHTON	D606 L047
	1845 DENT	22 WEST ST	BRIGHTON	DA66 L011
	1846 DENT	22 WEST ST	BRIGHTON	D601 L047
	1848 DENT	22 WEST ST	BRIGHTON	D602 L047
	1850 DENT	22 WEST ST	BRIGHTON	D603 L047
	1852 DENT	22 WEST ST	BRIGHTON	D604 L047
	1854 DENT	22 WEST ST	BRIGHTON	D605 L047
SINGLETON & BOWDEN & BROTHERS	1833 SURDENT	WELLINGTON PL	BRISTOL	D931 L075
	1833 SURDENT	17 LR MAUDLIN ST	BRISTOL	D931 L075
SINGLETON JOHN.AUGUSTUS	1830 DENT	25 HIGH STREET	WORCESTER	D006 L001
SINGLETON W	1840 DENT WHOMECH	1 FOREGATE STREET	WORCESTER*	D011 L001
SINGLETON WALTER (& W R H)DEN	1840 1 FOREGATE STREET WORCESTER			010 L001
SINGLETON WILLIAM.ROBERT.HENR	1840 DENTW	1 FOREGATE ST	WORCS	D010 L001
SLATER J MCQ	1854 DENT	ALBION ST	HANLEY	D015 L001
SMALE CHARLES	1848 DENT	18 BOND ST	MANCHESTER	D475 L020
	1848 DENT	18 BOND ST	MANCHESTER	D332 L016
	1850 DENT	59 PICCADILLY	MANCHESTER	D476 L020
	1851 DENT	59 PICCADILLY	MANCHESTER	D567 L020
	1852 DENT	59 PICCADILLY	MANCHESTER	D477 L020
	1852 DENT	59 PICCADILLY	MANCHESTER	D216 L009
	1855 DENT	59 PICCADILLY	MANCHESTER	D478 L020
SMART J S	1855 DENT		CARDIFF (OCC)	DC47 L085
SMARTT G G	1851 DENT	BAKER ST	ENFIELD	DA77 L011
SMARTT T	1850 DENT	48 HARMER ST	GRAVESEND	DC17 L084
SMITH (& FATH R)	1834 DENT	61 ST JAMES ST	LIVERPOOL	D236 L009
	1834 DENT	125 TITHEBARN ST	LIVERPOOL	D236 L009
SMITH E (& H)	1855 DENT	16 PORTLAND PL	NEWCASTLE	D223 L009
SMITH FREDERICK	1847 SURDENT	22B BOND ST	LEEDS	D276 L015
SMITH H & E	1855 DENT	16 PORTLAND PL	NEWCASTLE	D223 L009
SMITH ISAAC	1839 DENT	40 ALL SAINTS ST	HASTINGS	D584 L011
SMITH J C	1855 DENT	1 HAMOND PL	CHATHAM	D594 L046
SMITH ROWLAND	1846 DENT	MILL ST	LIVERPOOL	D303 L014
	1848 DENT	3 HILL ST & MILL ST	LIVERPOOL	D332 L016
SMITH ROWLAND & SON	1834 DENT	125 TITHEBARN ST	LIVERPOOL	D236 L009
	1834 DENT	61 ST JAMES ST	LIVERPOOL	D236 L009
SMITH S E	1850 DENT	48 BLACKETT ST	NEWCASTLE	D214 L009
SMITH WILLIAM	1828 DENT	36 BOLD ST	LIVERPOOL	D025 L020
	1828 DENT	36 BOLD ST	LIVERPOOL	D403 L016
	1829 DENT	30 BOLD ST	LIVERPOOL	D404 L016
	1832 DENT	41 BOLD ST	LIVERPOOL	D445 L016
	1834 DENT	43 BOLD ST	LIVERPOOL	D405 L016
	1834 DENT	41 BOLD ST	LIVERPOOL	D236 L009
	1835 DENT	44 BOLD ST	LIVERPOOL	D406 L016
	1837 DENT	44 BOLD ST	LIVERPOOL	D566 L020
	1837 DENT	45 BOLD ST	LIVERPOOL	D407 L016
	1839 DENT	89 BOLD ST	LIVERPOOL	D408 L016

SMITH WILLIAM	1841 DENT	89 BOLD ST	LIVERPOOL	D409 L016
	1843 DENT	89 BOLD ST	LIVERPOOL	D410 L016
	1843 DENT	12 HAMILTON ST	BIRKENHEAD	D410 L016
	1843 DENT		BIRKENHEAD	D434 L019
	1843 DENT	89 BOLD ST	LIVERPOOL	D434 L019
	1843 DENT	PRICE ST	BIRKENHEAD	D964 L076
	1845 DENT	34 CHURCH ST	BIRKENHEAD	D965 L076
	1845 DENT	34 CHURCH ST	BIRKENHEAD	D411 L016
	1845 DENT	89 BOLD ST	LIVERPOOL	D411 L016
	1846 DENT	89 BOLD ST	LIVERPOOL	D303 L014
	1846 DENT	89 BOLD ST	LIVERPOOL	D879 L072
	1847 DENT	89 BOLD ST	LIVERPOOL	D412 L016
	1848 DENT	12 COLQUITT ST	LIVERPOOL	D332 L016
	1849 DENT	12 COLQUITT ST	LIVERPOOL	D413 L016
	1849 DENT	34 CHURCH ST	BIRKENHEAD	D413 L016
	1851 DENT	12 COLQUITT ST	LIVERPOOL	D414 L016
	1851 DENT	12 COLQUITT ST	LIVERPOOL	D438 L020
	1852 DENT	12 COLQUITT ST	LIVERPOOL	D216 L009
	1853 DENT	62 BOLD ST	LIVERPOOL	D415 L016
SMITH WILLIAM G	1855 DENT	62 BOLD ST	LIVERPOOL	D416 L016
SNAPE	1840 DENT	NEWGATE ST	CHESTER	D718 L061
SNAPE J	1840 DENT	NEWGATE ST	CHESTER	D734 L063
SNAPE JOSEPH	1843 DENT	NEWGATE ST	CHESTER	D434 L019
	1846 DENT	NEWGATE ST	CHESTER	D303 L014
	1846 DENT	NEWGATE ST	CHESTER	D713 L061
	1848 DENT	NEWGATE ST	CHESTER	D332 L016
	1850 DENT	LOWER BRIDGE ST	CHESTER	D709 L034
SNELL H B	1852 DENT	92 UNION ST	STONEHOUSE	D493 L022
SNELL HARRY B	1850 DENT	92 UNION ST	STONEHOUSE	D147 L008
SOUTHAM	1840 DENT	36 BATH ST	LEAMINGTON	D307 L014
	1841 DENT	36 BATH ST	LEAMINGTON	D306 L014
	1842 CUPPER SURDENT	36 BATH ST	LEAMINGTON	D305 L014
SOUTHAM HENRY	1841 DENT CUPPER	36 BATH ST	LEAMINGTON *	D028 L002
SPENCE DAVID	1845 DENT		TURNHAM GREEN	DA66 L011
SPENCER JOHN N	1847 SURDENT	CORN MARKET ST	OXFORD	D815 L002
SPENCER JOHN NORMAN	1846 SURDENT	141 HIGH ST	OXFORD	D640 L050
SPENCER NORMAN	1851 DENT	63 HIGH ST	OXFORD	DA42 L011
	1852 SURDENT	63 HIGH ST	OXFORD	D645 L050
SPICER HENRY	1845 DENT		STOCKWELL PLACE	DA66 L011
SPURGIN J C	1849 DENT	1 WELLINGTON ST	LEAMINGTON	D310 L014
SPURGIN JOSEPH CAKEBREAD	1850 DENT CUPPER	1 WELLINGTON ST	LEAMINGTON *	D013 L002A
SPURR (& LUKYN)	1850 DENT	7 BROAD ST	NOTTINGHAM	D013 L020
SPURR JOSEPH	1834 DENT	BROAD ST	NOTTINGHAM	D502 L023
	1840 DENT	BROAD ST	NOTTINGHAM	D503 L023
	1841 DENT	BROAD ST	NOTTINGHAM	D331 L016
SQUIRE W	1855 DENT		HANWELL	D594 L046
ST CROIX DUNCAN & ROGERS	1843 DENT	29 DICKINSON ST	MANCHESTER	D473 L020
ST MARC M	1851 DENT	116 HIGH ST	CROYDON	D611 L048
	1851 DENT	116 HIGH ST	CROYDON	DA77 L011
STAMBURY N	1851 DENT	40 OLD STEINE	BRIGHTON	DA77 L011
	1852 DENT	40 OLD STEINE	BRIGHTON	D604 L047
	1854 DENT	40 OLD STEINE	BRIGHTON	D605 L047
	1855 SURDENT	40 OLD STEYNE	BRIGHTON	D594 L046
STANLEY WILLIAM	1846 SURDENT	HIGH ST	RUNCORN	D713 L061
STANLEY WILLIAM STAMER	1843 DENT	8 RUSSELL ST	CHORLTON	D473 L020
STANSFIELD JOHN	1806 SURDENT MD	26 UPPER PARK ST	BRISTOL *	D905 L075
STAVELEY	1847 DENT	MARKET PL	READING	D884 L049

STAVELEY W H	1847 DENT	23 MARKET PL	READING	D815 L011
	1854 DENT	10 MARKET PL	READING	DA71 L011
STAVELEY W H W	1853 DENT	10 MARKET PL	READING	D627 L049
STAVELEY WILLIAM H W	1854 DENT	10 MARKET PL	READING	D628 L049
STAVELEY WILLIAM HENRY	1852 DENT	10 MARKET PL	READING	D788 L020
STEER WILLIAM HOOKE	1844 DENT	26 ABOVE BAR ST	SOUTHAMPTON	D144 L068
STEERE W H	1848 DENT	26 ABOVE BAR ST	SOUTHAMPTON	D357 L017
	1849 DENT	26 ABOVE BAR	SOUTHAMPTON	D341 L017
	1849 DENT	26 ABOVE BAR	SOUTHAMPTON	D345 L017
STEERE WILLIAM H	1847 DENT	26 ABOVE BAR	SOUTHAMPTON	D340 L017
STEPHENS (& WHITE)	1851 SURDENT	5 NELSON ST	BRISTOL	D896 L075
	1852 SURDENT	5 NELSON ST	BRISTOL	D897 L075
	1853 DENT	5 NELSON ST	BRISTOL	D951 L075
	1853 SURDENT	5 NELSON ST	BRISTOL	D898 L075
	1854 SURDENT	15 COLLEGE GREEN	BRISTOL	D899 L075
	1855 SURDENT	15 COLLEGE GREEN	BRISTOL	D947 L075
STEPHENS J C	1852 DENT	35 ST AUBYN ST	DEVONPORT	D493 L022
STEPHENS JAMES C	1844 DENT	35 ST AUBYN ST	DEVONPORT	D144 L008
	1844 DENT	35 ST AUBYN ST	DEVONPORT	D492 L022
	1850 SURDENT	35 ST AUBYN ST	DEVONPORT	D147 L008
	1852 DENT	35 ST AUBYN ST	DEVONPORT	D788 L020
	1852 DENT	35 ST AUBYN ST	DEVONPORT	D145 L008
STEPHENS JOHN C	1840 SURDENT	9 PRINCES ST	DEVONPORT	D143 L020
STEPHENS JOHN HARRIS	1850 DENT	16 ST ANDREWS ST	PLYMOUTH	D147 L008
	1852 DENT	BUCKWELL ST	PLYMOUTH	D145 L008
	1852 DENT	BUCKWELL ST	PLYMOUTH	D788 L020
STEPHENS NATHANIEL	1847 SURDENT	ST MARY ST	TRURO	DC64 L067
STEPHENS NATHANIEL COOPER	1852 DENT	ST MARY ST	TRURO	D788 L020
STEVENS (& WHITE)	1853 DENT	5 NELSON ST	BRISTOL	D802 L020
STEVENS AUGUSTUS	1831 DENT	GRANBY ST	LEICESTER	D501 L024
STEWARD	1843 DENT		SOUTHAMPTON	D338 L017
STEWART C	1840 SURDENT	6 NICHOLAS ST	BRISTOL	D945 L075
	1841 SURDENT	NICHOLAS ST	BRISTOL	D937 L075
	1842 SURDENT	NICHOLAS ST	BRISTOL	D938 L075
	1843 SURDENT	NICHOLAS ST	BRISTOL	D939 L075
	1844 SURDENT	NICHOLAS ST	BRISTOL	D940 L075
	1845 SURDENT	NICHOLAS ST	BRISTOL	D822 L002
	1847 SURDENT	KING SQ AVE	BRISTOL	D942 L075
	1848 SURDENT	KING SQ AVE	BRISTOL	D943 L075
	1849 SURDENT	KING SQ AVE	BRISTOL	D944 L075
	1850 SURDENT	KING SQ AVE	BRISTOL	D946 L075
	1851 SURDENT	KING SQ AVE	BRISTOL	D896 L075
	1852 SURDENT	KING SQ AVE	BRISTOL	D897 L075
	1853 SURDENT	KING SQ AVE	BRISTOL	D898 L075
	1854 SURDENT	KING SQ AVE	BRISTOL	D899 L075
	1855 SURDENT	KING SQ AVE	BRISTOL	D947 L075
STEWART CHARLES	1838 SURDENT	6 NICHOLAS ST	BRISTOL	D935 L075
	1839 SURDENT	6 NICHOLAS ST	BRISTOL	D936 L075
	1842 DENT	6 NICHOLAS ST	BRISTOL	DB46 L049
	1846 SURDENT	16 WILSON ST	BRISTOL	D879 L072
	1848 DENT	KING SQ AVE	BRISTOL	DA50 L011
	1848 DENT	KING SQ AVE	BRISTOL	D125 L075
	1849 DENT	KING SQ AVE	BRISTOL	D891 L068
	1850 DENT	KING SQ AVE	BRISTOL	D960 L075
	1850 SURDENT	POWIS ST	WOOLWICH	DA75 L011
	1852 DENT	KING'S SQ AVENUE	BRISTOL	D788 L020
	1853 DENT	KING SQ AVE	BRISTOL	D951 L075

STEWART CHARLES	1853 DENT	KING SG AVE	BRISTOL	D802 L020
STEWART M	1833 SURDENT	6 NICHOLAS ST	BRISTOL	D931 L075
	1834 SURDENT	6 NICHOLAS ST	BRISTOL	D932 L075
	1835 SURDENT	6 NICHOLAS ST	BRISTOL	D820 L002
	1836 SURDENT	6 NICHOLAS ST	BRISTOL	D933 L075
STEWART MARK	1828 SURDENT	6 NICHOLAS ST	BRISTOL	D927 L075
	1829 SURDENT	6 NICHOLAS ST	BRISTOL	D821 L002
	1830 SURDENT	6 NICHOLAS ST	BRISTOL	D928 L075
	1831 SURDENT	6 NICHOLAS ST	BRISTOL	D929 L075
	1832 SURDENT	6 NICHOLAS ST	BRISTOL	D930 L075
STEWART ROBERT E	1855 DENT	3 MONA ST	LIVERPOOL	D416 L016
STOKES	1848 SURDENT	HIGH ST	BANBURY	DA93 L011
STOKES & PHILLIPS	1851 SURDENT	51 BLACKETT ST	NEWCASTLE	D215 L009
	1855 DENT	51 BLACKETT ST	NEWCASTLE	D222 L009
STOKES H C	1841 SUR DENT	51 BLACKETT ST	NEWCASTLE*	D241 L009
	1844 DENT	51 BLACKETT ST	NEWCASTLE	D213 L009
	1850 DENT	51 BLACKETT ST	NEWCASTLE	D214 L009
	1853 DENT	51 BLACKETT ST	NEWCASTLE	D243 L009
	1855 DENT	43 BLACKETT ST	NEWCASTLE	D223 L009
	1855 DENT	51 BLACKETT ST	NEWCASTLE	D219 L009
STOKES HENRY	1836 DENT	40 BLACKETT ST	NEWCASTLE	D834 L011
	1838 SURDENT	40 BLACKETT ST	NEWCASTLE	D239 L009
STOKES HENRY C	1833 DENT	SAVILLE ROW	NEWCASTLE	D246 L009
	1834 DENT	35 BLACKETT ST	NEWCASTLE	D236 L009
	1837 DENT	40 BLACKETT ST	NEWCASTLE	D566 L020
	1839 SURDENT	40 BLACKETT ST	NEWCASTLE	D240 L009
	1847 SURDENT	51 BLACKETT ST	NEWCASTLE	D242 L009
STOKES HENRY COLLIER	1848 DENT	51 BLACKETT ST	NEWCASTLE	D332 L016
STOKES HENRY COLLIN	1852 DENT	51 BLACKETT ST	NEWCASTLE	D216 L009
STOKES STANLEY	1847 SURDENT	63 HIGH ST	OXFORD	D815 L002
	1849 SURDENT	HIGH ST	BANBURY	DA94 L011
	1850 SURDENT	HIGH ST	BANBURY	DA95 L011
	1851 SURDENT	HIGH ST	BANBURY	DA96 L011
STOKES THOMAS	1847 DENT	11 GOSTA GREEN	BIRMINGHAM	D061 L002
	1849 SURDENT	11 GOSTA GREEN	BIRMINGHAM	D062 L002
	1850 SURDENT	11 GOSTA GREEN	BIRMINGHAM	D063 L002
	1850 DENT	11 GOSTA GREEN	BHAM	D013 L002
	1852 DENT SUR	11 GOSTA GREEN	BIRMINGHAM *	D078 L002
	1855 SURDENT	11 GOSTA GREEN	BIRMINGHAM	D064 L002
STONER H	1855 SURDENT	162 WESTERN RD	BRIGHTON	D594 L046
STONER H W	1852 DENT	35 TEMPLE ST	BRIGHTON	D604 L047
STONER HARRY	1854 DENT	162 WESTERN RD	BRIGHTON	D605 L047
STRANGE CHARLES	1852 DENT	112 STRETFORD RD HULME	MANCHESTER	D216 L009
	1855 DENT	122 STRETFORD NEW RD	MANCHESTER	D478 L020
STREET F	1840 DENT	HIGH ST	POOLE	D143 L020
STRINGER JAMES	1849 SURDENT BRICKLAYER	FARM STREET	BIRMINGHAM *	D062 L002
	1850 DENT	FARM ST	BHAM	D013 L002
	1850 SURDENT BRICKLAYER	FARM STREET	BIRMINGHAM *	D063 L002
STUART C	1855 SURDENT	43 POWIS ST	WOOLWICH	D594 L046
STUART CHARLES	1839 SUR DENT	NICHOLAS ST	BRISTOL *	D654 L068
	1840 DENT	NICHOLAS ST	BRISTOL	D143 L020
	1845 DENT	43 POWIS ST	WOOLWICH	DA66 L011
STYAN JAMES	1845 SURDENT	124 EAST ST	LEEDS	D275 L015
	1846 SURDENT	124 EAST ST	LEEDS	D713 L061
	1847 SURDENT	147 EAST ST	LEEDS	D276 L015
STYER	1845 SURDENT	ST GILES ST	NORTHAMPTON	D700 L060
	1847 SURDENT	ST GILES SQ	NORTHAMPTON	D701 L060

STYER A S	1839 SURDENT	ST GILES SQ	NORTHAMPTON	D584 L020
STYER ABRAHAM	1849 SURDENT	ST GILES SQ	NORTHAMPTON	DA79 L011
	1850 DENT	ST GILES SQ	NORTHAMPTON	D013 L020
	1852 DENT	ST GILES SQ	NORTHAMPTON	D702 L060
SUGGETT (& DUNSFORD)	1850 DENT	17 ST GILES ST	NORWICH	D652 L051
	1852 SURDENT	ST GILES ST	NORWICH	D653 L051
	1853 DENT	17 ST GILES ST	NORWICH	D655 L051
	1854 DENT	17 ST GILES ST	NORWICH	D651 L051
	1854 DENT	70 HIGH ST	KING'S LYNN	D651 L051
SUGGETT J	1853 DENT	TUESDAY MKT PL	KING'S LYNN	D655 L051
SULLIVAN CHARLES	1836 DENT	BROAD ST	NORWICH	D649 L051
	1839 DENT	POST OFFICE ST	NORWICH	D654 L011
SUMMERS J	1811 DENT	NUNGATE	NEWCASTLE	D237 L009
SUTCLIFFE JAMES	1853 SURDENT	26 WESTGATE	BRADFORD	D261 L010
SUTTON GEORGE WILLIAM	1849 DENT PATMEDDEALER	LEE ST	LOUTH *	D870 L056
SUTTON R C	1855 DENT	CANNON ST	LOUTH	D682 L056
SWINSON T	1845 DENT	12 DORVILLES ROW	HAMMERSMITH	DA66 L011
	1855 DENT	9 GROVE PL HAMMERSMITH	LONDON	D594 L046
SWINSON THOMAS	1839 DENT	12 DORVILL ROW FULHAM	LONDON	D584 L020
SYDER JOSEPH	1851 DENT	51 MT PLEASANT	LIVERPOOL	D438 L020
	1852 DENT	51 MT PLEASANT	LIVERPOOL	D216 L009
	1853 DENT	51 MT PLEASANT	LIVERPOOL	D415 L016
	1855 DENT	51 MT PLEASANT	LIVERPOOL	D416 L016
SYLVESTER G J	1850 DENT	9 FOREGATE ST	WORCESTER	D099 L011
SYLVESTER G.I	1837 DENT	57 HIGH STREET	WORCESTER	D009 L001
SYLVESTER G.J	1838 SURDENT	59 BROAD STREET	WORCESTER	D032 L005
SYLVESTER GEORGE	1855 SURDENT	AND	GREAT MALVERN	D016 L001
	1855 SURDENT	14 FOREGATE STREET	WORCESTER	D016 L001
SYLVESTER GEORGE JOSEPH	1840 DENT	59 BROAD STREET	WORCESTER	D010 L001
	1847 DENT	59 BROAD STREET	WORCESTER	D012 L001
	1850 DENT	9 FOREGATE STREET	WORCESTER	D013 L001
	1851 SURDENT	9 FOREGATE STREET	WORCESTER	D014 L001
SYLVESTER GEORGE.J	1853 DENT	14 FOREGATE STREET	WORCESTER	D031 L004
SYLVESTER GEORGE.JOSEPH	1841 DENT	59 BROAD STREET	WORCESTER	D028 L002
	1854 DENT	14 FOREGATE STREET	WORCESTER	D015 L001
SYLVESTER JOHN	1850 DENT	GREAT MALVERN	WORCESTERSHIRE	D013 L001
SYMONDS J W	1833 DENT	BATH ST	ST HELIER	DA80 L011
SYMONS JOHN	1836 DENT	11 OXFORD ST	NEWCASTLE	DB34 L011
	1838 SURDENT	11 OXFORD ST	NEWCASTLE	D239 L009
	1839 SUR DENT	11 OXFORD ST	NEWCASTLE	D240 L009

TALMA ARMAN	1793 DENT	WATERGATE	CHESTER	D281 L011
	1795 DENT	WATERGATE ST	CHESTER	D712 L061
TARRATT WILLIAM	1850 DENT	87 UNION ST	STONEHOUSE	D147 L008
	1852 DENT	87 UNION ST	STONEHOUSE	D493 L022
TAYLOR	1852 SURDENT	31 CHURCH ST	DURHAM	D287 L013
TAYLOR (& CHAMBERLAIN)	1855 DENT	124 HIGH ST	SUNDERLAND	D223 L009
TAYLOR JOHN	1853 DENT (SUR)	MARKET PL	NEWARK	D507 L023
TAYLOR THOMAS	1832 DENT	50 STAFFORD ST	LIVERPOOL	D445 L016
	1835 SUR DENT	BYE ST	HEREFORD *	D007 L014
	1850 DENT AURIST OCULIST	ASHBY RD	LOUGHBOROUGH *	D013 L020
	1855 DENT	ASHBY RD	LOUGHBOROUGH	D511 L023
TEARNE C.M	1820 SUR DENT	BRIDGE STREET	WORCESTER*	D004 L001
	1840 DENT	65 FOREGATE STREET	WORCESTER	D010 L001
TEARNE CHARLES	1798 DENT	TYTHING	WORCESTER	D279 L011
TEARNE CHARLES (JUN)	1788 DENT	HIGH ST	WORCESTER	DA46 L011
	1790 DENT	HIGH STREET	WORCESTER	D001 L001
	1792 DENT	HIGH STREET	WORCESTER	D002 L001
	1794 DENT	COOKEN STREET	WORCESTER	D003 L001
	1798 DENT	HIGH ST	WORCESTER	D279 L011
TEARNE CHARLES (SEN)	1788 DENT	TYTHING	WORCESTER	DA46 L011
	1790 DENT	TYTHING	WORCESTER	D001 L001
	1792 DENT	TYTHING	WORCESTER	D002 L001
	1794 DENT	TYTHING	WORCESTER	D003 L001
TEARNE CHARLES M	1828 SUR SURDENT	BALCONY HOUSE BRIDGE ST	WORCS*	D025 L002
TEARNE CHARLES.M	1822 PHY SUR SURDENT	5 BRIDGE ST	WORCESTER*	D005 L001
	1830 DENT	BALCONY HOUSE BRIDGE STREET	WORCS	D006 L001
	1835 DENT	HENWICK	WORCESTER	D007 L001
	1837 DENT	HENWICK	WORCESTER	D009 L001
	1837 DENT	HENWICK	WORCESTER	D008 L001
	1840 DENT	65 FOREGATE STREET	WORCESTER	D011 L001
	1840 DENT	HENWICK	WORCESTER	D011 L001
TEARNE T S	1850 DENT	54 FOREGATE ST	WORCESTER	D099 L011
TEARNE THEODORE	1851 SURDENT	BROAD STREET	WORCESTER	D014 L001
TEARNE THEODORE.S	1850 DENT	53 FOREGATE STREET	WORCESTER	D013 L001
	1853 DENT	BRIDGE STREET	WORCESTER	D031 L004
TEARNE THEODORE.SHELDON	1847 DENT MRCSL	63 FOREGATE ST	WORCS	D012 L001
THIRKETTLE T	1855 DENT	1 RICHMOND ST	BRIGHTON	D594 L046
THOM JOHN	1840 DENT	BELLEVUE TCE	DODBROOK	D143 L008
THOMAS C	1829 DENT	19 HATTON GDNS	LIVERPOOL	D404 L016
THOMAS CONOLLY	1827 DENT	37 SIR THOMAS BDGS	LIVERPOOL	D402 L016
	1828 DENT	19 HATTON GDNS	LIVERPOOL	D403 L016
THOMAS CONOLY	1824 DENT	37 SIR THOMAS BDGS	LIVERPOOL	D401 L016
THOMAS JAMES	1838 DENT	TYTHING	WORCESTER	D032 L005
THOMAS WILLIAM	1825 DENT	37 SIR THOMAS BDGS	LIVERPOOL	D444 L016
	1828 DENT	PRINCESS ST	SHREWSBURY	D025 L006
THOMPSON & HCPDURN	1853 GURDENT	LOW PAVEMENT	NOTTINGHAM	D507 L023
THOMPSON F	1855 DENT	NEW RD HAMMERSMITH	LONDON	D594 L046
THOMPSON JOHN N	1847 DENT	MIDDLE PAVEMENT	NOTTINGHAM	D505 L023
THOMPSON MS	1811 DENT	73 HIGH ST	SOUTHAMPTON	D334 L017
THOMPSON W	1840 DENT SUR	LOW PAVEMENT	NOTTINGHAM *	D503 L023
	1848 DENT	LOW PAVEMENT	NOTTINGHAM	D800 L020
THOMPSON W C	1828 SURDENT	1 ST MARY ST	WEYMOUTH	DA72 L011
THOMPSON WILLIAM	1823 DENT	BRUNSWICK PL	SOUTHAMPTON	D142 L017
	1825 DENT	LONG ROW	NOTTINGHAM	D500 L023
	1828 DENT	LONG ROW	NOTTINGHAM	D025 L020
	1830 DENT	ORCHARD ST	CHELTENHAM	D119 L020
	1831 DENT	LOW PAVEMENT	NOTTINGHAM	D501 L024

THOMPSON WILLIAM	1832 DENT	LOW PAVEMENT	NOTTINGHAM	D508 L023
	1834 DENT SUR	LOW PAVEMENT	NOTTINGHAM *	D502 L023
	1835 DENT	LOW PAVEMENT	NOTTINGHAM	D007 L014
	1841 DENT	LOW PAVEMENT	NOTTINGHAM	D331 L016
	1844 DENT	LOW PAVEMENT	NOTTINGHAM	D509 L023
	1844 SURDENT	LOW PAVEMENT	NOTTINGHAM	D504 L023
	1847 DENT	LOW PAVEMENT	NOTTINGHAM	D505 L023
	1848 DENT	LOW PAVEMENT	NOTTINGHAM	D506 L023
	1850 DENT	LOW PAVEMENT	NOTTINGHAM	D013 L020
THORN JOHN	1840 DENT	BELLE VUE TCE	DODBROOK	D143 L020
THORNE JOHN	1844 DENT	BELLEVUE TCE	DODBROKE	D144 L008
THORNTON FRANCIS	1825 DENT	PLATT ST	NOTTINGHAM	D500 L023
THORNTON WILLIAM	1837 SURAURIST DENT	SIDWELL ST	EXETER *	D166 L008
THWAITES J	1853 SURDENT	17 PARK ST	BRISTOL	D898 L075
	1854 SURDENT	17 PARK ST	BRISTOL	D899 L075
	1855 SURDENT	17 PARK ST	BRISTOL	D947 L075
THWAITES J H B	1850 DENT	48 PARK ST	BRISTOL	D960 L075
	1853 DENT	48 PARK ST	BRISTOL	D951 L075
	1853 DENT	48 PARK ST	BRISTOL	D802 L020
THWAITES JOHN H B	1848 DENT	2 KINGSDOWN PDE	BRISTOL	D125 L075
	1848 DENT	2 KINGSDOWN PDE	BRISTOL	D450 L011
	1849 DENT	2 KINGSDOWN PDE	BRISTOL	D891 L068
	1852 DENT	48 PARK ST	BRISTOL	D788 L020
TIBBS JOHN	1850 DENT	NELSON TCE	BARNSTAPLE	D147 L008
TIBBS JOHN MAY	1852 DENT	1 BEACH HOUSE	TEIGNMOUTH	D788 L020
	1852 DENT	26 STRAND	DAWLISH	D788 L020
TIBBS S	1839 SURDENT	REGENT ST	CHELTENHAM	D957 L068
	1839 DENT	58 REGENT ST	CHELTENHAM	D654 L068
	1839 SURDENT	58 REGENT ST	CHELTENHAM	D832 L069
	1840 SURDENT	58 REGENT ST	CHELTENHAM	D833 L069
	1840 DENT	59 REGENT ST	CHELTENHAM	D143 L020
	1841 SURDENT	58 REGENT ST	CHELTENHAM	D834 L069
	1841 DENT	10 NORTHGATE ST	GLOUCESTER	D830 L068
	1842 SURDENT	58 REGENT ST	CHELTENHAM	D835 L069
	1843 SURDENT	58 REGENT ST	CHELTENHAM	D836 L069
	1844 SURDENT	58 REGENT ST	CHELTENHAM	D837 L069
	1845 SURDENT	58 REGENT ST	CHELTENHAM	D838 L069
	1846 SURDENT	58 REGENT ST	CHELTENHAM	D839 L069
	1847 SURDENT	58 REGENT ST	CHELTENHAM	D840 L069
	1848 SURDENT	58 REGENT ST	CHELTENHAM	D841 L069
	1848 DENT	58 REGENT ST	CHELTENHAM	D954 L069
	1849 SURDENT	58 REGENT ST	CHELTENHAM	D842 L069
	1849 DENT	58 REGENT ST	CHELTENHAM	DB81 L082
	1850 SURDENT	58 REGENT ST	CHELTENHAM	D843 L069
	1851 SURDENT	58 REGENT ST	CHELTENHAM	D844 L069
	1852 SURDENT	58 REGENT ST	CHELTENHAM	D845 L069
	1853 SURDENT	58 REGENT ST	CHELTENHAM	D847 L069
	1853 SURDENT	58 REGENT ST	CHELTENHAM	D846 L069
TIBBS SOMERSET	1842 DENT	58 REGENT ST	CHELTENHAM	DB46 L049
	1843 DENT	58 REGENT ST	CHELTENHAM	D955 L068
	1844 SURDENT	58 REGENT ST	CHELTENHAM	D959 L069
	1847 DENT	58 REGENT ST	CHELTENHAM	D890 L068
	1850 DENT	58 REGENT ST	CHELTENHAM	DA74 L011
	1851 DENT	58 REGENT ST	CHELTENHAM	D953 L069
	1852 DENT	58 REGENT ST	CHELTENHAM	D952 L069
	1852 DENT	58 REGENT ST	CHELTENHAM	D788 L020
	1853 SURDENT	58 REGENT ST	CHELTENHAM	D956 L068

Name	Year	Type	Address		Town	Code	Code2
TINN G T	1850	DENT	4 NEW BRIDGE ST		NEWCASTLE	D214	L009
	1851	SURDENT	4 NEW BRIDGE ST		NEWCASTLE	D215	L009
	1853	DENT	4 NEW BRIDGE ST		NEWCASTLE	D243	L009
	1855	DENT	7 NEW BRIDGE ST		NEWCASTLE	D223	L009
	1855	DENT	4 NEW BRIDGE ST		NEWCASTLE	D219	L009
TINN GEO T	1847	SURDENT	74 GREY ST		NEWCASTLE	D242	L009
TINN GEORGE T	1852	DENT	4 NEW BRIDGE ST		NEWCASTLE	D216	L009
	1855	DENT	4 NEW BRIDGE ST		NEWCASTLE	D222	L009
TINN GEORGE TRISTRAM	1848	DENT	77 GREY ST		NEWCASTLE	D332	L016
TINN T	1844	DENT	75 GREY ST		NEWCASTLE	D213	L009
TITTERINGTON WILLIAM	1851	DENT	NEW RD		LANCASTER	D438	L019
	1855	DENT	NEW RD		LANCASTER	D222	L011
TITTERINTEN WILLIAM	1848	DENT	NEW RD		LANCASTER	D332	L016
TOMPSON F P	1851	DENT	SHEPHERD'S BUSH HAMMERSMITH		LONDON	DA77	L011
TOOTELL WILLIAM.HENRY	1852	DENT	6 HIGH STREET		BIRMINGHAM	D078	L002
TOWNSEND	1812	SURDENT	2 LOWER BOROUGH WALLS		BATH	D114	L007
TOWNSEND T	1819	SURDENT	2 LOWER BOROUGH WALLS		BATH	D115	L007
TOWNSEND THOMAS	1800	SURDENT	ABBEY CHURCHYARD		BATH	D111	L007
	1809	SURDENT	LOWER BOROUGH WALLS		BATH	D113	L007
TRACEY JOHN	1844	DENT	TACKET ST		IPSWICH	D667	L052
	1850	DENT	TACKET STT		IPSWICH	DA91	L011
TRACY J	1846	SURDENT	TACKET ST		IPSWICH	DA85	L011
	1853	DENT			IPSWICH	D655	L051
	1853	DENT	TACKET ST		IPSWICH	D655	L051
	1853	DENT	ABBEYGATE ST		BURY ST EDMUNDS	D655	L051
TRACY JOHN	1839	DENT	BROOK ST		IPSWICH	D654	L068
	1844	DENT	34 ABBEYGATE ST		BURY ST EDMUNDS	D667	L011
	1855	SURDENT	34 ABBEYGATE ST		BURY ST EDMUNDS TU	WD668	L011
	1855	DENT	TACKET ST		IPSWICH	D668	L052
TRIPE THOMAS	1840	DENT	19 GEORGE ST		PLYMOUTH	D143	L008
TROTTER F K	1855	DENT	GUILDHALL ST		LINCOLN	D682	L056
TUBBS C F	1850	DENT	3 PRINCESS PL		PLYMOUTH	D147	L008
TUBBS CHARLES F	1852	DENT	4 ATHENAEUM TCE		PLYMOUTH	D493	L022
TUBBS CHARLES FOULGER	1852	DENT	4 ATHENAEUM TCE		PLYMOUTH	D788	L020
	1852	DENT	4 ATHENAEUM TCE		PLYMOUTH	D145	L008
TUCK WILLIAM	1847	SURDENT	FORE ST		CAMBORNE	DC64	L067
	1852	DENT			CAMBORNE	D788	L020
TUPHOLME ANNE	1849	DENT	MARKET PL		SPILSBY	D870	L056
TURNBULL GEORGE	1850	DENT	3 VICTORIA PL		MANCHESTER	D476	L020
	1852	DENT	10 CHATHAM ST		MANCHESTER	D216	L009
	1855	DENT	12 CHATHAM ST		MANCHESTER	D478	L020
TURNER & WADE	1843	SURDENT	4 CONEY ST		YORK	D251	L010
	1846	DENT	4 CONEY ST		YORK	D258	L010
TURNER (& BLAIR)	1824	DENT	51 BOLD ST		LIVERPOOL	D401	L016
TURNER (& HORNER)	1822	DENT	CONEY ST		YORK	D255	L010
TURNER DANIEL	1828	DENT	77 NEWHALL STREET		BIRMINGHAM	D054	L002
	1828	DENT	77 NEWHALL ST		BIRMINGHAM	D023	L006
	1829	MECHDENT	77 NEWHALL STREET		BIRMINGHAM	D055	L002
	1830	MECHDENT	77 NEWHALL STREET		BIRMINGHAM	D056	L002
	1833	MECHDENT	77 NEWHALL STREET		BIRMINGHAM	D079	L002
	1835	MECHDENT	77 NEWHALL STREET		BIRMINGHAM	D057	L002
	1837	DENT (MECH)	77 NEWHALL ST		BIRMINGHAM	D566	L020
	1839	DENT	NEWHALL STREET		BIRMINGHAM	D083	L002
	1839	DENT	77 NEWHALL ST		BHAM	D301	L002
	1841	DENT	14 PARADISE STREET		BIRMINGHAM	D058	L002
	1842	DENT	14 PARADISE STREET		BIRMINGHAM	D075	L002
	1845	DENT	14 PARADISE STREET		BIRMINGHAM	D077	L002

TURNER DANIEL	1846 DENT		14 PARADISE ST	BIRMINGHAM	D879 L072
	1847 SURDENT		14 PARADISE STREET	BIRMINGHAM	D061 L002
TURNER JOHN	1828 DENT		4 CONEY ST	YORK	D025 L010
	1830 DENT		4 CONEY ST	YORK	D256 L010
	1834 DENT		4 CONEY ST	YORK	D236 L009
	1837 DENT		4 CONEY ST	YORK	D257 L010
	1840 DENT		4 CONEY ST	YORK	D734 L063
	1840 DENT		4 CONEY ST	YORK	D888 L006
	1841 DENT		4 CONEY ST	YORK	D241 L009
	1841 DENT		4 CONEY ST	YORK	D331 L016
	1851 SURDENT		39 GOODRAMGATE	YORK	D259 L010
TWEEDY JAMES	1839 DENT		5 KING'S PDE	CAMBRIDGE	D584 L020
	1839 DENT		KING'S PDE	CAMBRIDGE	D654 L068
TWYFORD THOMAS	1794 DENT PERF TOYMAN			LICHFIELD *	D282 L011
UNDERHILL S	1850 SURDENT BRICKLAYER		CHARLES HENRY STREET	BIRMINGHAM *	D063 L002
	1850 SURDENT BRICKLAYER		NEW THOMAS STREET	BIRMINGHAM *	D063 L002
UNDERHILL SAMUEL	1849 SURDENT BRICKLAYER		CHARLES HENRY ST	BIRMINGHAM *	D062 L002A
	1849 SURDENT BRICKLAYER		NEW THOMAS ST	BIRMINGHAM *	D062 L002
VANBUTCHELL MARTIN	1790 SURDENT		56 UPPER MOUNT ST	LONDON	D274 L011
VERNIER CHARLES	1835 DENT		69 MT PLEASANT	LIVERPOOL	D406 L016
	1839 DENT		13 ARCADE PASSAGE	LIVERPOOL	D408 L016
VIDGEN R	1846 SURDENT		BACK OF MARKET	BATH	D124 L007
VIDGEN ROBERT	1842 SURDENT		10 BARTON ST	BATH	D123 L007
	1854 DENT		8 UPPER BOROUGH WALLS	BATH	D129 L007
VINEN F A B	1851 DENT		184 HIGH ST	SOUTHAMPTON	D342 L017
VIRGIN HENRY J	1853 SURDENT		63 HIGH ST	OXFORD	DB80 L082
	1854 SURDENT		63 HIGH ST	OXFORD	D628 L049
VIZARD EDWARD	1855 DENT		BRUNSWICK PL	SCARBORO	D262 L010
	1855 DENT		10 VERNON PL	SCARBORO	D222 L009
	1855 DENT		BRUNSWICK PL	SCARBORO	D550 L031
WADE (& TURNER)	1843 SURDENT		4 CONEY ST	YORK	D251 L010
	1846 DENT		4 CONEY ST	YORK	D258 L010
WADE EDWIN	1848 DENT		4 CONEY ST	YORK	D332 L016
	1851 SURDENT		4 CONEY ST	YORK	D259 L010
	1855 DENT		4 CONEY ST	YORK	D222 L009
WADY JOHN	1798 DENT PRACT IN PHYSIC		LOWER MAUDLIN LANE	BRISTOL *	D900 L075
	1799 DENT PRACT IN PHYSIC		LOWER MAUDLIN LANE	BRISTOL *	D901 L075
	1801 DENT PRACT IN PHYSIC		LOWER MAUDLIN LANE	BRISTOL *	D902 L075
	1803 DENT PRACT IN PHYSIC		LOWER MAUDLIN ST	BRISTOL *	D903 L075
WAINWRIGHT JOHN	1845 SURDENT		3 PRICE ST	BIRKENHEAD	D965 L076
	1846 SURDENT		PRICE ST	BIRKENHEAD	D713 L061
	1847 DENT		44 PRICE ST	BIRKENHEAD	D412 L016
	1848 DENT		PRICE ST	BIRKENHEAD	D332 L016
	1849 DENT		44 PRICE ST	BIRKENHEAD	D413 L016
	1850 DENT		PRICE ST	BIRKENHEAD	D709 L034
	1851 SURDENT		3 PRICE ST	BIRKENHEAD	D799 L020
	1851 DENT		3 PRICE ST	BIRKENHEAD	D966 L076
	1851 DENT		44 PRICE ST	BIRKENHEAD	D414 L016
	1853 DENT		51 PRICE ST	BIRKENHEAD	D415 L016
	1854 DENT		3 PRICE ST	BIRKENHEAD	D967 L076
	1855 DENT		51 PRICE ST	BIRKENHEAD	D416 L016
WALKER F A	1851 SURDENT		BAXTERGATE	DONCASTER	D259 L056
	1855 DENT		GROVE ST	RETFORD	D511 L023
WALKER JOHN	1847 DENT		88 NORTHGATE ST	GLOUCESTER	D012 L001
	1849 DENT		88 NORTHGATE ST	GLOUCESTER	D891 L068
	1853 DENT (MECH)		88 NORTHGATE ST	GLOUCESTER	D951 L075
WALKER JOSEPH	1829 CHEM APOTH SURDENT		6 BROAD ST	BATH *	D118 L007

WALL R H	1853 DENT	OXFORD ST	READING	D627 L049
	1855 DENT		READING	DA90 L011
WALL ROBERT H	1854 DENT	13 OXFORD ST	READING	D628 L049
WALL ROBERT HENRY	1854 DENT (SUR & MECH)	13 OXFORD ST	READING	DA71 L011
WALLACE HENRY	1832 DENT	11 DUKE ST	LIVERPOOL	D445 L016
	1834 DENT	30 DUKE ST	LIVERPOOL	D405 L016
	1835 DENT	3 CORNWALLIS ST	LIVERPOOL	D406 L016
WALLER & MARTIN	1845 DENT	68 HIGH ST	GUILDFORD	DA66 L011
WALLER ROBERT	1854 DENT	PUMP ST	NORWICH	D651 L051
WAND JOHN	1828 DENT	GIBRALTAR ST	SHEFFIELD	D750 L066
WARD T	1854 DENT	HIGH ST	BEDFORD	DA71 L011
WARREN EDWARD P	1855 SURDENT	31 TEMPLE ROW	BIRMINGHAM	D064 L002
WARREN EDWARD PRITCHETT	1850 DENT	34 TEMPLE ROW	BHAM	D013 L002
WARREN EDWARD.P	1847 SURDENT	34 TEMPLE ROW	BIRMINGHAM	D061 L002
	1854 DENT	31 TEMPLE ROW	BIRMINGHAM	D069 L002
WARREN EDWARD.PRITCHETT	1849 SURDENT	34 TEMPLE ROW	BIRMINGHAM	D062 L002
	1850 SURDENT	34 TEMPLE ROW	BIRMINGHAM	D063 L002
	1852 DENT	31 TEMPLE ROW	BIRMINGHAM	D078 L002
WARRINGTON HENRY JAMES	1855 DENT	231 OXFORD ST	CHORLTON	D478 L020
WATFORD WILLIAM S	1845 DENT	31 BEDFORD SQ	BRIGHTON	DA66 L011
WATSON EDWARD	1790 SURDENT	12 LEICESTER ST	LONDON	D274 L011
WATSON JOHN	1830 DENT	63 WICKER	SHEFFIELD	D751 L066
WAWN & DOWNINGS	1820 SURDENT	NORTHUMBERLAND PL	NEWCASTLE	D787 L020
	1821 SURDENT	NORTHUMBERLAND PL	NEWCASTLE	D210 L009
WAWN C N	1824 SURDENT	NORTHUMBERLAND PL	NEWCASTLE	D238 L009
	1827 DENT SUR	1 NORTHUMBERLAND PL	NEWCASTLE*	D211 L009
	1833 DENT	1 NORTHUMBERLAND ST	NEWCASTLE	D246 L009
	1836 DENT	NORTHUMBERLAND PL	NEWCASTLE	DB34 L011
	1838 SURDENT	NORTHUMBERLAND PL	NEWCASTLE	D239 L009
WAWN CHARLES N	1811 SURDENT	NORTHUMBERLAND PL	NEWCASTLE	D237 L009
	1839 SURDENT	1 NORTHUMBERLAND PL	NEWCASTLE	D240 L009
WAWN CHARLES NEWBY	1828 DENT	1 NORTHUMBERLAND PL	NEWCASTLE	D025 L020
	1829 DENT	1 NORTHUMBERLAND PL	NEWCASTLE	D212 L009
	1834 DENT	1 NORTHUMBERLAND PL	NEWCASTLE	D236 L009
	1837 DENT	1 NORTHUMBERLAND PL	NEWCASTLE	D566 L020
WAY EDWARD	1849 DENT	BEDFORD HOUSE	TUNBRIDGE WELLS	DA69 L011
WAYLING G	1853 DENT	ANGEL HILL	BURY ST EDMUNDS	D655 L051
WAYLING GEORGE	1850 DENT	ANGEL HILL	BURY ST EDMUNDS	DA91 L011
	1855 SURDENT	ANGEL HILL	BURY ST EDMUNDS	D668 L011
WEALE THOMAS	1796 SUR DENT	61 CROSSHALL ST	LIVERPOOL *	D392 L016
	1800 SUR DENT	60 CROSSHALL ST	LIVERPOOL *	D389 L016
	1803 SUR DENT	60 CROSSHALL ST	LIVERPOOL *	D390 L016
WEBB J W	1855 SURDENT	ROBERTSON ST	HASTINGS	D594 L046
WEBOTE JAMES THOMAS	1837 DENT	30 NEWHALL ST	BIRMINGHAM	D566 L020
WEBOTE JAMES.THOMAS	1835 DENT	30 NEWHALL STREET	BIRMINGHAM	D057 L002
WEBSTER (& FATHER T)	1830 SURDENT	1 TEMPLAR'S ST	LEEDS	D256 L010
WEBSTER JAMES T	1832 DENT	17 SIR THOMAS BDGS	LIVERPOOL	D445 L016
WEBSTER THOMAS & SON	1830 SURDENT	1 TEMPLAR'S ST	LEEDS	D256 L010
WEEKES JOHN	1839 DENT	54 GEORGE ST	HASTINGS	D584 L011
WEIR J A	1855 DENT	56 PERCY ST	NEWCASTLE	D223 L009
WEIR JAMES ANTHONY	1855 DENT	56 PERCY ST	NEWCASTLE	D219 L009
WELCH W (JUN)	1851 DENT	WEST BY THAMES	KINGSTON UPON THAMESDA77 L011
WELCH W T	1855 DENT	WEST-BY-THAMES	KINGSTON	D594 L046
WELCH WILLIAM (JUN)	1851 DENT	WEST BY THAMES	KINGSTON ON THAMES DA83 L011
WEST WILLIAM WOOLLEY	1841 DENT	YORK ST	BOSTON	D331 L016
WESTALL FREDERICK	1846 DENT	62 BOLD ST	LIVERPOOL	D303 L014
	1846 DENT	16 GT GEORGE ST	LIVERPOOL	D879 L072

WESTALL FREDERICK	1847 DENT	62A BOLD ST	LIVERPOOL	D412 L016
WESTON W	1843 DENT	NORTHAMPTON ST	LEICESTER	D664 L024
WESTON WILLIAM	1842 DENT	NORTHAMPTON ST	LEICESTER	D662 L024
	1846 DENT	NORTHAMPTON ST	LEICESTER	D658 L024
	1849 SURDENT	NORTHAMPTON ST	LEICESTER	D661 L024
WHATFORD J T	1849 DENT	8 AMBROSE PL	WORTHING	D595 L046
	1850 DENT	8 AMBROSE PL	WORTHING	D596 L046
	1851 DENT	AMBROSE PL	WORTHING	DA77 L011
	1852 DENT	11 PRINCE ALBERT ST	BRIGHTON	D604 L047
	1854 DENT	13 PALACE PL	BRIGHTON	D605 L047
	1855 SURDENT	13 CASTLE SQ	BRIGHTON	D594 L046
WHATFORD W	1851 DENT	38 REGENCY SQ	BRIGHTON	DA77 L011
WHATFORD W S	1848 DENT	1 WESTERN TCE	BRIGHTON	D602 L047
	1850 DENT	38 REGENCY SQ	BRIGHTON	D603 L047
	1852 DENT	95 WESTERN RD	BRIGHTON	D604 L047
	1854 DENT	95 WESTERN RD	BRIGHTON	D605 L047
	1855 SURDENT	95 WESTERN RD	BRIGHTON	D594 L046
WHATFORD WILLIAM	1839 DENT	30 NORFOLK SQ	BRIGHTON	D584 L011
	1839 DENT	30 NORFOLK SQ	BRIGHTON	D607 L047
	1843 SURDENT	31 BEDFORD SQ	BRIGHTON	D600 L047
	1846 DENT	THE PRIORY WESTERN RD	BRIGHTON	D601 L047
WHATFORD WILLIAM S	1845 DENT	PRIORY LODGE WESTERN RD	BRIGHTON	D606 L047
WHITE & STEPHENS	1851 SURDENT	5 NELSON ST	BRISTOL	D896 L075
	1852 SURDENT	5 NELSON ST	BRISTOL	D897 L075
	1853 DENT	5 NELSON ST	BRISTOL	D951 L075
	1853 SURDENT	5 NELSON ST	BRISTOL	D898 L075
	1854 SURDENT	15 COLLEGE GREEN	BRISTOL	D899 L075
	1855 SURDENT	15 COLLEGE GREEN	BRISTOL	D947 L075
WHITE & STEVENS	1853 DENT	5 NELSON ST	BRISTOL	D802 L020
WHITE JOHN HAINES	1848 DENT	10 LEVER ST	MANCHESTER	D475 L020
	1848 DENT	10 LEVER ST	MANCHESTER	D332 L016
	1850 DENT	10 LEVER ST	MANCHESTER	D476 L020
	1851 DENT	70 LEVER ST	MANCHESTER	D567 L020
	1852 DENT	70 LEVER ST	MANCHESTER	D477 L020
	1852 DENT	10 LEVER ST	MANCHESTER	D216 L009
	1855 DENT	10 LEVER ST	MANCHESTER	D478 L020
WHITE R	1846 SURDENT	ST GILES ST	NORWICH	DA85 L011
	1846 SURDENT	THEATRE PLAIN	YARMOUTH	DA85 L011
WHITE RICHARD	1845 DENT	76 ST GILES ST	NORWICH	D650 L051
	1850 DENT	76 ST GILES ST	NORWICH	D652 L051
	1850 DENT	TUCK'S COURT ST GILES ST	NORWICH	DA91 L011
	1850 DENT	THEATRE ST	YARMOUTH	DA91 L011
	1852 SURDENT	ST GILES ST	NORWICH	D653 L051
	1854 DENT	ST GILES ST	NORWICH	D651 L051
WHITE W	1847 SURDENT	2 JOHN ST	BRISTOL	D942 L075
	1848 SURDENT	2 JOHN ST	BRISTOL	D943 L075
	1849 SURDENT	5 NELSON ST	BRISTOL	D944 L075
	1850 DENT	SOHO ST HANDSWORTH	BIRMINGHAM	D099 L011
	1850 SURDENT	5 NELSON ST	BRISTOL	D946 L075
WHITE WILLIAM	1848 DENT	5 NELSON ST	BRISTOL	DA50 L011
	1848 DENT	5 NELSON ST	BRISTOL	D125 L075
	1849 DENT	5 NELSON ST	BRISTOL	D891 L068
	1850 DENT	SOHO ST	BHAM	D013 L002
	1850 DENT	5 NELSON ST	BRISTOL	D960 L075
	1852 DENT CHEM	SOHO STREET HANDSWORTH	BIRMINGHAM ‡	D078 L002
	1852 DENT	5 NELSON ST	BRISTOL	D788 L020
	1854 DENT	SOHO STREET	BIRMINGHAM	D069 L002

WHITLOCK CHARLES	1811 SURDENT	NEWGATE ST	NEWCASTLE	D237 L009
WICKHAM W	1851 DENT	HIGH ST	TUNBRIDGE WELLS	DA77 L011
	1855 SURDENT	HIGH ST	TUNBRIDGE WELLS	D594 L046
WICKLAND FRANCIS	1795 DENT	CAPTAIN CAREY'S LANE	BRISTOL	D894 L075
	1797 DENT	CAPTAIN CAREY'S LANE	BRISTOL	D895 L075
	1798 DENT	CAPTAIN CAREY'S LANE	BRISTOL	D900 L075
	1799 DENT	CAPTAIN CAREY'S LANE	BRISTOL	D901 L075
WIGHTMAN ELLAM FOX	1846 DENT	143 FRIARGATE	PRESTON	D713 L072
WILCOCK J H	1838 SURDENT (MECH)	ST AUGUSTINE'S PL	BRISTOL	D935 L075
WILCOCK JOHN	1839 DENT CUPPER	30 HIGH ST	GUERNSEY *	D654 L011
WILCOCKS JOHN	1847 DENT	GEORGE ST	PLYMOUTH	D152 L008
WILDING THOMAS	1841 SURDENT	JOHN ST	STOCKPORT	D472 L020
WILDING THOMAS WILLIAM	1843 SURDENT	JOHN ST	STOCKPORT	D473 L020
WILDSMITH BENJAMIN	1788 PERR HD TDRAWER	HANGING DITCH	MANCHESTER *	D450 L020
	1794 DENT PERR HD	18 HUNTER'S LANE	MANCHESTER *	D451 L020
	1797 DENT PERR HD	18 HUNTER'S LANE	MANCHESTER *	D452 L020
WILKINSON COL	1840 DENT	13 TRAFALGAR ST	LEEDS	D734 L063
	1841 DENT	13 TRAFALGAR ST	LEEDS	D241 L009
WILKINSON MAJOR	1845 DENT	3 YORK ST	LIVERPOOL	D411 L016
	1849 DENT	3 YORK ST	LIVERPOOL	D413 L016
	1851 DENT	3 YORK ST	LIVERPOOL	D414 L016
WILKINSON WILLIAM	1854 DENT	CHARLES ST	LEICESTER	D660 L024
WILLIAMS C M	1842 DENT	GALLOWTREEGATE	LEICESTER	D662 L024
	1843 DENT	GALLOWTREEGATE	LEICESTER	D664 L024
WILLIAMS CHARLES MARCH	1835 DENT	GALLOWTREEGATE	LEICESTER	D007 L014
	1841 DENT	GALLOWTREEGATE	LEICESTER	D028 L002
WILLIAMS E	1854 DENT	ASPLEY GUISE	WOBURN	DA71 L011
WILLIAMS EDWIN	1850 DENT	ASPLEY	WOBURN	DA91 L011
WILLIAMS G S	1843 SURDENT	57 PARK ST	BRISTOL	D939 L075
	1844 SURDENT	57 PARK ST	BRISTOL	D940 L075
	1845 SURDENT	57 PARK ST	BRISTOL	D822 L002
	1846 SURDENT	57 PARK ST	BRISTOL	D941 L075
	1847 SURDENT	57 PARK ST	BRISTOL	D942 L075
	1848 SURDENT	57 PARK ST	BRISTOL	D943 L075
	1849 SURDENT	57 PARK ST	BRISTOL	D944 L075
	1850 SURDENT	57 PARK ST	BRISTOL	D946 L075
	1851 SURDENT	57 PARK ST	BRISTOL	D896 L075
	1852 SURDENT	57 PARK ST	BRISTOL	D897 L075
	1853 SURDENT	57 PARK ST	BRISTOL	D898 L075
	1854 SURDENT	3 CHESTERFIELD PL CLIFTON	BRISTOL	D899 L075
	1855 SURDENT	3 CHESTERFIELD PL CLIFTON	BRISTOL	D947 L075
WILLIAMS GEORGE S	1846 SURDENT	58 PARK ST	BRISTOL	D879 L072
	1848 DENT	57 PARK ST	BRISTOL	DA50 L011
	1848 DENT	57 PARK ST	BRISTOL	D125 L075
	1849 DENT	57 PARK ST	BRISTOL	D891 L068
	1850 DENT	57 PARK ST	BRISTOL	D960 L075
	1852 DENT	57 PARK ST	BRISTOL	D788 L020
	1853 DENT	57 PARK ST	BRISTOL	D951 L075
	1853 DENT	57 PARK ST	BRISTOL	D802 L020
WILLIAMSON W	1855 DENT	37 GALLOWTREEGATE	LEICESTER	D511 L023
WILLIAMSON WILLIAM	1846 DENT	16 GALLOWTREEGATE	LEICESTER	D658 L024
	1847 DENT	16 GALLOWTREEGATE	LEICESTER	D505 L025
	1849 SURDENT	GALLOWTREEGATE	LEICESTER	D661 L024
	1850 SURDENT	HO SPARKENHOE ST	LEICESTER	D013 L001
	1850 DENT	16 GALLOWTREEGATE	LEICESTER	D013 L001
	1854 DENT	GALLOWTREEGATE	LEICESTER	D660 L024
WILLIS WILLIAM E	1853 DENT	66 NORTHGATE ST	GLOUCESTER	D951 L075

WILLSON & SON	1841 SURDENT	12 PARAGON BDGS	BATH	D122 L007
	1842 SURDENT	12 PARAGON BDGS	BATH	D123 L007
	1846 SURDENT	12 PARAGON BDGS	BATH	D124 L007
	1848 SURDENT	12 PARAGON BDGS	BATH	D125 L007
	1850 SURDENT	12 PARAGON BDGS	BATH	D127 L007
WILLSON (& FATHER)	1841 SURDENT	12 PARAGON BDGS	BATH	D122 L007
	1842 SURDENT	12 PARAGON BDGS	BATH	D123 L007
	1846 SURDENT	12 PARAGON BDGS	BATH	D124 L007
	1848 SURDENT	12 PARAGON BDGS	BATH	D125 L007
	1850 SURDENT	12 PARAGON BDGS	BATH	D127 L007
WILLSON I	1833 SURDENT	13 PARAGON BDGS	BATH	D120 L007
WILLSON ISAAC	1822 SURDENT	13 PARAGON BDGS	BATH	D005 L020
	1837 SURDENT	12 PARAGON BDGS	BATH	D121 L007
	1849 SURDENT	12 PARAGON BDGS	BATH	D126 L007
WILLSON J	1840 DENT	PARAGON BDGS	BATH	D143 L020
WILLSON JOHN	1849 SURDENT	12 PARAGON BDGS	BATH	D126 L007
	1852 DENT	12 PARAGON BDGS	BATH	D128 L007
	1852 SURDENT	12 PARAGON BDGS	BATH	D788 L020
	1854 DENT	12 PARAGON BDGS	BATH	D129 L007
WILSON CHARLES	1837 DENT	57 BARKER'S POOL	SHEFFIELD	D566 L020
WILSON CHARLES W	1845 DENT	9 CLARENCE ST	LIVERPOOL	D411 L016
	1849 DENT	36 BOLD ST	LIVERPOOL	D413 L016
	1851 DENT	3 APPLE GROVE HIGH TRANMERE	BIRKENHEAD	D414 L016
	1853 DENT	1 BOLD PL	LIVERPOOL	D415 L016
	1855 DENT	1 BOLD PL	LIVERPOOL	D416 L016
WILSON CHARLES WILLIAM	1843 DENT	9 CLARENCE ST	LIVERPOOL	D434 L019
	1846 DENT	36 BOLD ST	LIVERPOOL	D303 L014
	1846 DENT	9 CLARENCE ST	LIVERPOOL	D879 L072
	1848 DENT	36 BOLD ST	LIVERPOOL	D332 L016
WILSON EDWARD	1849 SURDENT	160 SOUTH ST	SHEFFIELD	D756 L066
	1852 SURDENT		LITTLE SHEFFIELD	D260 L010
	1854 DENT	2 LITTLE SHEFFIELD	SHEFFIELD	D757 L066
WILSON GEORGE	1855 DENT	4 WHITEFRIARGATE	HULL	D222 L009
WILSON I	1819 DENT TO HRH DUKE OF	13 PARAGON BUILDINGS	BATH	D115 L007
WILSON ISAAC	1812 DENT	STANLEY PLACE	BATH	D114 L007
	1826 SURDENT	13 PARAGON BUILDINGS	BATH	D117 L007
	1829 DENT EXTR TO HRH DK	13 PARAGON BDGS	BATH	D118 L007A
	1830 SURDENT TO HRH DKE O	13 PARAGON BDGS	BATH	D119 L007
WILSON THOMAS	1850 DENT	19 BROAD ST	BHAM	D013 L002
WILSON W	1850 DENT	19 BROAD ST	BIRMINGHAM	D099 L011
WILSON WILLIAM	1843 DENT	10 CLARENCE ST	LIVERPOOL	D410 L016
	1852 SURDENT	25 ELDON ST	SHEFFIELD	D260 L010
	1852 DENT	5 CANNON STREET	BIRMINGHAM	D078 L002
	1852 DENT	25 ELDON ST	SHEFFIELD	D216 L009
	1853 DENT	71 KIRKGATE	WAKEFIELD	D261 L010
	1854 DENT	32 NORFOLK ST	SHEFFIELD	D757 L066
	1855 DENT	NORFOLK ST	SHEFFIELD	D222 L009
WILTON W	1855 DENT	10 FREDERICK ST	SUNDERLAND	D223 L009
WILTON W J	1857 SURDENT	6 VILLIERS ST	SUNDERLAND	D243 L009
WILTON WILLIAM JOSEPH	1855 DENT	10 FREDERICK ST	SUNDERLAND	D222 L009
WINCKWORTH & SON	1846 SURDENT	14 MILSOM ST	BATH	D124 L007
	1848 SURDENT	14 MILSOM ST	BATH	D125 L007
WINCKWORTH (& FATHER)	1846 SURDENT	14 MILSOM ST	BATH	D124 L007
	1848 SURDENT	14 MILSOM ST	BATH	D125 L007
WINCKWORTH (& HEATH)	1822 SURDENT	8 EDGAR BDGS	BATH	D005 L020
WINCKWORTH J	1833 SURDENT	3 EDGAR BDGS	BATH	D120 L007
WINCKWORTH JOHN	1829 SURDENT (SUCC TO SIG	3 EDGAR BUILDINGS	BATH	D118 L007

WINCKWORTH JOHN	1830	SURDENT	3 EDGAR BUILDINGS	BATH	D119 L007
	1837	SURDENT	3 EDGAR BDGS	BATH	D121 L007
	1840	DENT	14 MILSOM ST	BATH	D143 L020
	1841	SURDENT	14 MILSOM ST	BATH	D122 L007
	1842	SURDENT (FROM LONDON)	14 MILSOM ST	BATH	D123 L007
WINCKWORTH W D	1850	SURDENT	14 MILSOM ST	BATH	D127 L007
	1854	DENT	14 MILSON ST	BATH	D129 L007
WINCKWORTH WILLIAM	1849	SURDENT	14 MILSOM ST	BATH	D126 L007
	1852	SURDENT	14 MILSOM ST	BATH	D788 L020
WINCKWORTH WILLIAM DAWSON	1852	DENT	14 MILSOM ST	BATH	D128 L007
WINDER THOMAS	1845	DENT	142 LONG MILLGATE	MANCHESTER	D474 L020
	1848	DENT	1 ASHLEY LANE	MANCHESTER	D475 L020
	1848	DENT	1 ASHLEY LANE	MANCHESTER	D332 L016
	1850	DENT	1 ASHLEY LANE	MANCHESTER	D476 L020
WINDSOR THOMAS	1828	SUR DENT	65 LONG MILLGATE	MANCHESTER *	D464 L020
WINGATE	1826	SUR APOTH ACCOUCHEUR	9 YORK ST	BATH *	D117 L007
	1829	SUR APOTH ACCOUCHEUR	9 YORK ST	BATH *	D118 L007
WINKWORTH J	1819	DENT	3 RICHMOND PLACE BEACON HILL	BATH	D115 L007
WINKWORTH JOHN	1826	SURDENT	3 EDGAR BUILDINGS	BATH	D117 L007
WITHANALL EDWARD	1770	BLEEDER TOOTHDRAWER	16 LOWER PRIORY	BIRMINGHAM *	D033 L002A
WOLFF J	1855	DENT	5 SUSSEX ST	SUNDERLAND	D223 L009
WOOD	1845	DENT	127 ST JAMES ST	BRIGHTON	DB70 L025
WOOD BENJAMIN	1840	DENT	30 NORTH GATE	HALIFAX	D734 L063
	1841	DENT	30 NORTHGATE	HALIFAX	D241 L009
WOOD JOHN	1854	DENT	7 TRIM ST	BATH	D129 L007
WOOD R	1854	SURDENT	94 MILTON RD	GRAVESEND	DC35 L084
	1855	DENT	94 MILTON RD	GRAVESEND	D594 L046
	1855	SURDENT	94 MILTON RD	GRAVESEND	DC18 L084
WOOD RICHARD	1844	DENT	DOTWICH ST	NORTH SHIELDS	D213 L009
WOOD ROBERT	1848	DENT	7 GERMAN PL	BRIGHTON	D602 L047
	1850	DENT	7 GERMAN PL	BRIGHTON	D603 L047
	1852	DENT	3 PAVILION BDGS	BRIGHTON	D604 L047
WOOD W R	1851	DENT	38 HIGH ST	LEWES	DA77 L011
	1851	DENT	7 GERMAN PL	BRIGHTON	DA77 L011
	1854	DENT	3 PAVILION BDGS	BRIGHTON	D605 L047
	1855	DENT	3 PAVILION BDGS	BRIGHTON	D594 L046
WOOD WILLIAM ROBERT	1839	DENT	30 GRAND PDE	BRIGHTON	D607 L047
	1839	DENT	30 GRAND PDE	BRIGHTON	D584 L011
	1843	SURDENT	7 GERMAN PL	BRIGHTON	D600 L047
	1845	DENT	7 GERMAN PL	BRIGHTON	D606 L047
	1845	DENT	EAST ST	CHICHESTER	DA66 L011
	1845	DENT	27 NORTH ST	LEWES	DA66 L011
	1845	DENT	7 GERMAN PL	BRIGHTON	DA66 L011
	1846	DENT	7 GERMAN PL	BRIGHTON	D601 L047
WOODCOCK E	1849	DENT	2 OXFORD ROW	LEEDS	D277 L015
	1851	DENT	2 OXFORD ROW	LEEDS	D283 L015
WOODCOCK EDMUND	1843	SURDENT	54 ALBION ST	LEEDS	D275 L015
	1846	SURDENT	54 ALBION ST	LEEDS	D713 L061
	1847	SURDENT	22 PARK SQ	LEEDS	D276 L015
	1852	DENT	2 OXFORD RD	LEEDS	D216 L009
	1853	SURDENT	2 OXFORD ROW	LEEDS	D261 L010
	1855	DENT	2 OXFORD ROW	LEEDS	D222 L009
WOODCOCK H	1853	DENT	70 ST GILES ST	NORWICH	D655 L051
WOODCOCK HENRY	1830	DENT	24 ST GILES BROAD ST	NORWICH	D119 L020
	1836	DENT	8 TUESDAY MARKET PL	KING'S LYNN	D649 L051
	1836	DENT	BROAD ST	NORWICH	D649 L051
	1842	SURDENT	70 BROAD ST	NORWICH	D648 L051

WOODCOCK HENRY	1845 SURDENT	TUESDAY MARKET PL	KING'S LYNN	D650 L011
	1845 DENT	70 ST GILES ST	NORWICH	D650 L051
	1850 DENT	70 ST GILES ST	NORWICH	DA91 L011
	1850 DENT	70 ST GILES ST	NORWICH	D652 L051
	1852 SURDENT	70 ST GILES ST	NORWICH	D653 L051
WOODCOCK J	1853 DENT	GRANGE RD	GUERNSEY	DC68 L088
WOOFFENDALE ROBERT	1777 DENT	6 PARADISE ST	LIVERPOOL	D327 L016
	1781 DENT	6 PARADISE ST	LIVERPOOL	D328 L016
	1787 DENT	PARADISE ST	LIVERPOOL	D329 L016
WOOLFORD & CO	1853 SURDENT	541/2 KIRKGATE	LEEDS	D261 L010
WOOLFREYES HENRY	1850 DENT	ABINGTON ST	NORTHAMPTON	D013 L020
WOOLFRYES	1847 SURDENT	ABINGTON ST	NORTHAMPTON	D701 L060
WOOLFRYES HENRY	1849 SURDENT	ABINGTON ST	NORTHAMPTON	DA79 L011
	1852 DENT	ABINGTON ST	NORTHAMPTON	D702 L060
WOOLFRYES HENRY A	1847 SURDENT	ABINGTON ST	NORTHAMPTON	D815 L002
WOOLLEY W	1850 DENT	130 BROMSGROVE ST	BIRMINGHAM	D099 L011
WOOLLEY WILLIAM	1846 DENT	52 BROMSGROVE ST	BIRMINGHAM	D879 L072
	1847 DENT	130 BROMSGROVE STREET	BIRMINGHAM	D061 L002
	1849 SURDENT	130 BROMSGROVE STREET	BIRMINGHAM	D062 L002
	1850 DENT	130 BROMSGROVE ST	BHAM	D013 L002
	1850 SURDENT	130 BROMSGROVE STREET	BIRMINGHAM	D063 L002
	1852 DENT	130 BROMSGROVE STREET	BIRMINGHAM	D078 L002
WOOTTON WILLIAM	1853 SURDENT	6 HORTON ST	HALIFAX	D261 L010
WOOTTON WILLIAM TOW	1855 DENT	6 HORTON ST	HALIFAX	D222 L0099
WORFOLK GEORGE	1853 SURDENT	180 MARSH LANE	LEEDS	D261 L010
WORKMAN MAURICE	1842 DENT	150 FRIAR ST	READING	D625 L049
	1844 DENT	150 FRIAR ST	READING	D626 L049
	1847 DENT	150 FRIAR ST	READING	D884 L049
WRIGHT	1842 DENT	125 WARWICK ST	LEAMINGTON	D305 L014
	1845 SURDENT	125 WARWICK ST	LEAMINGTON	D309 L014
	1848 SURDENT	125 WARWICK ST	LEAMINGTON *	D308 L014
	1816 AUR ELECTR DENT CUPP13 BRIDGE ST		BRISTOL *	D915 L075
	1817 DENT	BRIDGE ST	BRISTOL	D949 L075
	1817 AUR ELECTR DENT CUPP13 BRIDGE ST		BRISTOL *	D916 L075
	1818 SUR AUR DENT	7 COLLEGE GREEN	BRISTOL *	D917 L075
	1818 DENT	COLLEGE GREEN	BRISTOL	D950 L075
WRIGHT (& FATH)	1816 AUR ELECTR DENT CUPP13 BRIDGE ST		BRISTOL *	D915 L075
	1817 AUR ELECTR DENT CUPP13 BRIDGE ST		BRISTOL *	D916 L075
	1817 DENT	BRIDGE ST	BRISTOL	D949 L075
	1818 DENT	COLLEGE GREEN	BRISTOL	D950 L075
	1818 SUR AUR DENT	7 COLLEGE GREEN	BRISTOL *	D917 L075
WRIGHT T	1845 DENT	CROSS CHEAPING	COVENTRY	D077 L006
WRIGHT T S (JUN)	1854 DENT	2 OSBORN PL	LEAMINGTON	D015 L001
WRIGHT THOMAS	1831 SURDENT	37 QUEEN ST	HULL	D380 L018
	1832 SURDENT	33 LOWER BYROM ST	MANCHESTER	D467 L020
	1833 SURDENT	33 LOWER BYROM ST	MANCHESTER	D468 L020
	1850 SURDENT	HERTFORD ST	COVENTRY	D063 L002
WRIGHT THOMAS SAMUEL	1850 DENT	HERTFORD ST	COVENTRY	D013 L002
	1850 SURDENT	HERTFORD ST	COVENTRY	D714 L002
YANIEWICZ FELIX	1832 DENT	44 BOLD ST	LIVERPOOL	D445 L016
	1834 DENT	54 BOLD ST	LIVERPOOL	D405 L016
	1834 DENT	43 BOLD ST	LIVERPOOL	D236 L009
	1835 DENT	51 BOLD ST	LIVERPOOL	D406 L016
	1837 DENT	51 BOLD ST	LIVERPOOL	D566 L020
	1837 DENT	56 BOLD ST	LIVERPOOL	D407 L016
	1839 DENT	130 BOLD ST	LIVERPOOL	D408 L016
	1841 DENT	60 MT PLEASANT	LIVERPOOL	D409 L016

YANIEWICZ FELIX	1843 DENT	60 MT PLEASANT	LIVERPOOL	D410 L016
	1843 DENT	60 MT PLEASANT	LIVERPOOL	D434 L019
	1845 DENT	60 MT PLEASANT	LIVERPOOL	D411 L016
	1846 DENT	60 MT PLEASANT	LIVERPOOL	D879 L072
	1846 DENT	60 MT PLEASANT	LIVERPOOL	D303 L014
	1848 DENT	60 MT PLEASANT	LIVERPOOL	D332 L016
	1849 DENT	60 MT PLEASANT	LIVERPOOL	D413 L016
	1851 DENT	60 MT PLEASANT	LIVERPOOL	D414 L016
	1851 DENT	60 MT PLEASANT	LIVERPOOL	D438 L020
	1852 DENT	60 MT PLEASANT	LIVERPOOL	D216 L009
	1853 DENT	60 MT PLEASANT	LIVERPOOL	D415 L016
	1855 DENT	60 MT PLEASANT	LIVERPOOL	D416 L016
YARNOLD THOMAS	1853 DENT	HIGH ST	CHEPSTOW	D951 L075
YOUNG	1855 DENT	CROCKHERBTOWN	CARDIFF (OCC)	DC46 L085
YOUNG F	1850 SURDENT	1 BELMONT CLIFTON	BRISTOL	D946 L075
	1851 SURDENT	1 BELMONT CLIFTON	BRISTOL	D896 L075
YOUNG F G	1854 SURDENT	5 UNITY ST	BRISTOL	D899 L075
	1855 SURDENT	5 UNITY ST	BRISTOL	D947 L075
YOUNG FREDERICK C	1853 DENT	53 PARK ST	BRISTOL	D802 L020
	1853 DENT	53 PARK ST	BRISTOL	D951 L075
YOUNG FREDERICK G	1850 DENT	1 BELMONT CLIFTON	BRISTOL	D960 L075
	1852 DENT	1 BELMONT CLIFTON	BRISTOL	D788 L020
YOUNG FREDERICK GRAHAM	1848 DENT	50 PARK ST	BRISTOL	DA50 L011
	1848 DENT	50 PARK ST	BRISTOL	D125 L075
	1849 DENT	50 PARK ST	BRISTOL	D891 L068
YOUNG G	1852 SURDENT	57 PARK ST	BRISTOL	D897 L075
	1853 SURDENT	5 UNITY ST	BRISTOL	D898 L075
YOUNG GRAHAM	1852 DENT	COMMERCIAL ST	NEWPORT	DA76 L011
	1853 DENT	5 UNITY ST	BRISTOL	D802 L020
	1855 DENT	64 CROCKHERBTOWN	CARDIFF (OCC)	DC47 L085

2.2 Directory codes

D	Date	Publisher	Norton Number	Short Title	Location
001	1790	Grundy	779	The Worcester Royal Directory	001
002	1792	Grundy	780	The Worcester Royal Directory	001
003	1794	Grundy	781	The Worcester Royal Directory	001
004	1820	Lewis	762	Worcestershire General & Comm. Directory For 1820	001
005	1822	Pigot	35	London & Provincial New Comm. Directory (Chesh, Derbys, Glos, Heref, Lancs, Leics, Lincs, Monm, Norf, Notts, Rutl, Shrops, Som, Staffs, Warw, Wilts, Worcs, Yorks, Wales)	020
006	1830	Pigot	738	Comm. Directories of Birmingham, Worcester and their environs	001
007	1835	Pigot	62	Directory of Derbys, Heref, Leics, Lincs, Monm, Notts, Rutl, Shrops, Staffs, Warw, Worcs, N & S Wales	014
008	1837	Pigot	-	Worcestershire Directory	001
009	1837	Stratford	783	Guide & Directory to...Worcester for 1837	001
010	1840	Bentley	768 775	History, Gazetteer, Directory and Statistics of Worcestershire	001
011	1840	Haywood	784	Directory of Worcester	001
012	1847	Hunt	370	Comm. Directory for Gloucester, Hereford, & Worcester....also of [other places in Glos, Heref, & Worcs.]	001
013	1850	Slater	86	Directory of [Derby, Heref, Leics, Lincs, Monm, Nhants, Notts, Rutl, Shrops, Staffs, Warw, Worcs.]	001
014	1851	Lascelles	785	Directory...of Worcester & Neighbourhood	001
015	1854	Kelly	121	P. O. Directory of Birmingham, Warw, Worcs, & Staffs.	001
016	1855	Billings	777	Directory...of the County of Worcester	001
025	1828	Pigot	47	Nat. Comm. Directory for 1828-9 (Chesh, Cumb, Derby, Dur, Lancs, Leics, Lincs, Nthumb, Notts, Rutl, Shrop, Staffs, Warw, Westm, Worcs, Yorks, N. Wales)	020
028	1841	Pigot	71	Nat. Comm. Directory of Warw, Leics, Rutl, [Nhants.], Staffs., Worcs.	002
029	1769	Gore	438	Liverpool Directory	016
030	1767	Gore	437	Liverpool Directory	016
031	1852	Slater	695	Classified Directory of the Manufacturing District 15 miles round Birmingham, incl. Worcester & the potteries	004
032	1838	Robson	107	Directory of the Western Counties [Glos, Heref, Monm, Shrops, Worcs, N & S Wales]	005
033	1770	Sketchley	700	Universal Directory for the Towns of Birmingham, Wolverhampton, Walsall, Dudley	002
034	1773	Swinney	701	The New Birmingham Directory	002
035	1776	Swinney	702	Birmingham Directory	002
036	1785	Pye	708	A New Directory for the Town of Birmingham and the hamlet of Deritend	002
037	1787	Pye	709	Birmingham Directory	002
038	1817	Baines	837	Directory, General and Commercial of Leeds	015
039	1791	Pye	711	Birmingham Directory	002
040	1826	Parson	838	General and Commercial Directory of Leeds	015
041	1800	Chapman	717	Birmingham Directory	002
042	1834	Baines & Newsome	840	General and Commercial Directory of Leeds	015

D	Date	Publisher	Norton Number	Short Title	Location
043	1803	Chapman	719	Birmingham Directory	002
044	1805	Holden	21	Triennial Directory for 1805, 1806, 1807	002
045	1808	Chapman	721	Annual Directory of Birmingham and its vicinity	002
046	1809	Holden	23	Triennial Directory for 1809, 1810, 1811	011
047	1812	Wrightson	724	New Triennial Directory of Birmingham	002
048	1815	Wrightson	725	Triennial Directory of Birmingham	002
049	1816	Wardle & Pratt	30	The Commercial Directory for 1816-17 containing [31 places in Lancs, Chesh, Yorks, and Leek, Birmingham and Wolverhampton]	002
050	1818	Wrightson	726	Triennial Directory of Birmingham	002
051	1821	Wrightson	727	Triennial Directory of Birmingham	002
052	1823	Wrightson	728	Triennial Directory of Birmingham	002
053	1825	Wrightson	729	Triennial Directory of Birmingham	002
054	1829	Pigot	737	Comm. Directory of Birmingham and its environs	002
055	1829	Wrightson	730	Annual Directory of Birmingham	002
056	1830	West	693	History, Topography and Directory of Warkswickshire	002
057	as 007				
058	as 028				
059	1772	Gore	439	Liverpool Directory	016
060	1842	White	796	Directory and Topography of Leeds and the Clothing District of Yorkshire	015
061	1847	Wrightson/Webb	735	Annual Directory of Birmingham	002
062	1849	White, F.	741	History & Geneneral Directory of Birmingham	002
063	1850	White, F.	694	History, Gazetteer & Directory of Warwickshire	002
064	1855	White, F.	696	General & Comm. Directory & Topography of... Birmingham including Aston etc. with Wolverhampton (etc.) & Dudley & Oldbury...	002
069	1854	Shalder	744	Birmingham Directory	002
075	1842	Wrightson/Webb	734	Directory of Birmingham	002
077	1845	Kelly	109	P.O. Directory of Birmingham, Warks., & part of Staffs.	002
078	1852	Slater	742	General & Classified Directory of Birmingham and its vicinities for 1852-3	
079	1833	Wrightson/Webb	731	Directory of Birmingham	002
081	1797	Pye	713	Birmingham Directory	002
082	1839	Haigh	841	General & Comm. Directory of Leeds	015
083	1839	Wrightson/Webb	733	Directory of Birmingham	002
098	1855	White	-	Directory of S. Staffordshire	006
099	1850	Kelly	116	P.O. Directory of Birmingham, Staffs., Worcs.	006
104	1851	White	650	History, Gazetteer & Directory of Staffs	006
105	1774	Gore	440	Liverpool Directory	016
109	1846	Williams	649	Comm. Directory for Staffordshire and the Potteries	006
110	1787	Bailey	253	The Bristol & Bath Directory	007
111	1800	Robbins	625	Bath Directory	007
112	1805	Browne	626	New Bath Directory for 1805	007
113	1809	Browne	627	New Bath Directory for..1809	007
114	1812	Wood & Cunningham	628	New Bath Directory	007
115	1819	Gye	629	Bath Directory	007
116	1824	Keene	630	Improved Bath Directory	007
117	1826	Keene	631	Bath Directory	007
118	1829	Keene	633	Bath Directory	007

D	Date	Publisher	Norton Number	Short Title	Location
119	1830	Pigot	53	Nat. Comm. Directory [Beds, Berks, Bucks, Cambs, Corn, Devon, Dorset, Glos. Hants, Heref, Hunts, Monm, Norf, Nhants, Oxon, Som, Suff, Wilts, S Wales]	007
120	1833	Silverthorne	634	Bath Directory	007
121	1837	Silverthorne	635	Bath Directory	007
122	1841	Silverthorne	636	Bath Directory	007
123	1842	Pigot & Slater	74	Nat. & Comm. Directory of Dorset, Gloucs, Heref, Monm, Oxf, Som, Wilts, with Derby, Shrops, Staffs, Warw, Worcs.	
124	1846	Silverthorne	637	Bath Directory	007
125	1848	Hunt	760	Dir. & Court Guide for the cities of Bath, Bristol, & Wells...	007
126	1849	Clark	638	Bath Annual Directory & Almanach	007
127	1850	Erith	639	Bath Annual Directory	007
128	1852	Vivian	640	A Directory of the City & Boro' of Bath	007
129	1854	Vivian	623	A Directory for the city & boro' of Bath, city of Wells, & towns of Bradford, Chippenham, Corsham & Lacock, Frome, Keynsham, Marshfield, Melksham & Trowbridge	007
142	1823	Pigot	36	London & Prov. New Comm. Directory [Lond., Middlesex, 300pl. in Beds, Berks, Bucks, Cambs, Corn, Devon, Dorset, Ex, Hants, Herts, Hunts, Kent, Nhants, Oxon, Suff, Surr, Suss.]	008
143	1840	Robson	105	Comm. Directory of London & the Western Counties [Berks, Corn, Devon, Dorset, Glos, with Bristol, Heref, Som, Monm, S. Wales]	020
144	1844	Slater	78	Royal Nat. Comm. Directory [Berks, Bucks, Corn, Devon, Dorset, Glos, Hants, Heref, Monm, Som, Wilts, N & S Wales]	068
147	1850	White	174	History, Gazetteer & Directory of Devonshire	008
149	1827	Trewman	178	Exeter Journal	008
150	1828	Besley	207	Exeter Itinerary & General Directory	008
151	1839	Trewman	189	Exeter Journal	008
152	1847	Besley	210	West of England Pocket Book	008
153	1853	Besley	211	West of England Pocket Book	008
154	1791	Trewman	-	Exeter Pocket Journal	008
155	1796	Trewman	-	Exeter Pocket Journal	008
156	1816	Trewman	176	Exeter Pocket Journal	008
157	1822	Trewman	-	Exeter Pocket Journal	008
158	1825	Trewman	177	Exeter Pocket Journal	008
159	1828	Trewman	179	Exeter Journal	008
160	1830	Trewman	180	Exeter Journal	008
161	1831	Trewman	181	Exeter Journal	008
162	1832	Trewman	182	Exeter Journal	008
163	1833	Trewman	183	Exeter Journal	008
164	1834	Trewman	184	Exeter Journal	008
165	1836	Trewman	186	Exeter Journal	000
166	1837	Trewman	187	Exeter Journal	008
167	1838	Trewman	188	Exeter Journal	008
168	1840	Trewman	190	Exeter Journal	008
169	1841	Trewman	191	Exeter Journal	008
170	1842	Trewman	192	Exeter Journal	008

D	Date	Publisher	Norton Number	Short Title	Location
171	1843	Trewman	193	Exeter Journal	008
172	1844	Trewman	194	Exeter Journal	008
173	1845	Trewman	195	Exeter Journal	008
174	1846	Trewman	196	Exeter Journal	008
175	1847	Trewman	197	Exeter Journal	008
176	1848	Trewman	198	Exeter Journal	008
177	1849	Trewman	199	Exeter Journal	008
178	1850	Trewman	200	Exeter Journal	008
179	1851	Trewman	201	Exeter Journal	008
180	1852	Trewman	202	Exeter Journal	008
181	1853	Trewman	203	Exeter Journal	008
182	1854	Trewman	204	Exeter Journal	008
183	1855	Trewman	205	Exeter Journal	008
210	1821	Pigot	34	Comm. Directory of Ireland, Scotland & 4 most northern counties of England for 1821-2 & 1823	009
211	1827	Parson & White	234	History, Directory & Gazetteer of...Durham & Northumberland	009
212	as 025				
213	1844	Williams	595	Comm. Directory of Newcastle upon Tyne, N. & S. Shields, Sunderland, etc.	009
214	1850	Ward	576	Northumberland & Durham Directory	009
215	1851	Ward	577	North of England Directory (Brampton, Carlisle, Darlington, Gateshead, Hartlepool, Middlesborough, Newcastle, N. Shields, Seaham, S. Shields, Stockton, Sunderland, Wigtown, Yarmouth)	009
216	1852	Slater	96	Royal, Nat. & Comm. Directory & Topography of Scotland and... Manchester, Liverpool, Birmingham, Leeds, Hull, Sheffield, Carlisle & Newcastle upon Tyne	009
217	1852	Ward	578	North of England Directory	009
218	1854	Ward	580	North of England Directory	009
219	1855	Whellan	582	History, Topography & Directory of Northumberland... Gateshead, Berwick on Tweed	009
222	1855	Slater	99	Royal, Nat. & Comm. Directory of the Northern Counties	020
223	1855	Ward	581	North of England Directory	009
236	1834	Pigot	61	Nat. Comm. Directory of the counties of Chester, Cumberland, Durham, Lancashire, Northumberland, Westmorland and Yorkshire	009
237	1811	McKenzie & Dent	590	Triennial Directory for Newcastle upon Tyne, Gateshead, etc.	009
238	1824	Humble	591	A General Directory for Newcastle upon Tyne, Gateshead [etc.]	009
239	1838	Richardson	593	Directory of Newcastle & Gateshead	009
240	1839	Richardson	594	Newcastle & Gateshead Dir. Advertiser; Supplement for 1839	009
242	1847	White	575	General Directory of Newcastle upon Tyne, Blyth, N. & S. Shields, Tynemouth, Durham [Co. & towns] & Berwick on Tweed	009
243	1853	Ward	579	North of England Directory	009
246	1833	Ihler	592	A Directory of the towns of Newcastle, Gateshead and their suburbs	009
251	1843	Williams	862	City of York Directory	010

D	Date	Publisher	Norton Number	Short Title	Location
255	1822	Baines	786	History, Directory & Gazetteer of the County of York	010
256	1830	Parson & White	788	Directory...of Leeds...York, and the Clothing District of Yorkshire	010
257	1837	White	790	History, Gazetteer & Directory of the W. Riding of Yorkshire with York and Hull	010
258	1846	White, F.	799	General Directory of Kingston on Hull & the City of York, with Scarborough	010
259	1851	White, F.	801	General Directory of Kingston on Hull & the City of York	010
260	1852	White	803	Gazetteer and Directory of Sheffield...20 miles round	010
261	1853	White	804	Directory & Gazetteer of Leeds...and the Clothing Districts of...Yorkshire	010
262	1855	Gillbanks	809	Directory & Gazetteer...of Scarborough etc. ...	010
272	1783	Bailey	2	Western & Midland Directory	011
273	1784	Bailey	3	British Directory	011
274	1790	Wilkes	8	Universal British Directory, Vol. 1	011
275	1845	Williams	842	Directory of Leeds	015
276	1847	White	800	Directory & Topography of Leeds, Bradford [etc.] & the Clothing Districts of the West Riding	015
277	1849	Charlton & Archdeacon	844	Directory of Leeds	015
279	1798	Wilkes	18	Universal British Directory Vol. 4	011
280	1847	Charlton	843	Directory of Leeds	015
281	1793	Wilkes	13	Universal British Directory Vol. 2	011
282	1794	Wilkes	15	Universal British Directory Vol. 3	011
283	1851	Slade & Roebuck	845	Directory of the Borough & Neighbourhood of Leeds	015
284	1811	Holden	24	Annual London & Country Directory of the United Kingdom & Wales in 3 vols.	011
285	1809	Robinson	836	Leeds Directory	015
286	1853	Walker	244	Durham Directory & Almanach	013
287	1852	Walker	243	Durham Directory & Almanach	013
289	1854	Walker	245	Durham Directory & Almanach	013
292	1851	Hagar	235	Directory of the County of Durham	013
297	1847	Walker	238	Durham Directory & Almanach	013
299	1800	Bisset	716	Poetic Survey round Birmingham	002
300	1800-08	Bisset	20	Grand Nat. Directory or Literary & Comm. Iconography	002
301	1839	Robson	739	Birmingham and Sheffield Directory	002
302	1818	Pigot	31	Comm. Directory for 1818-19-20 containing [about 52 towns in Midlands]	002
303	1846	Williams	754	Guide & Directory of Royal Leamington Spa, Warwick, [etc.]	014
305	1842	Beck	-	Leamington Guide	014
306	1841	Beck	-	Leamington Guide	014
307	1840	Beck	-	Leamington Guide	014
308	1848	Beck	-	Leamington Guide	014
309	1845	Beck	-	Leamington Guide	014
310	1849	Dewhurst	755	Directory of Royal Leamington Spa	014
311	1835	Fairfax	751	New Guide to Leamington Spa and its environs	014
312	1833	Fairfax	749	New Guide & Directory to Leamington Spa	014
313	1834	Fairfax	-	New Guide & Directory to Leamington Spa	014
314	1838	Fairfax	753	Guide, Directory and Almanach to Leamington Spa	014
315	1832	Fairfax	748	New Leamington Guide	014

D	Date	Publisher	Norton Number	Short Title	Location
316	1833	Merridew	750	Moncrieff's Guide to Leamington Spa	014
317	1837	Merridew	752	Improved Edition of Moncrieff's Guide to Leamington Spa	014
318	1822	Moncrieff	-	Visitors' New Guide	014
319	1824	Moncrieff	-	Visitors' New Guide	014
320	1829	Moncrieff	-	Visitors' New Guide	014
321	1822	Smith	-	Leamington Guide	014
322	1823	Sharpe	-	New Guide of Leamington & Warwick	014
323	1817	Sharpe	-	New Guide of Leamington & Warwick	014
324	1818	Sharpe	-	New Guide of Leamington & Warwick	014
325	1825	Sharpe	-	New Guide of Warwick & Leamington	014
326	1839	Reeve	-	Guide to Royal Leamington Spa	014
327	1777	Gore	441	Liverpool Directory	016
328	1781	Gore	442	Liverpool Directory	016
329	1787	Gore	443	Liverpool Directory	016
330	1814	Wardle & Bentham	29	Comm. Directory for 1814-15 containing...[31 places in Lancs, Ches, & Yorks and Leek in Staffs.]	016
331	1841	Pigot	70	Directory ...of [Yorks, Leics, Rutl, Lincs, Nhants, Notts, with Manchester and Salford etc.]	016
332	1848	Slater	83	Directory of [Ches, Cumb, Dur, Lancs, North, and Westm, and Yorks]	016
333	1849	Slater	84	Directory of Yorkshire & Lincolnshire	015
334	1811	Cunningham	358	Directory for Southampton	017
335	1834	Fletcher	359	Southampton Directory	017
336	1836	Fletcher	360	Directory of Southampton	017
337	1839	Fletcher	-	Directory of Southampton	017
338	1843	Cooper	361	P. O. Directory of Southampton	017
339	1845	Cooper	362	P. O. Directory of Southampton	017
340	1847	Forbes & Knibb	363	P. O. Directory of Southampton	017
341	1849	Forbes & Knibb	364	P. O. Directory of Southampton	017
342	1851	Forbes & Knibb	365	P. O. Directory of Southampton	017
343	1853	Forbes & Knibb	366	P. O. Directory of Southampton	017
344	1855	Forbes & Knibb	367	P. O. Directory of Southampton	017
345	1849	Rayner	368	Directory of Southampton	017
346	1852	Hunt	356	Directory of Hampshire & Dorset [with] Isle of Wight	017
357	1848	Kelly	113	P. O. Directory of Hampshire, Dorset, Wiltshire	011
365	1835	Craggs	826	New Triennial Directory & Guide of Kingston-upon-Hull	018
369	1823	Baines	-	Directory of Hull	018
371	1792	Battle	817	Appendix to the Hull & Beverley Directory	018
374	1826	White	825	Directory, Guide & Annals of Kingston-upon-Hull	018
375	1838	Noble	827	Directory of Kingston-upon-Hull	018
376	1839	Purdon	828	Directory of Kingston-upon-Hull	018
377	1842	Stephenson	829	Directory of Kingston-upon-Hull and its environs	018
378	1848	Stephenson	830	Directory of Kingston-upon-Hull	018
379	1851	Freebody	831	Directory of Kingston-upon-Hull	018
380	1831	White	789	Directory, Guide & Annals of Kingston-upon-Hull	018
389	1800	Gore	448	Liverpool Directory	016
390	1803	Gore	450	Liverpool Directory	016
391	1804	Woodward	451	New Liverpool Directory	016
392	1796	Gore	447	Liverpool Directory	016
393	1805	Gore	453	Liverpool Directory	016
394	1807	Gore	454	Liverpool Directory	016
395	1810	Gore	455	Liverpool Directory	016

D	Date	Publisher	Norton Number	Short Title	Location
396	1811	Gore	456	Liverpool Directory	016
397	1813	Gore	457	Liverpool Directory	016
398	1814	Gore	458	Liverpool Directory	016
399	1821	Gore	461	Liverpool Directory	016
400	1823	Gore	462	Liverpool Directory	016
401	1824	Baines	422	History, Directory & Gazetteer of the County of Lancaster	016
402	1827	Gore	464	Liverpool Directory	016
403	1828	Gore	465	Liverpool Directory	016
404	1829	Gore	466	Liverpool Directory	016
405	1834	Gore	469	Liverpool Directory	016
406	1835	Gore	470	Liverpool Directory	016
407	1837	Gore	471	Liverpool Directory	016
408	1839	Gore	472	Liverpool Directory	016
409	1841	Gore	473	Liverpool Directory	016
410	1843	Gore	474	Liverpool Directory	016
411	1845	Gore	475	Liverpool Directory	016
412	1847	Gore	476	Liverpool Directory	016
413	1849	Gore	477	Liverpool Directory	016
414	1851	Gore	478	Liverpool Directory	016
415	1853	Gore	479	Liverpool Directory	016
416	1855	Gore	480	Liverpool Directory	016
431	1816	Gore	459	Liverpool Directory	016
432	1818	Gore	460	Liverpool Directory	016
434	1843	Pigot & Slater	484	General & Classified Directory & Street Register of Liverpool	019
436	1844	Slater	77	Directory of an extensive manufacturing district around Manchester with...towns in Cheshire & Lancashire and the whole of N. Wales	019
437	1851	Mannex	757	History & Directory of Westmorland	019
438	1851	Slater	93	Classified Directory of Lancashire & the manufacturing district excepting Manchester	020
439	1854	Mannex	430	History, topography and directory of mid-Lancashire	019
440	1829	Parson & White	158	History, Directory & Gazetteer of Cumberland & Westmorland	019
441	1849	Mannex	756	History, Topography & Directory of Westmorland & Lonsdale	019
443	1847	Mannex	159	History, Gazetteer & Directory of Cumberland	019
444	1825	Gore	463	Liverpool Directory	016
445	1832	Gore	468	Liverpool Directory	016
449	1781	Raffald	489	Manchester & Salford Directory	020
450	1788	Holme	490	A Directory for Manchester & Salford	020
451	1794	Scholes	491	Manchester & Salford Directory	020
452	1797	Scholes	492	Manchester & Salford Directory	020
453	1800	Bancks	493	Manchester & Salford Directory	020
454	1802	Bancks	494	Manchester & Salford Directory	020
455	1804	Dean	495	Manchester & Salford Directory	020
456	1808	Dean	496	Manchester & Salford Directory	020
457	1811	Dean	497	Manchester & Salford Directory	020
458	1813	Pigot	499	Manchester & Salford Directory	020
459	1815	Pigot & Dean	500	Manchester & Salford Directory	020
460	1817	Pigot & Dean	501	Manchester & Salford Directory	020

D	Date	Publisher	Norton Number	Short Title	Location
461	1819	Pigot & Dean	502	Manchester & Salford Directory	020
462	1821	Pigot & Dean	503	New Directory of Manchester [with places] twelve miles round	020
463	1824	Pigot & Dean	504	Directory for Manchester etc. [with places] within twenty-four miles	020
464	1828	Wardle	505	Manchester & Salford Director & Memorandum Book	020
465	1829	Pigot	507	General Directory of Manchester	020
466	1830	Pigot	508	General Directory of Manchester	020
467	1832	Pigot	509	General & Classified Directory of Manchester...also [places] within twelve miles	020
468	1833	Pigot	510	General & Classified Directory of Manchester...also [places] within twelve miles with an addenda for 1833	020
469	1836	Pigot	512	General & Classified Directory of Manchester...also [places] within twelve miles	020
470	1838	Pigot	513	General, Classified and Street Directory of Manchester [with places] within twelve miles & some others...more distant	020
471	1840	Pigot & Slater	514	General, Classified & Street Directory of Manchester	020
472	1841	Pigot & Slater	515	General, Classified & Street Directory of Manchester [with places] within twelve miles & some others	020
473	1843	Pigot & Slater	517	General & Classified Directory & Street Register of Manchester	020
474	1845	Slater	521	General & Classified Directory & Street Register of Manchester & Salford	020
475	1848	Slater	523	General & Classified Directory & Street Register of Manchester & Salford	020
476	1850	Slater	524	General & Classified Directory & Street Register of Manchester & Salford	020
477	1852	Whellan	427	New Alphabetical & Classified Directory of Manchester & Salford, Bolton [etc.]	020
478	1855	Slater	528	General & Classified Directory & Street Register of Manchester & Salford	020
489	1854	Gilmour	369	Winchester Almanach & P. O. Directory	021
491	1830	Brindley	219	Plymouth, Stonehouse & Devonport Directory	022
492	1844	Flintoff	222	Directory & Guide to Plymouth, Devonport [etc.]	022
493	1852	Brendon	224	Directory of Plymouth, Stonehouse [etc.]	022
499	1799	Willoughby	600	Nottingham Directory	023
500	1825	Glover	604	Nottingham Directory	023
501	1831	Pigot	56	Directory for [Derby, Leics, Notts, Rutl]	024
502	1834	Dearden	605	History, Topography & Directory of Nottingham & the adjacent villages	023
503	1840	Orange	606	Nottingham Annual Register	023
504	1844	Glover	607	History & Directory of Nottingham	023
505	1847	Slater	82	Directory of Ireland & Isle of Man	023
506	1848	Lascelles & Hagar	608	Comm. Directory of Nottingham	023
507	1853	White, F.	598	History, Directory & Gazetteer for the County of Nottingham	023
508	1832	White	596	History, Gazetteer & Directory of Nottinghamshire	023
509	1844	White, F. & J.	597	History, Directory & Gazetteer of the County of Nottingham [with] Gainsborough	023
510	1854	Wright	609	Nottingham Directory	023
511	1855	Kelly	126	P.O. Directory of [Derby, Leics, Notts, Rutl]	023

D	Date	Publisher	Norton Number	Short Title	Location
524	1818	Rogerson	419	Lancashire General Directory for 1818	020
525	1811	Pigot	498	Manchester & Salford Directory	020
533	1853	Oakey	-	Comm. & Trade Directory of Preston	028
534	1841	Whittle	-	Comm. Directory of Preston & Its Environs	028
537	1852	-	-	Wigan Directory	029
538	1845	Williams	814	Directory of Huddersfield	030
539	1850	Charlton	815	Directory of Huddersfield, Leeds, Dewsbury, & the adjacent villages	030
550	1855	-	-	Directory of Scarborough	031
565	1829	Wardle & Wilkinson	506	Manchester & Salford Director	020
566	1837	Pigot	64	Directory of Scotland & the Isle of Man	020
567	1851	Slater	525	Alphabetical & Classified Directory of Manchester [with places] within twelve miles & some others	020
569	1845	Ibbetson	810	Directory of Bradford	041
570	1845	Walker	812	Directory of Halifax	041
571	1850	Burton	813	Directory of Halifax, Huddersfield, Holmfirth and adjacent villages	041
576	1844	Slater	79	Directory of Shropshire [& N & S Wales, Liverpool & towns in Ches & Lancs]	002
582	1831	Hinton	400	The Watering Places of Great Britain & Fashionable Directory	044
583	1833	Robins	401	The Watering Places of Great Britain & Fashionable Directory	044
584	1839	Pigot	67	Directory of [Beds, Cambs, Essex, Herts, Hunts, Kent, Mdsx, Norf, Suff, Surrey, Suss, & London]	011
585	1840	Fry	403	Fashionable Guide & Directory to the Public Places of Resort in Great Britain	044
586	1847	Bagshaw	404	History, Gazetteer & Directory of Kent	044
587	1849	Williams	405	South-eastern coast Directory	044
591	1839	Smith	411	Topography of Maidstone & its environs	045
592	1850	Phippen	412	New & enlarged directory for Maidstone & its environs	045
594	1855	Kelly	123	P.O. Directory of [Essex, Herts, Kent, Mdsx, Surrey, & Sussex]	046
595	1849	Phillips	691	Handbook & Directory of Worthing	046
596	1850	Phillips	692	Handbook & Directory of Worthing	046
597	1826	Pigot	43	London & Provincial Directory for 1826-7 [London, Mdsx, Ess, Herts, Kent, Surr, Suss.]	011
598	1822	Baxter	673	The Stranger in Brighton & Baxter's New Brighton Directory	047
599	1824	Baxter	674	Stranger in Brighton & Directory	047
600	1843	Leppard	678	Brighton & Hove Directory	047
601	1846	Kelly	681	P.O. Brighton Directory	047
602	1848	Folthorp	682	Court Guide & General Directory for Brighton	047
603	1850	Folthorp	683	Court Guide & General Directory for Brighton	047
604	1852	Folthorp	684	Court Directory & General Directory for Brighton including Hove	047
605	1854	Taylor	606	Original Brighton & Hove Directory, including Cliftonville	047
606	1845	Leppard	680	Brighton & Hove Directory	047
607	1839	Leppard	677	Brighton Directory	047
611	1851	Gray	664	A New Commercial & General Directory of...Croydon	048
612	1853	Gray	665	Comm. & General Directory of...Croydon	048

D	Date	Publisher	Norton Number	Short Title	Location
613	1855	Gray & Warren	666	Comm. & General Directory of...Croydon	048
623	1827	Horniman	. 132.	Reading Directory	049
624	1837	Ingall	133	Reading Directory	049
625	1842	Snare	128	P.O. Directory [Berkshire]	049
626	1844	Snare	-	Berkshire Advertiser	049
627	1853	Macaulay	130	Berkshire Directory	049
628	1854	Billing	131	Directory & Gazetteer of Berkshire & Oxfordshire	049
639	1835	Vincent	613	The Oxford University, City & County Directory for 1835	050
640	1846	Hunt	610	Oxford Directory[with] Abingdon, Banbury [etc.]	050
645	1852	Gardner	611	History, Gazetteer & Directory of the County of Oxford	050
648	1842	Blyth	568	Norwich Guide & Directory	051
649	1836	White	559	History, Gazetteer & Directory of Norfolk	051
650	1845	White	560	History, Gazetteer & Directory of Norfolk	051
651	1854	White, F.	562	History, Gazetteer & Directory of Norfolk	051
652	1850	Hunt	561	Directory of East Norfolk with part of Suffolk	051
653	1852	Mason	570	Norwich General & Comm. Directory & Handbook	051
654	1839	Robson	101	Comm. Directory of London & the 9 counties of [Beds, parts of Berks & Bucks, Camb, Glos with Bristol, Hunts, Norf, Suff, Wilts] with Guernsey & Jersey	068
655	1853	Kelly	120	P.O. Directory of Cambridgeshire, Norfolk & Suffolk	051
658	1846	White	541	History, Gazetteer & Directory of Leicestershire & ...Rutland..[with] Grantham & Stamford	024
660	1854	Melville	543	Directory & Gazetteer of Derbyshire & Leicestershire	057
661	1849	Hagar	542	Comm. Directory of the County of Leicester	024
662	1842	Cook	540	Leicestershire Almanack, Directory & Advertiser	024
663	1827	Combe	546	Leicester Directory	024
664	1843	Cook	547	A Guide to Leicester containing...a directory with an Almanack for 1843	024
667	1844	White	661	History, Gazetteer & Directory of Suffolk & the towns near its borders	052
668	1855	White	662	History, Gazetteer & Directory of Suffolk	052
673	1851	Oakey	-	Comm. Directory of Preston	053
676	1840	Bragg	621	General Directory for the County of Somerset	055
680	1794	Weston	544	Leicester Directory	024
681	1849	Kelly	115	P.O. Directory of Lincolnshire	056
682	1855	Kelly	125	P.O. Directory of Lincolnshire	056
685	1843	Victor & Baker	553	Lincoln Comm. Directory & Private Residents' Guide	056
690	1852	Freebody	168	Directory of...Derby, Chesterfield, [other towns in Derbyshire]...Burton-on-Trent	057
693	1846	Bagshaw	167	History, Gazetteer & Directory of Derbyshire, with Burton-on-Trent	057
694	1843	Glover	170	History & Directory of...Derby	057
696	1838	Bridgen	657	Directory of Wolverhampton	058
697	1839		-	Wolverhampton Directory	058
699	1851	Melville	660	Directory of Wolverhampton, with Bilston [etc.]	059
700	1845	Burgess	-	Directory of Northampton	060
701	1847	Hickman	-	Directory of Northampton	060
702	1852	Phillips	572	Directory of Northampton	060
709	1850	Bagshaw	142	History, Gazetteer & Directory of the County Palatine of Chester	034
712	1795	Broster	148	Chester Guide...to which is added a directory	061
713	1846	Williams	141	Comm. Directory of...Chester [etc.]	061
714	1850	Lascelles	745	Directory & Gazetteer of Coventry & Neighbourhood	002
718	1840	Parry	151	Chester General Guide	061

D	Date	Publisher	Norton Number	Short Title	Location
727	1851	Mannex	532	History, topography & directory of the borough of Preston & 7 miles around, with Chorley	020
728	1850	Heap	434	Bury Directory	020
732	1855	Mannex	-	History, topography & directory of mid-Lancashire	064
734	1840	Robson	106	Comm. Directory of London & the counties of [Ches, Derby, Durham, Shrops, Worcs, Yorks & N. Wales]	063
735	1819	Pigot	32	Comm. Directory for 1819-20	064
747	1817	Brownell	851	Sheffield General Directory	066
748	1821	Gell & Bennett	852	Sheffield General & Comm. Directory	066
749	1825	Gell	853	New General & Comm. Directory of Sheffield & its vicinity	066
750	1828	Blackwell	854	Sheffield Directory & Guide	066
751	1830	Pigot	-	Comm. Directory of Birmingham, Sheffield & their environs	066
752	1833	White	855	History & General Directory of...Sheffield	066
753	1841	White	856	General Directory of Sheffield with Rotherham [& places within 6 miles]	066
754	1841	Rodgers	857	Sheffield & Rotherham Directory	066
755	1845	White	858	General Directory of Sheffield with Rotherham, Chesterfield [& places within 12 miles]	066
756	1849	White	859	General Directory of Sheffield with Rotherham, Chesterfield [& places within 12 miles]	066
757	1854	Kelly	860	P.O. Directory of Sheffield with the neighbouring towns & villages	066
774	1829	Glover	166	Directory of the County of Derby	066
778	1833	White	-	Directory & topography of Leeds, Bradford, Halifax, Huddersfield, Wakefield & the whole of the clothing district of the West Riding	066
780	1851	Bagshaw	615	History, Gazetteer & Directory of Shropshire	043
786	1845	Williams	423	Directory of Bolton, Rochdale, Bury, Oldham, Burnley,	020
			424	Bacup etc. ...also classified lists of merchants & manufacturers of Manchester & Leeds	
787	1820	Pigot	33	Comm. Directory of Ireland, Scotland & the most north-ern counties of England	020
788	1852-3	Slater	97	Royal National Comm. Directory & Topography of [Berks, Corn, Devon, Dorset, Gloucs, Hants., Som, Wilts & S. Wales]	020
799	1851	Pinkney	145	Directory of Birkenhead & its environs	020
800	1848	Kelly	114	P.O. Directory of [Derby, Leics, Notts, Rutl]	020
801	1852	Whittle	431	Blackburn as it is...including...a directory for 1852	020
802	1853	Scammell	318	Bristol General Directory	020
803	1849	Glover	171	History & Directory of Derby	057
809	1850	Glover	172	History & Directory of...Derby	057
815	1847	Kelly	112	P.O. Directory [Berks, Nhants, Oxon, Beds, Bucks, Hunts]	002
819	1832	Pigot	57	London & Provincial Directory for 1832-3-4 [London, Ess, Herts, Kent, Mdsx, Surrey, Suss]	002
820	1835	Mathews	292	Bristol Directory	002
821	1829	Matthews	286	Bristol Directory	002
822	1845	Mathews	302	Bristol Directory	002
830	1841	Bryant	352	A directory for Gloucester	068
832	1839	Davies	323	Cheltenham Annuaire	069

D	Date	Publisher	Norton Number	Short Title	Location
833	1840	Davies	324	Cheltenham Annuaire	069
834	1841	Davies	325	Cheltenham Annuaire	069
835	1842	Davies	326	Cheltenham Annuaire	069
836	1843	Davies	327	Cheltenham Annuaire	069
837	1844	Davies	328	Cheltenham Annuaire	069
838	1845	Davies	329	Cheltenham Annuaire	069
839	1846	Davies	330	Cheltenham Annuaire	069
840	1847	Davies	331	Cheltenham Annuaire	069
841	1848	Davies	332	Cheltenham Annuaire	069
842	1849	Davies	333	Cheltenham Annuaire	069
843	1850	Davies	334	Cheltenham Annuaire	069
844	1851	Davies	335	Cheltenham Annuaire	069
845	1852	Davies	336	Cheltenham Annuaire	069
846	1853	Davies	337	Cheltenham Annuaire	069
847	1854	Davies	338	Cheltenham Annuaire	069
864	1826	White & Parson	548	History & Directory of...the county of Lincoln, in-cluding Kingston-upon-Hull & adjacent towns & villages	070
865	1842	White	550	History, Gazetteer & Directory of Lincolnshire	070
870	1849	Hagar	551	Comm. Directory of the market towns in Lincolnshire	056
875	1810	Berry	567	Concise History & Directory of...Norwich	051
876	1814	Rowe	216	Plymouth, Plymouth dock & Stonehouse General Directory	022
877	1822	Taperell	217	Plymouth, Plymouth dock, Stonehouse..Directory	022
878	1783	Chase	563	The Norwich Directory	072
879	1846	Slater	81	Directory of Ireland...[with Birmingham, W. Bromwich, Bristol, Leeds, Manchester, Sheffield & towns in Scotland]	072
887	1814	Hodson	601	Nottingham directory	023
888	1840	White	795	History, Gazetteer & Directory of the E. & N. Ridings [with Hull & York]	006
890	1847	Hunt	249	City of Gloucester & Cheltenham Directory	068
891	1849	Hunt	250	Directory & Topography for Gloucester, Bristol [with] Berkeley, Cirencester [& other places in Gloucs.]... with Aberavon, Aberdare [& other places in S. Wales & Monm.]	068
892	1792	Reed	254	Bristol Directory	075
893	1793	Matthews	255	Bristol Directory	075
894	1795	Matthews	256	Bristol Directory	075
895	1797	Matthews	257	Bristol Directory	075
896	1851	Mathews	308	Bristol & Clifton Directory	075
897	1852	Mathews	309	Bristol & Clifton Directory	075
898	1853	Mathews	310	Bristol & Clifton Directory	075
899	1854	Mathews	311	Bristol & Clifton Directory	075
900	1798	Matthews	258	Bristol Directory	075
901	1799	Matthews	259	Bristol Directory	075
902	1801	Matthews	260	Bristol Directory	075
903	1803	Mathews	261	Bristol Directory	075
904	1805	Mathews	262	Bristol Directory	075
905	1806	Mathews	263	Bristol Directory	075
906	1807	Mathews	264	Bristol Directory	075
907	1808	Mathews	265	Bristol Directory	075
908	1809	Mathews	266	Bristol Directory	075
909	1810	Mathews	267	Bristol Directory	075

D	Date	Publisher	Norton Number	Short Title	Location
910	1811	Mathews	268	Bristol Directory	075
911	1812	Mathews	269	Bristol Directory	075
912	1813	Mathews	270	Bristol Directory	075
913	1814	Mathews	271	Bristol Directory	075
914	1815	Mathews	272	Bristol Directory	075
915	1816	Mathews	273	Bristol Directory	075
916	1817	Mathews	274	Bristol Directory	075
917	1818	Mathews	275	Bristol Directory	075
918	1819	Mathews	276	Bristol Directory	075
919	1820	Mathews	277	Bristol Directory	075
920	1821	Mathews	278	Bristol Directory	075
921	1822	Mathews	279	Bristol Directory	075
922	1823	Mathews	280	Bristol Directory	075
923	1824	Mathews	281	Bristol Directory	075
924	1825	Mathews	282	Bristol Directory	075
925	1826	Mathews	283	Bristol Directory	075
926	1827	Mathews	284	Bristol Directory	075
927	1828	Mathews	285	Bristol Directory	075
928	1830	Mathews	287	Bristol Directory	075
929	1831	Mathews	288	Bristol Directory	075
930	1832	Mathews	289	Bristol Directory	075
931	1833	Mathews	290	Bristol Directory	075
932	1834	Mathews	291	Bristol Directory	075
933	1836	Mathews	293	Bristol Directory	075
934	1837	Mathews	294	Bristol Directory	075
935	1838	Mathews	295	Bristol Directory	075
936	1839	Mathews	296	Bristol Directory	075
937	1841	Mathews	298	Bristol Directory	075
938	1842	Mathews	299	Bristol Directory	075
939	1843	Mathews	300	Bristol Directory	075
940	1844	Mathews	301	Bristol Directory	075
941	1846	Mathews	303	Bristol Directory	075
942	1847	Mathews	304	Bristol Directory	075
943	1848	Mathews	305	Bristol Directory	075
944	1849	Mathews	306	Bristol Directory	075
945	1040	Mathews	297	Bristol Directory	075
946	1850	Mathews	307	Bristol & Clifton Directory	075
947	1855	Mathews	312	Bristol Directory	075
948	1816	Evans	313	Bristol Index or Evans's Directory	075
949	1817	Evans	314	Bristol Index or Evans's Directory	075
950	1818	Browne	315	Bristol Index & Evans's Directory	075
951	1853	Scammell	353	Gloucester, Bristol & S. Wales Directory	075
952	1852	Edwards	348	Cheltenham Directory	069
953	1851	Edwards	347	Cheltenham Directory	069
954	1848	Edwards	344	Cheltenham Directory	069
955	1843	Harper	341	Comm. & Fashionable Guide for Cheltenham	068
956	1853	Harper	349	Cheltenham Directory	068
957	1839	Weller	340	The Original Cheltenham Directory	068
958	1845	Rowe	343	Illustrated Cheltenham Guide	068
959	1844	Harper	342	Comm. & Fashionable Guide for Cheltenham	069
960	1850	Hunt	867	Directory & Topography for the city of Bristol and... Axbridge, Burnham, Clevedon, Weston-super-Mare	075

D	Date	Publisher	Norton Number	Short Title	Location
964	1843	Mortimer & Harwood	144	Directory of Birkenhead	076
965	1845	Law	-	Directory of Birkenhead	076
966	1851	Osborne	-	Birkenhead Directory	076
967	1854	Osborne	-	Directory of Birkenhead	076
A42	1851	Slater	91	Directory of [Berks, Bucks, Glocs, Hants, Heref, Monm, Oxon, Warks, Wilts, Worcs, S. Wales]	011
A43	1833	Pigot	59	London & Provincial..Directory for 1833-4	011
A44	1836	Thomas	221	Director: Being an alphabetical list of the inhabitants of Plymouth	011
A45	1855	Craven	374	Comm. Directory of the County of Huntingdon and the town of Cambridge	011
A46	1788	Grundy	778	Worcester Directory	011
A47	1853	Musson & Craven	134	Comm. directory of the County of Buckinghamshire and the town of Windsor	011
A48	1851	Gardner	135	History, Gazetteer & Directory of Cambridgeshire	011
A49	1837	Steel	164	Carlisle Directory	011
A50	1848	Hunt	173	Directory & Topography for Exeter & Bristol and Bridgewater, Collumpton [& other towns in Devon & Somerset]	011
A51	1807	Trewman	175	Exeter Pocket Journal	011
A52	1850	Colbran	418	Handbook & directory for Tunbridge Wells & its vicinity	011
A53	1848	White	247	History, Gazetteer & Directory of Essex	011
A54	1852	Osborne	689	Stranger's Guide & Comm. directory to Hastings & St. Leonard's	011
A66	1845	Kelly	108	P.O. Directory of Essex, Herts, Kent, Mdsx, Surrey, Sussex	011
A68	1822	Boore	672	Brighton Annual Directory & Fashionable Guide	011
A69	1849	Colbran	417	Handbook & Directory for Tunbridge Wells & its neighbourhood	011
A70	1840	Taite	165	Carlisle Directory	011
A71	1854	Kelly	122	P.O. Directory of [Berks, Nhants, Oxon, Beds, Bucks, Hunts]	011
A72	1828	Benson	233	Weymouth Guide & Comm. Directory	011
A73	1838	Wright	414	Topography of Rochester, Chatham, Strood...etc.	011
A74	1850	Edwards	346	Cheltenham Directory	011
A75	1850	Williams	372	Directory of the principal market towns in Hertfordshire	011
A76	1852	Lascelles	556	Directory & Gazetteer of Monmouth	011
A77	1851	Kelly	117	P.O. Directory of the six Home Counties	011
A78	1850	Hunt	622	Directory & Topography of Axbridge, Bruton [etc. in Somerset]...[&] Bristol	011
A79	1849	Whellan	571	History, Gazetteer & Directory of Northamptonshire	011
A80	1833	Collins	376	Strangers' Guide to Guernsey & Jersey	011
A81	1840	Payn	379	The Priveleged Islands, being a companion to... Guernsey, Jersey, Alderney, Serk [etc.]	011
A82	1845	Naftel	380	British Press Royal Almanac...for the island of Jersey	011
A83	1851	Archdeacon	663	Directory for Richmond, Kew, Twickenham, Kingston, Hampton, Staines, Windsor, Eton, Egham, Wingfield, Maidenhead, Cookham, Slough, etc.	011
A84	1855	Kelly	124	P.O. Directory of [Hants, Wilts, Dors]	011
A85	1846	Kelly	110	P.O. Directory of [the Norfolk Counties - Cambs, Norf, Suff]	011

D	Date	Publisher	Norton Number	Short Title	Location
A86	1848	Mackie	433	Bolton Directory	011
A87	1841	Rusher	-	Reading Guide & Berkshire Directory	011
A88	1844	Rusher	-	Reading Guide & Berkshire Directory	011
A89	1852	Rusher	-	Reading Guide & Berkshire Directory	011
A90	1855	Rusher	-	Reading Guide & Berkshire Directory	011
A91	1850	Slater	85	...Directory of..[Beds, Cambs, Hunts, Lincs, Norf, Nhants,Suff]	011
A93	1848	Rusher	612	Banbury List & Directory	011
A94	1849	Rusher	612	Banbury List & Directory	011
A95	1850	Rusher	612	Banbury List & Directory	011
A96	1851	Rusher	612	Banbury List & Directory	011
A97	1852	Rusher	612	Banbury List & Directory	011
A98	1853	Rusher	612	Banbury List & Directory	011
A99	1854	Rusher	612	Banbury List & Directory	011
B01	1855	Rusher	612	Banbury List & Directory	011
B19	1821	Rusher	-	Reading Guide & Berkshire Directory	011
B20	1823	Rusher	-	Reading Guide & Berkshire Directory	011
B21	1793	Cruttwell	-	Bath Guide	011
B22	1794	Cruttwell	-	Bath Guide	011
B23	1796	Cruttwell	-	Bath Guide	011
B24	1848	Quiggin	392	Illustrated Guide & Visitor's Companion through the Isle of Man...with a directory for Douglas	011
B25	1839	Quiggin	386	Illustrated Guide...through the Isle of Man... [with] a directory of Douglas	011
B26	1818	Wright	-	Brighton ambulator	011
B28	1852	Lascelles	371	Directory & Gazetteer of Herefordshire	011
B32	1843	Lucas	-	Paddington Directory	011
B33	1855	Trounce	-	Islington Directory	011
B34	1836	Richardson	-	Directory of the towns of Newcastle & Gateshead	011
B35	1850	Ibbetson	811	General & Classified Directory of Bradford	078
B43	1839	Robson	102	Comm. Directory of the eight counties of [Beds, Bucks, Cambs, Hants, Hunts, Norf, Suff, Wilts, with Guernsey & Jersey]	078
B44	1847	Turner	-	Directory for Islington, Holloway & Pentonville	011
B45	1848	Whetstone	-	Directory of Richmond, Kingston, Hampton, Petersham, Mortlake, Sheen, Kew, Brentford, etc.	011
B46	1842	Pigot & Slater	76	Nat. Comm. Directory of [Berks, Bucks, Dors, Glos, Oxon, Som, Wilts]	049
B48	1838	Stapleton	402	Topography, History & Directory of Canterbury, Faversham [& other places in E. Kent]	025
B49	1801	Robbins	625a	Bath Directory	025
B50	1853	Bass	-	Deptford Guide	025
B51	1823	Longman, Hurst, Rees etc.	218	Tourist's companion being a guide to Plymouth...with a directory...	025
B52	1844	Quiggin	390	Illustrated Guide...through the Isle of Man	025
B53	1847	Naftel	381	British Press Royal Almanac...for the Island of Jersey	025
B54	1851	White, F.	802	General Directory & Topography of Kingston-upon-Hull & ...York [etc.] with Lincoln, Boston [etc.]	025
B68	1837	Whittle	-	History of the borough of Preston	078
B69	1845	Stapley	416	Tunbridge Wells Guide & Directory	025
B70	1845	Mason	877	Fashionable handbook for visitors to Brighton	025
B71	1854	Besley	212	West of England Pocket Book	025

D	Date	Publisher	Norton Number	Short Title	Location
B72	1852	Kelly	118	P.O. Directory of [Jersey, Guernsey etc. & Hampshire]	025
B73	1852	Quiggin	393	Illustrated guide...through the Isle of Man	079
B74	1837	Payn	378	Royal Almanack or Daily Calendar..for..Jersey, Guernsey, etc.	080
B75	1853	Childers	382	Royal Jersey Almanac	080
B76	1855	Walker	246	Durham Directory & Almanach	081
B78	1844	Vint & Carr	-	Directory of the borough of Sunderland	081
B79	1846	Hunt	129	Royal Windsor Directory	082
B80	1853	Lascelles	-	Directory & Gazetteer of the county of Oxford	082
B81	1849	Edwards	345	Cheltenham Directory for 1849	082
B82	1854	Monckton	413	Directory for Maidstone	082
B83	1834	Cowslade	-	Directory & Gazetteer for the county of Berkshire	049
B84	1847	Snare	-	Berkshire P.O. Directory	049
B86	1822	Rusher	-	Reading Guide & Berkshire Directory	049
B87	1829	Rusher	-	Reading Guide & Berkshire Directory	049
B88	1830	Rusher	-	Reading Guide & Berkshire Directory	049
B89	1831	Rusher	-	Reading Guide & Berkshire Directory	049
B90	1832	Rusher	-	Reading Guide & Berkshire Directory	049
B91	1833	Rusher	-	Reading Guide & Berkshire Directory	049
B92	1834	Rusher	-	Reading Guide & Berkshire Directory	049
B93	1835	Rusher	-	Reading Guide & Berkshire Directory	049
B94	1836	Rusher	-	Reading Guide & Berkshire Directory	049
B95	1837	Rusher	-	Reading Guide & Berkshire Directory	049
B96	1843	Rusher	-	Reading Guide & Berkshire Directory	049
B97	1845	Rusher	-	Reading Guide & Berkshire Directory	049
C03	1838	Rusher	-	Reading Guide & Berkshire Directory	049
C04	1839	Rusher	-	Reading Guide & Berkshire Directory	049
C05	1840	Rusher	-	Reading Guide & Berkshire Directory	049
C06	1846	Rusher	-	Reading Guide & Berkshire Directory	049
C07	1847	Rusher	-	Reading Guide & Berkshire Directory	049
C08	1848	Rusher	-	Reading Guide & Berkshire Directory	049
C12	1841	Johnston	-	Gravesend & Milton Directory	084
C13	1842	Johnston	409	New Guide to Gravesend	084
C14	1844	Johnston	-	Gravesend Advertiser	084
C15	1847	Johnston	-	Gravesend & Milton Directory	084
C16	1849	Large	-	Gravesend, Milton & Northfleet Directory	084
C17	1850	Large	-	Gravesend, Milton & Northfleet Directory	084
C18	1855	Hall	-	Gravesend & Northfleet Directory	084
C34	1846	Johnston	-	Gravesend & Milton Directory	084
C35	1854	Hall	-	Gravesend & Northfleet Directory	084
C46	1855	Ewen	872	Guide & Directory for...Cardiff	085
C47	1855	Wakeford	873	Cardiff Directory...embracing Llandaff...	085
C49	1848	Hunt	863	Bristol, Newport & Welch towns Directory	085
C50	1850	Slater	89	Directory of [Glocs, Her, Monm, Worcs, N & S Wales]	085
C55	1843	Pigot & Slater	518	General & Classified Directories & street registers of Manchester and Liverpool with the Isle of Man	087
C56	1852	Slater	95	Comm. directory of the Isle of Man [with] Manchester, Birmingham, Carlisle, Hull, Leeds, Liverpool, Newcastle upon Tyne, & Sheffield	087
C57	1832	Le Cras		Englishman's Almanack [Jersey]	088

D	Date	Publisher	Norton Number	Short Title	Location
C58	1843	Naftel	-	British Press Royal Jersey Almanac	088
C59	1848	Naftel	-	British Press Royal Jersey Almanac	088
C60	1849	Naftel	-	British Press Royal Jersey Almanac	088
C61	1852	Naftel	-	British Press Royal Jersey Almanac	088
C62	1854	Naftel	-	British Press Royal Jersey Almanac	088
C63	1855	Naftel	-	British Press Royal Jersey Almanac	088
C64	1847	Williams	154	Comm. Directory of the Principal market towns in Cornwall	067
C68	1853	Barbet	-	Almanack for the Channel Islands	089

2.3 Location codes

Public libraries unless otherwise stated
L   Library   L   Library

001	Worcester	
002	Birmingham	
003	Dudley	
004	Stourbridge	
005	Malvern	
006	William Salt Library, Stafford	
007	Bath	
008	Exeter	
009	Newcastle	
010	York	
011	Guildhall, London	
012	Hereford & Worcester County Library	
013	Durham	
014	Leamington	
015	Leeds	
016	Liverpool	
017	Southampton	
018	Hull	
019	Lancaster	
020	Manchester	
021	Winchester	
022	Plymouth	
023	Nottingham	
024	Leicester	
025	British Library	
026	Rochdale	
027	Rawtenstall	
028	Preston	
029	Wigan	
030	Huddersfield	
031	Scarborough	
032	Bury	
033	Bolton	
034	Stalybridge	
035	Burnley	
036	Chorley	

037	Haslingden
038	Blackburn
039	Stockport
040	Salford
041	Halifax
042	Accrington
043	Shrewsbury
044	Margate
045	Maidstone
046	Worthing
047	Brighton
048	Croydon
049	Reading
050	Oxford
051	Norwich
052	Ipswich
053	Lancashire County Record Office
054	Barrow-in-Furness
055	Taunton
056	Lincoln
057	Derby
058	Wolverhampton
059	Hanley
060	Northampton
061	Chester
062	Oldham
063	Warrington
064	St Helens
065	Southport
066	Sheffield
067	Redruth
068	Gloucester
069	Cheltenham
070	Grimsby
071	Society of Genealogists
072	Chetham's Library

L   Library

073 Lancashire County Library, Preston

074 Colne

075 Bristol

076 Birkenhead

077 IPC Business Press Ltd.

078 Institute of Historical Research

079 Douglas, Isle of Man

080 Jersey

081 Durham University Library

082 Bodleian Library

083 Salisbury

084 Gravesend

085 Cardiff

086 Newport

087 Manx Museum

088 Société Jersiaise

089 Guille-Allès Library, Guernsey

2.4 Biographical notes

These notes are not exhaustive but are intended as an aid to confirming the identity of individuals listed in the register (appendix 2.1). Appearances in journals and advertisements are omitted. Individuals mentioned are dentists unless otherwise stated.

Abbreviations used:

CD	Member of the College of Dentists
OSL	Member of the Odontological Society of London
OSGB	Member of the Odontological Society of Great Britain in 1863
P(date)	known to be in practice in (date), for dentists in practice after 1855. Not necessarily the end of a dentist's career. 'P1879' is in some cases an indication that the dentist appears in the first *Dentists Register* but subsequent entries have not been followed.
R	entry in the first *Dentists Register*
BDA	member of the British Dental Association in 1881-2
LDS	Licence in Dental Surgery of the Royal College of Surgeons of England
LSA	Licence of the Society of Apothecaries
MRCS	Member of the Royal College of Surgeons of England
W	Probate, with value; civil probate (post-1858), court named if pre-1858
WX	apparently no will proved
adm.	administration of estate
chd	chemist and druggist
b	brother
b-in-l	brother-in-law
f	father
f-in-l	father-in-law
h	husband
n	nephew
s	son
s-in-l	son-in-law
u	uncle

ABBOTT John
surgeon

ALABONE Alfred
CD1859 OSGB1863 P1879 R

ALEX & Jones
P1871

ALEX J
London connection
f of Montague Alex

ALEX Montague
1816-76(Southampton)
CD1857 P1868
W under £5,000
s of J. Alex

ALLAWAY William
P1863
WX

ALLDRIDGE John Lumley
1814-80(Portsea)
P1878
WX

ALLEN William Hart
P1879 R
Chd London connection

ALLEN William
bleeder

ALMOND William
LSA1842

ALSOP Edward
barber-surgeon, perfumer

ANDREWS Alfred
P1868

ARANSON Pasco
-1843(Birmingham)

ASPINWALL Joseph
P1865

ATKINSON(& fath J)= ATKINSON John Hastings
1819(Leeds)-89(Leeds)
CD1859 OSGB1863 P1875
LDS1863
W £15,226
s of John Hastings

ATKINSON John(Leeds)=ATKINSON John(Manchester)
1794(Halton)-1865(Leeds)
P1865
MRCS
W under £30,000
f of John Hastings Atkinson

AYTON Jacob
P1859
LDS1863 MD
Member of University College, London 1848

BAKER Stephen
cupper
in practice with James Prew, 1823

BALLANTYNE George
P1858

BALLARD George
P1875

BANNISTER William F
cupper

BARCLAY James
P1858

BARNARD J F (Southampton)=? J F(Bristol)
=? John Frederick
(Dover)

BARNES J W
apothecary,chd

BARRON William Henry
cupper
author

BARTLETT H N
P1873 Cloyton

BATE Charles
f of Charles Spence Bate

BATE Charles Spence
1814-89(South Brent)
OSL1857Pres. OSGB1863 P1889 R BDAPres.
LDS1860 FRS
W £4,668
zoologist, painter, associated with Plymouth
Dental Dispensary
s of Charles Bate whose practice he joined
in the late 1850s

BATE James Joseph Rogers
CD1857 P1881 R BDA
Tiverton

BAYNTUN Francis alias Power
1818-78(Sheffield)
P1856 as Bayntun, 1871 as Power
adm.1890 £150

BEACALL Edwin
P1860

BEAL Mary Ann
?widow of Richard Beal

BEAUMONT Alfonso Rodolph
MD
oculist

BELL & Jones
P1878

BELLABY G(oodman) Wood
1826-1909(Nottingham)
CD1857 OSGB1863 P1879 R

BELLAMY John Cremer
LSA1833
cupper

BENNETT James
?LSA1839

BEREND Louis
(Hanover)-1863(Göttingen)
P1858
W under £3,000
b of Samuel Salmom Berend

BEREND Samuel S(almon)
(Hanover)-1865(Chester)
OSL1857
W under £18,000
b of Louis Berend

BESWICK John
musician=?instrument maker

BEVERS Edmund
CD1859 P1903 R
WX

BEW Charles
trained with Spence of Edinburgh
former actor
dentist to Royal Household in Brighton
author

BICKLEY Francis
P1856

BINGHAM Charles
LSA1816

BIRD W = Bird M

BISHOP T
P1859
chd

BLACKMORE (& fath E) =? John Blackmore
P1879
s of Edward Blackmore

BLACKMORE Edward
P1870
f of dentist son (? John)

BLACKMORE Julia Anna Harriet
P1879 R

BLACKMORE Richard
Collumpton 1818

BLAIR James
1747(Blairgowrie)-1817(Liverpool)
WX
employed Thomas Whitfield Lloyd
f in l/uncle of William Robertson
gf of Henry Blair Robertson
ggf of James Blair
see Hillam,bibl.

BLAIR James & Lloyd = Mrs.Martha Blair
(widow of James) & Thomas Whitfield Lloyd

BLAIR James & Turner = Mrs.Martha Blair
(widow of James) & Turner

BOARDMAN (Plymouth) =? Boardman William
(Exeter)

BOARDMAN Mrs. =? widow of Boardman (Plymouth)

BOOTH Isaac
surgeon

BORLASE William Grenfell
   -1876(Exeter)
P1868
LDS1863

BOTT George (jun)
1772(Nottingham)-1804(Birmingham)
WX
trained Peter Flint
s of George Bott (sen)
b of Parker Bott
h of Sophia Bott
see Hillam, D G & C, bibl.

BOTT George (sen)
1748-1820(Nottingham)
W PCY £9,700
patent medicine vendor
f of George Bott (jun) & Parker Bott
f in l of Sophia Bott
see Hillam, D G & C, bibl.

BOTT Parker
1787(Nottingham)-1827(Nottingham)
W PCY under £5,000
s of George Bott (sen)
b of George Bott (jun)

b in l of Sophia Bott
see Hillam, D G & C, bibl.

BOTT Sophia
1768(Bushley)-1859(Birmingham)
WX
trained by father-in-law, George Bott (sen)
widow of George Bott (jun)
s in l of Parker Bott
see Hillam, D G & C, bibl.

BOULGER Patrick Joseph
CD1857 OSGB1863 P1858
WX

BOULNOIS James Joseph de
f of John de Boulnois

BOULNOIS John de
s of James Joseph de Boulnois

BOULTON R(ichard) B(ryant)
P1881 R BDA

BOWMER George
CD1857 OSGB1863 P1879 R

BRADLEY T(homas) D(unstall)
P1866
chd

BRADSHAW Francis
LSA1832

BRAE Andrew Edmund
1801(Ireland)-81(London)
OSL1858 P1871
W estate in England £609
successor to Joseph Murphy
retired to Guernsey

BREWER James
apothecary
s of Theodore Brewer

BREWER Theodore
apothecary, midwife, surgeon
f of James Brewer

BRIDGES Thomas Bartlett
P1881 Whitby R BDA

BRIDGMAN William Keneely (Kencely)
1812-83(Norwich)
OSL1857 OSGB1863 P1864
LDS1861
W £7,639
f of John Brooks Bridgman

BROMLEY Charles
OSL1857 OSGB1863 P1871
LDS1860
WX
trained Thomas Gill Palmer
employed T.P.Payne high reputation
f of Charles Henry Bromley (1839-90)

BROOKHOUSE Robert
1817(Derby)-1905(Knutsford)
OSL1857 OSGB1863 P1884 R
LDS1860
friend of John Dalton,advocate of the Manchester Ship Canal scheme

BROOKS John
from London
b in l & successor to trainer James Rose

BROOKS John & Rose = John Brooks & Elizabeth Rose (widow of James Rose)

BROOKS Robert Heygate
P1881 R BDA
f of Henry Reginald Fryer Brooks

BROOKSBANK Michael
CD1857 P1872

BROOMFIELD George
-1859(Scarborough)
P1857
W under £5,000

BROWN C = Brown Charles

BROWN Charles
1812-69(Woolwich)
P1869
W under £100

BROWN George
1804-71(Leamington)
P1868
W under £200

BROWN Henry S
P1863
WX

BROWNE John Crow
1823(Lowestoft)-
P1879 R
chd

BUCHANAN Alfred Daniel
CD1857 P1863

BUCK William
P1879 R
LDS1863 MRCS1843
f LSA1816

BUNTER George
P1879 R

BURCH R(obert)
P1879 R
chd

BURLEY John
P1871

BUTCHER Richard
P1879

BUTTERS James Hall
P1877

CAFFERATA James Lewis
1797-1870(Sunderland)
CD1857 P1870
W under £100
f of Phillip Cafferata

CALDCLEUGH John
OSL1859 P1879 R
LDS1863

CANTON
may be a branch of a London practice

CARR John
LSA1824

CARTER John Henry (Manchester) =? Carter
John Henry (Wakefield)

CARTER John Henry (Wakefield)
1811-93(Knaresborough)
CD1857 P1881 R BDA
most of practice in Leeds

f of John Henry Carter & Thomas Scales Carter

CARTWRIGHT & DAVIS
may be trading name of James Mallan

CATTLIN William Alfred
1814-87(Bournemouth)
LSA1836 FRCS
f of a dentist

CAUDLE William
LSA1828 MRCS1829

CAWLEY George
P1869

CHAMBERLAIN & TAYLOR
P1856

CHAMBERS Thomas
P1879

CHARLTON
from London

CHERRIMAN John V
1807-91(Brighton)
P1891 R
W £3,255
trained with Rothwell, assistant to Reale
London practice

CHILD William (Liverpool) =? Child William
(Leeds)

CHILD William (Leeds)
CD1857 P1876
?chd

CLARK Andrew
P1878

CLARK Ebenezer
1798-1875(Walthamstow)
W under £12,000

CLARKE (& fath E) = Clarke Isaiah William
(Bristol)
1826-95(Bristol)
P1895 R
W £300
s of E Clarke (Bristol)

CLARKE (& fath I)
P1879

CLARKE B J
P1868

CLARKE E
f of Isaiah William Clarke (Bristol)

CLARKE Isaiah William (Nottingham)
P1869
WX
preacher
f of dentists

CLARKE James (Brighton) =? James Clarke
(Nottingham)

CLARKE James (Nottingham)
-1885(Belfast)
P1885 R
LDS1862
W estate in England £11,761
f of James Clough Clarke
gf of 2 dentists
see Stoy, bibl.

CLARKE John Edward
chd

CLARKE T(homas) M(eadows)
P1879 R
chd cupper

CLOUGH Edward (Halifax)
P1879 Leeds R

CLOUGH Edward (Lincoln)=? Clough Edward
(Halifax)

COBB J(ohn) S(wanston)
P1879 R
LDS1861

COGAN John Daniel
WX
medical electrician

COGAN Samuel W
-1850(Taunton)
adm. under £200 1874

COKER Thomas
1810-77(Taunton)
P1879
W under £3,000
f of Thomas Voysey Coker (Bristol)

COLEMAN Alfred
P1881 R BDA
LDS1860
London practice

COLES Stratton J(ames)
1820-90(London)
CD1857 OSL1857 OSGB1863 P1887 R
W £21,078
associated with Plymouth Dental Dispensary

COMPTON Samuel
P1859

COPPEL Charles
P1871
WX

COREY Charles
P1861

CORNISH Henry Roberts
chd

CRAWCOUR Barnett
1776-1835(Norwich)
from a family of dentists

CRAWSHAW Henry
P1879
chd

CULLIS George Henry
1807/11-
P1879
WX
author

CUMBER Henry
cupper

CUNNINGHAM Patrick Gregson
1815-66(Salisbury)
P1859
W under £700

CURPHEY William
1805(Douglas)
watchmaker

CURTIS William B(rydges)
1813-73(Bristol)
P1870
W under £100

CUTTRISS W
P1877
f of Thomas Cuttriss (1846-1909)

DALE Henry
-1863(Leamington)
P1863
W under £1,500

DASH James
P1866

DAVENPORT Joseph Wilde
1819-77(Stoke Damerel)
CD1857 P1878
WX
author

DAVIDSON William
P1858

DAVIS J O (jun)
P1859
chd

DE BERRY Samuel
f of dentist
may be part of firm of Le Dray, alias John
Jordan

DE LESSERT Charles Grierson
1818(Ireland)-86(Wolverhampton)
OSL1858 P1886 R
LDS1860
W £304
s of A A de Lessert (Dublin)

DE LOUDE Louis Charles
author
f of dentist

DEANE Henry Edward
1820-1900(Manchester)
P1899 R
WX

DEARLE George
CD1857 P1879 R

DELABARRE Anthony Bernasconi
1805-69(London)
P1863
W under £20
claimed to be French Royal dentist

DICKER William Joseph
1815-83(Plymouth)
P1877
W £162
dispenser of medicine cupper

DICKIN Joseph Pearson
P1872

DINSDALE Cuthbert
P1857

DIXON & PICNOT = Mrs.Ruth Dixon (widow of
John Dixon) & Theodore Picnot q.v.

DIXON James Browne
1825-89(London)
P1889 R
W £319
chd
moved to London
s of a cleric

DIXON John
h of Ruth Dixon

DIXON Ruth
1792/96-
widow of John Dixon

DIXON Thomas
1818(Leeds)-
P1861
WX

DOLEMAN John
jeweller

DON B
P1857

DOWNES E Y
chd

DOWNING B =? Downing R

DOWNING E = Downing Edward

DOWNING Edward
1811/16-
P1873
s of Richard Downing(1772/76-1860)
b of Richard Downing(d.1861)

DOWNING R = Downing Rchard (jun)

DOWNING Richard (jun)
-1861(Newcastle upon Tyne)
W under £300
s of Richard Downing(1772/76-1860)
b of Edward Downing(1811/16-   )

DOWNING Richard
1772/76-1860(Newcastle upon Tyne)
P1860
W under £20
f of Edward and Richard Downing

DRABBLE Robert Charles
P1881 R BDA

DRAKE (Hull) =?Drake (Wolverhampton)

DRESCHFELD Leopold
1822(Bavaria)-97(Manchester)
P1881 R BDA
LDSIreland 1878
revolutionary activist in Bavaria; a founder
of Manchester Dental Hospital; involved in
Jewish congregation in Manchester
f of Hugh Dreschfeld
b of Professor Dreschfeld (Manchester Univ.)

DUFF John
P1863

DUNCAN Richard
P1863
LDS1863

DUNSFORD (James)
P1879 R

DURANT E
OSGB1863 P1879 R
chd

DURLACHER Abraham
1757(Germany)-1845
corn operator
see J C Dagnall, 'A history of chiropody-
podiatry and foot care', British Journal
of Chiropody, 44(1983), p.153

DUTTON William Henry
P1861
WX

DYASON Tassell
WX

EDEN Thomas Edward
1812-70(Brighton)
OSL1857 OSGB1863 P1866
MRCS1835 FRCS1863
s of Thomas Eden

EDWARDS Edward (Bath) =? Edwards Edward
(Exeter)

EDWARDS H
P1879 R

EDWARDS James
1815(Uxbridge)-
P1866
trained by James Prew
cousin of William Moore

ELLIOTT John
LSA1828

ELLIS Thomas
LSA1825 MRCS
accoucheur, surgeon apothecary

ENGLISH Thomas
MRCS
f of Thomas Robert Mairis English

ENGLISH Thomas Robert M(airis)
1819(Birmingham)-93(Birmingham)
OSL1857 OSGB1863 P1892 R
W £2301
s of Thomas English
consultant dentist at Birmingham Dental
Hospital

ENSOR Silas
P1856
WX
druggist, surgeon, apothecary

ESKELL Abraham
1824(Scotland)-
P1876

ESKELL Albert
1810-88(London)
P1879 R
W £1886
London practice
f of Edward & Harry Eskell
Eskells extensively involved in dentistry
both in Britain and colonies

ESKELL Francis =? Eskell Frederick

ESKELL Frederick
1818-74(London)
P1874
W under £2,000

ESKELL Frederick A
P1877

ESKELL Louis
P1869

ESKILL A =? Eskell Abraham

EVATT Henry Royle
1814(Derbyshire)-
P1876
medicine dealer

EVATT James
s of William Evatt

EVATT James
s of William Evatt

EVATT William
razor maker
f of James Evatt

FARTHING
all entries under this surname may possibly
refer to one individual, John Farthing of
Southampton

FARTHING John (Southampton)
practised in New York & London

FARTHING John (Cardiff)
P1858

FAULKNER John (jun)
1784(Manchester)-1842(Manchester)
W Chester under £450
s of Thomas Faulkner
f of Thomas John Faulkner
b in l of John Faulkner (sen)

FAULKNER Thomas
-1819(Manchester)
W Chester under £600
former fustian cutter
trained William Robertson
f of John Faulkner (jun)
f in l of John Faulkner (sen)
gf of Thomas John Faulkner

FAULKNER Thomas J(ohn)
P1864
WX
s of John Faulkner (jun)
gs of Thomas Faulkner
n of John Faulkner (sen)

FAULKNER J(ohn) (sen)
-1856(Manchester)
W Chester under £200
s in l of Thomas Faulkner
b in l of John Faulkner (jun)
u of Thomas John Faulkner

FAY =? Tullius Priest Fay

FAY Tullius Priest
1816-70(Liverpool)
P1870
W under £1500
? s of Cyrus Fay
f of Tullius William Ward Fay

FELTHAM
CD1857
P1879 R

FISHER Frederick
cupper

FISHER George
cupper

FLETCHER
chiropodist

FLINT Peter
apprenticed to George Bott (jun) 1798

FORBES John Luke
bleeder

FORT William
P1879
LDS1861
n of William Titterington

FOTHERGILL Alexander
1824-92(Darlington)
CD1857 OSGB1863 P1891 R BDAPres.1891
LDS1863
b of William Fothergill who trained him
s of railway surgeon

FOTHERGILL William
CD1857 OSGB1863 P1881 BDA
LDS1863
b of Alexander Fothergill whom he trained
f of John A Fothergill(d.1906)
s of railway surgeon

FOX Charles Prideaux
1820(Kingsbridge)-1905(Lowell, Mass.,USA)
s of Robert.Were Fox)1792-1872) q.v. for
brothers
until 1843 member of Society of Friends
became RC priest, later years in Canada &
US
Intimate friend of Charles Dickens

FOX Cornelius Willes
1811(Devonport)-51(Plymouth)
f of eminent doctor, Cornelius Benjamin Fox
(b.1839)

FOX George (Birmingham)
chd

FOX George F(rederick)
1822(Kingsbridge)-76(Southport)
OSL1857 OSGB1863 P1876
LDS1863
s of Robert Were Fox(1792-1872) q.v. for
brothers
pupil of brother Robert Were Fox(1816-59)
f of Walter Henry Fox(1854-1942)
     Ernest William Fox(1859-1939)
     Charles Herbert Fox(1861-1939)
gf of Frederick Neidhart Fox(1881-1923)
ggf of George Enthony Fox (1935-   )

FOX Robert Were
1792(Wadebridge)-1872(Kingsbridge)
P1856
W under £4000
f of Robert Were Fox, Charles Prideaux Fox,
George Frederick Fox, Sylvanus Bevan Fox,
Octavius Annesley Fox
gf of 3 dentists (see G F Fox)
ggf of Frederick Neidhart Fox(1881-1923)
     Lancelot E C Peckover, Hugh Douglas
     Peckover
gggf of George Enthony Fox(b.1935)
f of Francis Fox(1818-1914) railway engineer,
designer of Temple Meads Station after
working for I K Brunel

FOX Robert Were (jun)
1816(Plymouth)-59(London)
P1859
W under £3000
s of Robert Were Fox(1792-1872) q.v. for
brothers
trained by father

FOX Silvanus Bevan
1825(London)-1912(Exmouth)
P1910 R BDA
LDS1863
trained by father
s of Robert Were Fox(1792-1872) q.v. for
brothers
associated with Exeter Dental Dispensary &
Brighton & Hove Dental Dispensary
beekeeper

FOX Thomas
trained by Stewart of Bristol

FOX George (Kingsbridge)
P1858

GABRIEL Arnold
P1869

GABRIEL John
P1879 R

GACHES Daniel
P1864
WX

GALLEN John Jardine
demonstrator in morbid anatomy, Univ.of
Glasgow
cupper at Glasgow & Edinburgh Infirmaries

GAMBLE J G
OSGB1863 P1881 R BDA

GANTHERRY Robert
P1863

GARNER Joseph Samuel
s of a London dentist

GARNETT George Belk
P1877

GARNETT Henry William
1804-71(Scarborough)
P1865
W under £1,000

GARRETT Phillip L
CD1857 OSGB1863 P1857

GIDNEY Eleazer
1797(New York State)-1876(London)
author
see J M Campbell, bibl.

GILBARD James
P1865

GILBERT George
P1859
chd

GILL Seth
OSL1859 P1871
LDS1863

GOEPEL John Robert
P1884 R BDA
LDSIreland 1878

GOLDSTONE =? Goldstone George
apothecary

GOLDSTONE C
apothecary

GOLDSTONE George
MRCS1815 LSA1828

GOLDSTONE. =? Goldstone Richard
apothecary, surgeon

GOODMAN James
P1879 R
goldsmith

GOODMAN Samuel
P1856

GORDON James
1795(Nairn)-1864(Nairn)

P1857
former watchmaker, worked for a Bristol
dentist before opening own practice
virtuoso carver of ivory, exhibited at 1851
Great Exhibition
b of William Gordon (London)
see Schiach, bibl.

GOULD Frederick
P1879 R
chd
prosecuted for using 'surgeon-dentist' in
1859

GOULSON Benjamin
surgeon,man-midwife, bleeder

GRAY John
1815-66(Sheffield)
CD1857 P1865
W under £3,000

GRAYSON John
CD1857 P1858
f of F C(1845-1911) & A E Grayson

GREEN Thomas
bleeder

GREENSILL Edward
P1857
chd

GREGORY Edward James
-1903
CD1857 P1903 R BDA
LDSIreland 1878

GROVES =? Groves Anthony N

GROVES Anthony N(orris)
1795(Newton, Hants)-1853(Bristol)
a founder of Plymouth Brethren,1828
missionary in India 1833-34, 36-48,49-52
author
f of Edwin & John Groves
see Boase, bibl.

GROVES Edwin
P1866
WX
s of Anthony Norris Groves
b of John Groves

GROVES John
P1862
WX
s of Anthony Norris Groves
b of Edwin Groves

GUNTON Alfred
P1879 R

HAGREEN James Thomas
P1864

HAIR Quintin B(urns)
1812-75
P1874
WX
appointment to the Duchess of Kent

HAMILTON Horatio
P1859
chd

HAMMOND Thomas Cundale
P1877
WX

HARDING George
P1859

HARDING Thomas Henry
LDS1866
London practice
chd

HARGREAVES Charles
P1879 R

HARRINGTON George Fellowes
1812-95(Isle of Wight)
CD1857 OSGB1863 P1867
LDS1860
W £452
Mayor of Ryde twice. Inventor of clockwork
drill inter alia.
see Campbell, bibe.

HARRISON Henry
P1856

HARRISON Robert
P1879
f of Robert Eunson Harrison

HARRISON Robert Eunson
CD1857 P1879 R
LDS1863
s of Robert Harrison

HART =? Joseph or A.S. Hart

HART A(braham) S(eptimus)
-1865(London)
adm. under £2,000
London practice
s of Hammett Hart
b of Joseph Hart

HART Hammett
f of A S Hart & Joseph Hart
h of Mrs Hart

HART Joseph
1792(Bristol)-1868(Bristol)
P1867
WX
s of Hammett Hart
b of A S Hart

HART Mrs
widow of Hammett Hart
m of A S Hart & Joseph Hart

HARTLEY Francis William =? Hartley
William

HARVEY Charles Greaves =? Harvey
Christopher George
cupper

HARVER Christopher George
chd

HASLAM Simeon
chd

HAWKER Henry
P1864

HAY John
P1892 R BDA
bankrupt 1847

HAYMAN =? Hayman Samuel Augustine
          Hayman George John
Samuel Augustine - CD1857 P1879 R
                f of Alfred George &
                S J Hayman
George John - 1820-75 W under £600

HEARNE Edward
MRCS1842 LSA1843 MB1844
House surgeon UCH

HEATH George
CD1857 P1857
WX

HEATHCOAT Joseph =? Heathcote Joseph F

HELE Samuel
-1850(Exeter)
W Exeter under £1500
Resident dispenser Exeter dispensary

HELSBY Charles
-1861(Baguely)
P1861
W under £300

HELSBY Richard
1803-68(Penrith)
P1865
W under £1500
bought practice of John Robinson
(Manchester)

HEPBURN Duncan D(ewar)
CD1857 OSGB1863 P1866
LDS1860
b of David & Robert Hepburn

HESKETH Birch
-1788(Liverpool)
W Chester £3-600

HESLOP Richard
1813-77(Huddersfield)
P1867
W under £7,000
jeweller goldsmith

HIAM C
P1879

HICKMAN Henry
P1875

HIGGINBOTTOM John
1783-1867(Liverpool)
P1867
W under £200

HIGMAN H R
P1857

HILDYARD Charles =? Hillyard Charles
P1859

HUCKLEY Anthony
P1879 R
LDSIreland 1878

HODGSON Joseph
P1856

HOGARTH Thomas
chd

HOOTON Jonathan
P1879 R
LDSIreland 1878

HOPKINSON William
1821-71(Salford)
CD1857 OSGB1863
P1871

HOPTON & Co
P1856

HORDERN John James
P1863
WX

HORNOR Benjamin
1772-1836(York)

HOWARD John
LSA1834

HUDSON T
P1879 R
chd

HIGGINS J
P1879 R
chd

HUGHES James A(ustin)
CD1859
P1869

HUGO M
P1862

HUGO S (G)
1831-1912
OSL1858 P1881 R BDA

HULME J Hughes
chd

HUME W
former miniature picture framer
materials manufacturer

HUMPHREY George Edward
P1869
WX

HUNT William
1812(Yeovil)-1905(Yeovil)
CD1857 OSL1857 OSGB1863 P1881 R BDA
LDS1861
W £14,725
s of dentist
f of William Alfred Hunt (1845-1929)
gave 1st demonstration of ether outside
London
1st dentist to Yeovil general dispensary

HUSSEY Edward William
P1863

HUTCHINSON Massey =? Hutchinson Matthew

HUTCHINSON Thomas
phlebotomist cupper

HYDEN David
hairdresser

IMRIE Robert Marshall
assistant to Cartwright

JACOB Henry Long
CD1857 OSL1857 P1879 R
LSA1840
later career in Birkenhead

JAMES John
P1873
WX
cupper

JARDINE Marsh Robert
1805(London)-
chd

JAY Thomas Edward
P1861

JEFFERIES T
later assistant to James Robertson
(Worcester)
P1857

JEFFERSON William
P1879 R

JENKINS H M
P1873
chd

JEWERS Frederick Arthur
OSL1857 OSGB1863 P1879 R
associated with Plymouth Dental Dispensary

JOEL Edward G
P1879 R

JOHNSON George F
P1859
chd

JONES (& ALEX) = Jones A B
OSL1857

JONES Edwin
1809(Birmingham)-
P1879
WX
1830s in London

JONES F(rederick) (Hart)
P1879 Stamford

JONES Grenville
1804-44(Shrewsbury)
1st obituary in *Jewish chronicle*
b of Horatio Jones

JONES Henry
P1866
WX

JONES Henry Micholls
P1875
WX

JONES Horatio
1819-
CD1857 P1879 R
trained Michael Edwards (Liverpool) 1874-77
b of Grenville Jones

JONES James Gibb
chd

JONES John (Manchester)
cupper chd

JONES John (Liverpool)
P1879 R
chd

JONES Morris
P1866

JONES Robert
P1873

JONES Samuel Aaron
P1888 R
WX

JONES John (Cambridge)
-1878(Chesterton)
P1864
W under £10,000
f of Alfred Jones
gf of Alfred Jones

JONES John(Birmingham)
herbalist

JORDAN Charles
P1879 R
WX

JORDAN Henry
author

JORDAN Henry Edward
-1864
P1863
WX

JUDSON B(enjamin) R(obert) G(lydden)
chd

KARRAN James
1820(Peel)-
CD1857 P1879 R
pupil & assistant of William Smith (Liverpool)

KELLY Thomas Moore
CD1857 OSGB1863 P1881 BDA
WX

KERNOTT C(harles) M(iddleton)
MRCS1839

KING Edward (Brecon)
1808-73(Talgarth)
CD1857
P1871
W under £300

KING Edward (Oxford)
assistant to William Lukyn

KING Joseph
OSL1857 OSGB1863 P1876
LDS1860
W £20,072
f of T E King

KING Norman
1811-80(Exeter)
CD1857(VP) OSL1857(VP) OSGB1863 P1879 R
W under £14,000
f of 2 dentists

KING Richard Swit =? King Richard Shaw

KIRKBY James
-1864(Sheffield)
W under £600

KYAN J Howard
OSL1859 P1881Preston R BDA
LDS1860

L'ESTRANGE Francis
P1879 R

LAMBERT Peter
jeweller

LAMBERT William
1803-87(East Grinstead)
P1878
W£13

LANSDALE Ralph
P1864

LAVENS Thomas Howard = LAVERS
P1879 R

chd
London practice

LE BRUN P
-1907(St.Helier)
W £101

LE DRAY
all entries refer to John Jordan(London)

LEADBETTER Edward
goldsmith

LEIGH Edward Philip
P1858
London practice

LEIGH Samuel George
1802(Brigstock)-
P1877
LDS1860
documents relating to career held by the
museum of the School of Dental Surgery,
University of Liverpool

LEVANDER James
P1857
WX

LEVASON Joseph
-1853(Hereford)
adm. under £800
Whitehaven in 1830s
f of Arthur Gre(n)ville Levason

LEVASON Lewis
1800-76(Liverpool)
W under £200
London practice 1852-53

LEVISON Jacob Leslie
1799-1874(London)
WX
London practice
connected with Birmingham Hebrew National
School, 1844
author

LEWIS James(Exeter) =? Lewis James (Cheltenham)

LEWIS James(Cheltenham)
surgeon-dentist in ordinary to King

LIDDON George
P1862

LITTLE (& HAYMAN) =? Little Stephen
                    ? Little Edward
                    ? Little Henry q.v.
Stephen Little CD1857 OSGB1863
Edward Little   P1879 R LDSIreland1878

LITTLE Henry
MRCS
trained in Paris

LLOYD E
chd (Savory & Lloyd)

LLOYD George Fieldhouse
CD1857 OSGB1863 P1879 R
London practice

LLOYD Richard
1817(Liverpool)-68(Liverpool)
P1864
W under £70,000
s of Thomas Whitfield Lloyd
b of James Blair Lloyd & Thomas Bridge
Lloyd
u of E J M Phillips

LLOYD Thomas Bridge
1808(Liverpool)-45(Manchester)
adm. Chester under £1,000
s of Thomas Whitfield Lloyd
b of Richard Lloyd & James Blair Lloyd
u of E J M Phillips

LLOYD Thomas W(hitfield)
1783(Liverpool)-1861(Birkenhead)
former instrument maker
assistant to James Blair
continued Blair's practice as Blair & Lloyd
f of Thomas Bridge Lloyd, Richard Lloyd &
James Blair Lloyd
gf of E J M Phillips

LOMAX James Wood
1822-94(Amersham)
P1889 R
W £23,031

LOWE Edwin
London practice

LOWS Andrew
P1879 R
LDS1860
London practice

LUKYN Christopher
P1879 R(LUKYER in 1879 Register)
? son of William Lukyn

LUKYN John
    -1849(Nottingham)
adm. 1859 under £300
s of William Lukyn

LUKYN W(Nottingham) = Lukyn William

LUKYN William
    -1863(Nottingham)
P1863
W under £450
London & Nottingham addresses
author
f of John Lukyn, ? of Christopher Lukyn

LYON William
P1864
chd

LYONS Morris
1811(Coventry)-
P1887 R
WX
?medical man
also lived Plymouth, Jersey, Norwich, Retford between 1834 & 1843

MACGREGOR Richard =? McGregor Richard H G

MAGOR Martin
OSL1860 P1881 R BDA
LDS1860
chd

MAISH E B
P1877
chd

MALLAN James
P1885 R
WX
from Holland
?bankrupt 1844, fled to America
prosecuted for fraud 1858
operated under a number of pseudonyms in
London
author
s of dentist

MALLAN Messrs = Moseley Abraham

MALLAN T(homas) H(ill)
P1872

MALLORY T(homas T(oft)
    -1865(Portsmouth)
W under £4,000

MANNE Elizabeth
widow of George Arthur Manne

MANNE George Arthur
    -1850(Hull)
h of Elizabeth Manne
succeeded by Robert Marks

MARDEN J(ames) W
P1875

MARGETSON William
1829-85(Dewsbury)
OSGB1863 P1881 R BDA
LDS1863

MARKHAM Henry
P1879 R

MARKHAM J(ohn)
chd

MARKLAND Edwin
P1858
WX
chd

MARKS Robert
P1859
successor to G A Manne

MARLEY J
P1867
chd

MARTIN (& Waller)
chd

MARTIN John
    -1873(Nice)
OSL1857 OSGB1863 P1867
LDS1860
W £40,000

MASON James
P1879 R

MASON William(Exeter)
CD1857 P1878

MASSEY John
    -1852(Hanley)
adm. Chester under £2,000
?f of William Massey(Hanley)

MASSEY William
P1873
?s of John Massey

MATTHEWS Alfred M
CD1857 P1881 R BDA
LDS1863

McADAM George C
1811-78(Hereford)
OSL1857 OSGB1863 P1879 R
W under £4,000
f of George Christopher McAdam(1845-98)
who treated Francis Kilvert

McGREGOR Richard H G
P1872

McOWEN William Henry
P1867

MEACHAM James
1818(Halesowen)-99(Birmingham)
P1892 R
W £1,829

MEADOWS J(Leicester)
P1863
chd

MEDD Joseph
chd

MEDWIN Aaron
P1881 R BDA
LDS1863
London practice
chd

MEREDITH Joseph
1806(Birmingham)-71(Shrewsbury)
P1867
WX
some time in Canada in 1840s

MERRICK Thomas
1806-66(Hull)
P1865
W under £100

MERRYWEATHER
London 1848-54

MESSENGER William
LSA1821

MICHEL Peter
WX

MIDDLETON Thomas Patchett
London 1855

MILLER Charles
barber

MILLIDGE William Henry
chd

MILNER James
chd

MITCHELL J W
London 1835-55

MITCHELL John
P1875

MOLINEUX Henry
cupper

MOORE Edward(Falmouth)
P1859

MOORE Henry
-1860(Windsor)
CD1857
W under £1,500

MOORE William Vanderkamp
1816-88(Plymouth)
OSL1862 P1881 R BDA
LDS1863
chd
associated with Plymouth Dental Dispensary

MORGAN
P1863

MORGAN William
LSA1840

MORLEY Henry
-1900(Derby)
OSL1857 OSGB1863 P1879 R
LDS1863

MORTIMER Henry Thomas
chd

MOSELEY Abraham
1817(Birmingham)-89(London)
CD1857 P1889 R
W £1,196
London practice
trained by James Mallan, practised at Bristol as 'Messrs.Mallan'
f of Alfred Mosely[sic](1855-1919), diamond
speculator & member of the Jewish Board of
Guardians

MOSELEY Gillam
1829-80(Sheffield)
OSGB1863 P1879 R
LDS1863
W under £4,000

MOSELY sometimes spelled in trade directories as MOSELEY
MOSLEY

MOSELY(& fath E) =Alfred Isaiah Mosely
P1879
s of Ephraim Mosely

MOSELY B =? Moseley Bedford
P1866

MOSELY Charles
-1861(Preston)
P1861
W under £2,000
London practice from 1847
b of Ephraim, Lewin & Simeon Mosely

MOSELY Ephraim
-1873(Paris)
P1873
W under £12,000
London practice from 1840
Paris practice
b of Charles, Lewin & Simeon Mosely
f of Benjamin Ephraim Mosely, Alexander
Mosely Morley[sic], Alfred Isaiah Mosely
(LDS 1862, d.1879 Newcastle upon Tyne)

MOSELY H(Lincoln)= Mosel(e)y Henry B
=? Mosely H(arry) B(enj-
amin)
P1863

MOSELY H(arry) B(enjamin)
P1879 Leeds

MOSELY Lewin
1807-75(London)
P1872
W under £2,000
London practice from 1841
b of Charles, Ephraim & Simeon Mosely

MOSELY Simeon
1815-88(Hull)
CD1857 P1888 R
W £591
London practice from 1840
secretary of Hull Synagogue

MOSLEY L =? Mosely Lewin

MOSS Barnett
-1845(Manchester)
WX
committed suicide over debt

MOSS Isaac
London practice 1844-49

MOULD Thomas
P1857
WX

MUMMERY John Rigden
1809-85(London)
OSL1857 P1884 R BDA
W £21,551
anthropologist, fellow of the Linnaean
Society
f of John Howard Mummery

MURPHY J K(Hull) =? Murphy Joseph Kinnaird

MURPHY James(Hull) =? Murphy James(Nottingham)

MURPHY James Brabazon
CD1857 OSL1857 P1866

MURPHY John Lother
1813(Dublin)-
P1879
WX
author

MURPHY Joseph
formerly with Le Sec, successor to A E Brae

MURPHY Joseph Kinnaird
1811(Leeds)-

NAILER William
bleeder

NEEP William Edward John
CD1857 P1879
WX

NELSON George
LSA1837

NELSON Nathaniel
P1867
WX

NEWMAN William John
-1888(Liverpool)
OSGB1863 P1887 R BDA
LDSIreland 1878
associated with the founding of Liverpool
Dental Dispensary

NICHOLSON Joseph
P1864
LDS before 1870

NIGHTINGALE (& f D & bro 1) = Nightingale
Charles OR Nightingale Daniel Thomas

NIGHTINGALE (& f D & bro 2) = Nightingale
Charles OR Nightingale Daniel Thomas

NIGHTINGALE C(harles)
P1881 R BDA
London practice
s of Daniel Nightingale
b of Daniel Thomas Nightingale

NIGHTINGALE Daniel
1800-69(Tynemouth)
P1859
W ubder £3,000
f of Charles Nightingale & Daniel Thomas
Nightingale
? related to Charles Gibbs Nightingale
(Shrewsbury 1863-75)

NIGHTINGALE Daniel Thomas
CD1859 OSGB1863 P1879 R
s of Daniel Nightingale
b of Charles Nightingale

NORMAN Richard R(obert) B(owles)
LSA1841 MRCS1840

NOWELL Charles
P1879 R

ORMROD Mary
? widow of John Ormrod

ORROCK James
1830(Edinburgh)-1913
CD1857 OSL1857 OSGB1863 P1865
LDS1860 MRCS
left dentistry for art
s of James Orrock(Edinburgh)
see Webber, bibl.

ORVISS R W
P1858
WX

OWEN Henry
P1874

OWEN Richard
P1881 R BDA
chd

OXLEY Thomas Louis
-1883(Paris)
CD1857 P1861
W £7,355

PALK E(dward)
chd

PALMER G = Palmer Joseph Gunn

PALMER J(ames) E(dwin)
OSL1859 P1881 R BDA
Peterborough
b of Thomas Gill Palmer with whom he was in
practice in Peterborough in the 1830s

PALMER Joseph Gunn
1787(London)-1860(Birmingham)
W under £1,500
member of the Society of Friends

PALMER Robert
druggist

PALMER Thomas Gill
1811(London)-75(Cheltenham)
OSL1857 OSGB1863 P1873
LDS1860
pupil of Parmlly, assistant to Charles
Bromley
b of James Edwin Palmer with whom he practsed in Peterborough
f of Gasgoigne Palmer

PARKINSON Edward
OSL1857 OSGB1863 P1866
WX

PARKINSON F = Parkinson Felix

PARKINSON Felix
1802/06-?1848
member of the Parkinson family of Raquet Ct.
London
cousin of George Parkinson(Bath) who succeeded him

PARKINSON George =? Parkinson George Thomas
1817(London)-90(London)
OSL1857 OSGB1863 P1881 R BDA
?LDS1860
b of James Parkinson of Raquet Ct., London
s of George H Parkinson
gs of James Parkinson
cousin of Felix Parkinson

PARKINSON James
P1878

PARKINSON Samuel M =?Parkinson Solomon
P1857

PARSLEY James
apprenticed barber-surgeon 1741

PARSON Thomas C
1815(Manchester)-
OSGB1863 P?1879 R
WX
f of Thomas Cooke Parson(1842-91)

PARSONS Joseph Henry
1815-97(Southport)
P1879 R
W £2,310
Torquay practice
related to John Milner Parsons

PARSONS Joseph Henry(Halifax) =?Parsons
Joseph Henry(Liverpool)

PARSONS Robert
1810(York)-
OSL1857 P1867
LDS1860

PATRICK & son =?Patrick Robert

PATRICK Robert
1815-79(Southport)
CD1857 OSGB1863 P1879 R
W under £3,000
Southport

PAYNE Thomas Pibble (Piball)
1821-97(Southampton)
OSGB1863 P1897 R
W £2,708
assistant to Charles Bromley
related to Arthur George Payne

PEAL Joseph
P1879 R

PEARSALL Robert
1792(Gloucs)-1868(Torquay)
P1868
adm. under £100

PEATSON Henry Robert
P1879 R
chd

PENNY George Stothert
CD1857 P1879 R
LDS1860 MRCS1844
1847 doctor in Manchester

PERFECT G(eorge)
P1879 Landport R
chd

PERRY T A(Douglas) =? Perry T A(Stratford)
cupper

PERRY William(jun) =Perry William Duncan
s of William Perry(sen)

PERRY William(sen)
-1835(Liverpool)
MRCS
W Chester under £7,000
f of William Duncan Perry

PHILLIPS Thomas
1816(Chepstow)-
P1870
chd

PICNOT Theodore
1820(London)-1910(Hague)
P1901 R
see De Maar,bibl.

PIERREPO(I)NT John
-1860(Greenwich)
P1858
W under £100

PILLING Edmund
P1861
WX
surgical instrument maker

PILLING James
P1871

PINNOCK John
perfumer

PLATTIN Howard
P1858
chd

POINTING John
cupper

POULTON S
P1856

POUNDALL William Lloyd
1824-98
P1879 R
?LDS1872 (may be son)
claimed to be first to use nitrous oxide
anaesthesia in England
?connected with Brighton & Hove Dental
Dispensary

PRATT & SON =Pratt Charles John chd
              Pratt John chd
cuppers

PRATT R
P1862

PREBBLE James
P1859

PRESTWICH Wright
P1879Oldham R

PREW James
1792/96(Somerset)-1846(Bath)
W PCC
assistant to Joseph Sigmond
trained James Edwards & James Robertson
(his successor)
f in l of G S Williams
account books at Wellcome Institute

PRICHARD Augustin
LSA/MRCS1840 MDBerlin

PRIDEAUX Francis
P1879 R
Bridgewater

PRIDEAUX Thomas Sims
P1853London
phrenologist

PRYNN C T R
P1857

QUINTIN Adolphus Uriah
P1876

QUINTIN Augustus Theodore
P1859

QUINTIN Louis Charles
WX

RAMSDEN Henry
1816-70(Leeds)
P1870 R
W under £450

RANSOM Robert
OSL1858 P1879 R
LDS1860
London practice

RANSOM William =?Ranson William

RANSON William
1814(Shiney Row)-
P1866

READ T(homas)
P1881 R BDA
LDS1866
London 1848-55

READ W(illiam)
P1881 R BDA
London 1849-55

REDWARD William C(harles)
-1882(Southsea)
P1882 R
W £9,251

REILLY Maurice S(helton)
P1879 R
Uxbridge
chd

RICHARDSON Frank
P1879 R
LDSIreland1878
Derby

RICHARDSON George
P1863

RICHARDSON J
cupper

RICHARDSON John
1808-85(Hull)
P1885 R
WX
chd

RITSON Joseph
P1865
Birkenhead

ROBARTS George
P1857

ROBERTS =? Roberts Charles Duncan(Ramsgate)
CD1857 OSGB1863 P1874
LDS1860

ROBERTS Benjamin
P1871

ROBERTS Charles
cupper

ROBERTS. J B
chd

ROBERTSON Henry Blair
1826(Birmingham)-53(Gravesend)
MRCS1848
s of William Robertson
b of James Robertson(1817-67)
gs of James Blair
see Cohen et al., bibl.

ROBERTSON James(Sheffield) =? Robertson
James(Bath)

ROBERTSON James(Worcester)
1817(Blairgowrie)-67(Henley-in-Arden)
OSL1857 OSGB1863 P1867
employed Thomas Jeffries
s of William Robertson
b of Henry Blair Robertson
gn of James Blair
see Cohen et al., bibl.

ROBERTSON William
1794(Blairgowrie)-1870(Solihull)
OSL1857 OSGB1863 P1865
W under £14,000
former manufacturer(?of jute)
trained by Thomas Faulkner
n & s in 1 of James Blair
f of James Robertson(Worcester) & Henry
Blair Robertson
author
see Cohen et al., bibl.

ROBERTSON James(Bath)
1811(Perth)-64
CD1857 P1864
assistant to F Parkinson
assistant & successor to James Prew
trained by uncle William Imrie(Edinburgh)

ROBINSON George Moore
P1856

ROBINSON John
formerly banker
agitator for repeal of corn laws
sold practice to Richard Helsby
left dentistry for alum making & finally
accountancy
see Grindon, Manchester banks

ROBINSON S R
P1859

RODWAY Henry Barron
OSL1857 OSGB1863 P1878

ROGERS =?Rogers A McDonald
CD1857

ROGERS C(harles) D(eeble)
OSL1857 OSGB1863 P1869
LDS1860

ROGERS Joseph
P1876
former hairdresser/perfumer

ROGERS Thomas(Leicester) =? Rogers Thomas
(Halifax etc)
=? Rogers Thomas(Southampton)
from London

ROGERS Thomas(Halifax etc)
1812(Denby)-76(Bristol)
P1859

W under £600
fine art dealer at death

ROSE Donald
assistant to Fox(London)
b of James Rose & Robert Rose

ROSE Elizabeth
widow of James Rose

ROSE James
-1830(Liverpool)
W Chester under £600
b of Donald Rose & Robert Rose
b in 1 of John Brooks, whom trained
h of Elizabeth Rose
f of Harry Rose(US), John Frederick Rose,
James Edward Rose
gf of 4 dentists
ggf of dentists

ROSE James Edward
1820(Liverpool)-93(Liverpool)
CD1857 OSGB1863 P1893 R
W £4,250
apprenticed to uncle John Brooks
s of James Rose
b of Harry Rose & John Frederick Rose
n of Donald Rose & Robert Rose
f of Walter Rose(South Africa), Charles Rose
(1859-87), Frederick Rose(1856-1926)
u of Colin Rose Carroll

ROSE John Frederick
CD1857 P1861
London 1850
s of James Rose
b of Harry Rose & James Edward Rose
u of Walter, Charles & Frederick Rose

ROTHWELL James
-1862(Wigan)
P1858
W under £200
dental instrument maker

ROWE C A =Rowe Charles Reynolds
LSA/MRCS1835
P1859

ROWLAND (& fath S) =?Rowland Charles S
perfumer

ROWLAND Smith
perfumer

ROWNEY (& Davenport) =?Rowney Thomas Walter
Faraday
P1879 R
LDS1877

ROWNTREE Matthew
1807-77(Nottingham)
P1869
W under £3,000

RUMBLE G(eorge)
P1879 R
chd

RUSHFORTH John
bonesetter

RUSPINI Bartholomew
1728(Bergamo)-1813(London)
dentist to Prince Regent
founder of Royal Masonic Institute for
Girls
see Campbell, bibl.

RUST Jeremiah Anderson
P1864

RUTTER John
1831(Leeds)-
P1866

RYMER Samuel Lee
1832(Plymouth)-1909(croydon)
CD1857originator OSGB1863pres.1882 P1879 R
BDApres.1889
LDS1863
pupil of W Perkins
mayor of Croydon 1893
a founder of Croydon General Hospital
editor of Quarterly Journal of Dental Science
see Lindsay, 'Personalities of the past',
pp.69-70, bibl.

SAFFORD Thomas Jeffrey
watchmaker

SAUNDERS Josiah
London 1848-55

SAYLES Frederick Alban
1800-72(Lincoln)
CD1857 P1872
W under £1,000
f of Francis Austin Sayles
b of Lewis Charles Sayles

SAYLES Lewis Charles
1795-1881(Leamington)
former goldsmith
assistant to McLean
W £4,773
u of Francis Austin Sayles
b of Frederick Alban Sayles

SCHOFIELD William
P1879 R
Manchester

SCHOLEFIELD James
CD1859 OSGB1863 P1879 R
LDS1863
Rochdale

SCOTT(Bury St.Edmunds) =Scott G
CD1857

SEDMOND Joseph
WX

SEDMOND Mr & Mrs
from Berlin

SEDMOND Richard
P1858

SELVEY Joseph
1825(Birmingham)-
P1897 R

SHALE Thomas Wadson
P1865

SHAW John(Nottingham)
P1879 R

SHEFFIELD John
1820-73(Carlisle)
P1873
W under £1,500
worked for a period with brother Isaac in
London
s of Thomas Sheffield(Carlisle)
b of Thomas Sheffield(Exeter) & Isaac
Sheffield(London)

SHEFFIELD Thomas(Carlisle)
f of Thomas Sheffield(Exeter), Isaac Sheff-
ield(London) & John Sheffield(Carlisle)

SHEFFIELD Thomas(Exeter)
1804-84(London)
OSL1857 OSGB1863 P1879 R
s of Thomas Sheffield(Carlisle)
b of John Sheffield(Carlisle) & Isaac Sheffield(London)
trained A J Woodhouse

SHEPHERD Henry
P1859

SHERWIN James
-1872(Sheffield)
OSL1859 P1871
W under £800

SHEW (& fath R) =Shew Robert
1807(Birmingham)-
s of Robert Shew(Birmingham & Bath)

SHEW Charles (Weare)
1806(Bristol)-76(Bristol)
CD1857 P1868
W under £450
s of Henry Shew

SHEW George(Bath)
f of Robert Shew(d.1854)(Birmingham & Bath)
?u of Christopher Shew(London)

SHEW George(Cheltenham)
1797/1801(Gloucs)-

SHEW Henry
f of Charles Weare Shew

SHEW Henry W =? son of Shew Henry

SHEW Robert
-1854(Bath)
W PCC
s of George Shew(Bath)
f of Robert Shew(b.1807)(Bath)

SHILLOCK J(oseph) B(radley)
P1879 R
chd

SIEMINS Adolphus
P1856

SIGMOND Joseph
1750(Germany)-
see Brown, 'Advertising dentists in 18th century Bath', bibl.

SIMMONS Isaac
corn extractor

SIMPSON (& Rose) =Simpson John(Liverpool)
& Elizabeth Rose

SIMPSON James(Maidstone)
-1857(Maidstone)
CD1857
cupper

SIMS Robert
1802-71(Highgate, Worcs)
P1871
W under £3,000
f of Charles Sims

SINCLAIR Archibald
WX

SINGLETON Walter
silversmith/jeweller, wholesale mechanical
goods

SLATER J(ohn) McQ(uoid)
P1876

SMALE Charles
P1863
LDS1863

SMART J(ohn) S(herrard)
CD1857 OSGB1863 P1876

SMITH E(& H)
P1856

SMITH H(& E)
P1856

SMITH J(ohn) C(ox)
CD1857 P1866

SMITH William
P1857
WX
trained James Karran

SNAPE Joseph
1811-85(Liverpool)
CD1857 OSL1858 P1879 R
LDS1860
W £14,574
Liverpool
f of Joseph Snape, George Henry Snape &
one other dentist son

SNELL Harry B(ingham)
P1879 R
chd

SOUTHAM Henry
cupper

SPURGIN Joseph Cakebread
cupper

SQUIRE W(illiam)
P1879 R
chd

STAMBURY N
P1859
London 1849-51

STANLEY William =Stanley William Stamer
MRCS1838

STANSFIELD John
MD

STAVELEY William Henry W(ackerell)
P1879 R

STEPHENS (& White)
P1861

STEPHENS James C
P1878

STEPHENS John Harris
P1879 R
chd

STEPHENS Nathaniel Cooper
P1867

STEWART Charles
1815(Bristol)-
P1879 R
WX
Dover

STEWART Robert E(dward)
1832-86(Liverpool)
CD1857 OSGB1863 P1881 R BDA
LDS1863
a founder of Liverpool Dental Hospital

STOKES =Stokes Stanley

STOKES Henry C
Henry Collier =Stokes Henry Colin
1807/11-61(Newcastle)
CD1859 P1861
W under £3,000

STOKES Thomas
1794(Birmingham)-
P1877?
surgeon

STONER Harry W(est)
1822-92
P1879 R
f of 3 dentists

STRANGE Charles
P1864

STRINGER James
bricklayer

STUART Charles
P1862
WX

STYAN James
P1870

STYER Abraham S
P1858

SUGGETT J
P1864

SUTCLIFFE James
CD1857 OSGB1863 P1879 R
LDS1863

SUTTON George William
patent medicine dealer

SUTTON R C
P1861
SYDER Joseph
P1871

SYLVESTER George Joseph
1812-88(Worcester)
P1888 R
W £48

TALMA Arman
1767-1804
French
s of a dentist
see Cohen, 'The Talma family', bibl.

TARRATT William
P1857

TAYLOR (& Chamberlain)
P1856

TAYLOR John
chd

TAYLOR Thomas(Liverpool) =?Taylor Thomas
(Hereford)

TAYLOR Thomas(Loughborough)
P1863
aurist oculist

TEARNE Charles
s of Charles Tearne(sen)

TEARNE Charles(sen)
f of Charles Tearne(jun)

TEARNE Charles M
physician surgeon

TEARNE Theodore Sheldon
MRCS1847

THIRKETTLE T(homas)
P1874

THOMAS William(Liverpool) =?Thomas William
(Shrewsbury)

THOMPSON John N(orthon)
LSA1824

THOMPSON William
LSA1822
surgeon

THORNTON William
aurist

THWAITES J(ohn)
P1865

THWAITES John H B
CD1857 P1859

TIBBS John =?Tibbs John May

TIBBS John May
P1869

TIBBS Somerset
1809-68(Brixton)
BD1857vpres. OSL1857vpres. OSGB1863 P1868
W under £8,000
?f of Percival Tibbs

TINN George Tristram
P1879 R
f of dentists

TITTERINGTON William
-1857(Lancaster)
P1856
W Chester under £300
u of William Fort

TRACY John
1798-1873(Ipswich)
CD1857 P1865
W under £600
f of Humphrey Wingfield Tracy, Nathaniel
Tracy(1830-1902)
gf of Hugh Tracy

TROTTER F K
P1867

TUBBS Charles Foulger
OSL1860 P1879 R
associated with Plymouth Dental Dispensary

TUCK William
P1877?
LDS1863

TURNBULL George
P1865

TURNER John
1780(Selby)-

TWYFORD Thomas
pupil of George Bott(jun)
perfumer/toyman

UNDERHILL Samuel
bricklayer

VINEN F A B
chd?

VIRGIN Henry J(ames)
  -1881(Headington)
OSL1862 P1881 R
LDS1864
committed suicide
partner of Thomas James Bennett

VIZARD Edward
OSL1857 OSGB1863 P1867
LDS1860

WADE Edwin
1810(York)-89(York)
P1865
W £13,976
sheriff of York(1861-62) Lord Mayor(1864-
65) magistrate 1867 civic presentation 1875
f of Frederick John Wade

WADY John
practitioner in physic

WAINWRIGHT John =?Wainwright John(Oldham
             1879R)
           =?Wainwright John 1816-75
             d.Parkhurst Prison
             formerly of Sheffield
             W under £200
CD1857 P1860 Birkenhead

WALKER F A(Doncaster) =Walker F A(Retford)
                      =Walker Francis Drury
CD1857 OSGB1863 P1879 R

WALKER John
P1856

WALKER Joseph
chd apothecary

WALL Robert Hall
P1877

WALLER & Martin =Waller Charles
LSA1819

WARREN Edward Pritchett
1818(London)-81(Birmingham)
P1881 R
LDS1860

WARRINGTON Henry James
P1879 R

WAWN Charles Newby
  -1840(Newcastle)
apprenticed barber surgeon 1797

WAYLING George (Chaplin)
CD1857 P1879 R

WEALE Thomas
  -1803(Liverpool)
W Chester £2-5,000
from London
surgeon

WEBSTER James T
?LSA1828

WEIR James Anthony
P1879 R
chd

WELCH William T(jun)
P1859

WHATFORD J T =?Whatford Jack Thomas
P1879 R
LDSIreland1878
London

WHATFORD William S(tarr)
1796-1887(Brighton)
CD1857 P1887 R
WX

WHITE John Haines
P1871

WHITE Richard
1819-92(Dover)
OSL1857 OSGB1863 P1892 R
LDS1860
W £13,232
pupil of James Robinson
author
f of dentists, including Percy White(d.1893)
& Richard Wentworth White(1847-1924)

WHITE William(Bristol)
P1865

WHITE William(Birmingham)
P1870
chd

WHITLOCK Charles
actor manager
married to Elizabeth Kemble
see Boyes, bibl.

WILCOCK John
cupper

WILDSMITH Benjamin
  -1799(Manchester)
W Chester under £40
perrukier/hairdresser

WILKINSON Colonel =Wilkinson Major

WILLIAMS Edwin
1820-84(Croydon)
CD1859 P1879 R

WILLIAMS George S(alusbury)
1821(Bath)-85(Winterbourne,Gloucs)
OSL1857 OSGB1863 P1879
LDS1860
W £49,196
s in l of James Prew
s of a surgeon

WILLIAMSON William
CD1857
WX
worked as mechanic for James Orrock(Edinburgh)
master of James Orrock(jun) q.v.

WILLSON Isaac
1778(Longnor)-1853(Bath)
W Bath
dentist to William IV
f of John Willson

WILLSON John
1813(Bath)-93(Bath)
P1878
W £3,259
s of Isaac Willson

WILSON Charles =?Wilson Charles William

WILSON Charles William
P1863
WX

WILSON Edward
P1865

WILSON George
-1909(Hull)
P1879 R
LDSIreland

WILSON Thomas
1806(Birmingham)-
watchmaker

WILSON William(Birmingham) =?Wilson William
(Sheffield)
1830(Birmingham)-
s of watchmaker

WILSON William(Sheffield)
P1879 R

WILTON William Joseph
P1879 R

WINCKWORTH (& fath J) =Winckworth William
Dawson

WINCKWORTH John
1792/96-1855(Bath)
W Bristol & Bath
successor to Joseph Sigmond
from London
f of William Dawson Winckworth

WINCKWORTH William Dawson
1822(Bath)-
P1910 R
s of John Winckworth

WINDSOR Thomas =?Winder Thomas

WINGATE
apothecary accoucheur

WITHANALL Edward
bleeder

WOLFF J
P1857

WOOD =?Wood John b of William Robert Wood

WOOD John
P1861

WOOD William Robert
CD1857 OSGB1863 P1893 R
LDS1863
?associated with Brighton & Hove Dental
Dispensary
trained nephew William Robert Wood(1842-90)
b of John Wood(Brighton)(d.1840s)

WOODCOCK Edmund
1819(Shoreditch)-
CD1857 OSGB1863 P1895 R
WX

WOODCOCK Henry
1790-1879(Norwich)
P1858
former watchmaker

WOOFFENDALE Robert
1742(Sheffield)-1828(New York State)
apprenticed druggist 1757
short period as assistant to Thomas Berdmore
practised Sheffield, Liverpool, London &
United States
author
f of John Wooffendale
much written about: e.g. B W Weinberger,
An introduction to the history of dentistry

in America(Chicago,1948), vol.2, pp.99-111

WOOLFRYES Henry A
LDS1860
London
former pupil & assistant of Normansell &
Slade

WOOLLEY William
1789(Worcester)-
P1876

WORFOLK George
P1879 R
chd

WORKMAN Maurice
MRCS1812

WRIGHT & son =Wright William
1773-1860
aurist electrician cupper
s in same trades

WRIGHT T(homas) S(amuel) (jun)
1821-1902(Leamington)
P1868
W £605
s of Thomas Samuel Wright q.v.

WRIGHT Thomas(Hull) =?Wright Thomas (Manchester)

WRIGHT Thomas Samuel
-1880(Leamington)
P1863
W under £150
f of Thomas Samuel Wright(1821-1902)

YANIEWICZ Felix
1805(Liverpool)-86(Upper Norwood)
P1874
MRCSEdinburgh
W 1886 £520, resworn 1900 £1120 (not in
1886 Calendar of Probates)
trained by Hutchins(Edinburgh)
trained Felix Weiss(1822-92)
gave first demonstration of inhalation
anaesthesia in Liverpool in Jan 1847 at
Liverpool Literary & Philosophical Society
of which he was for a period Secretary
s of Felix Yaniewicz, violinist of inter-
national repute
see C.Gray, bibl.

YOUNG Frederick Graham
CD1857 ?P1881 (directory entries to this
date but entries for Mrs.F Graham Young
1870-76) ?R ?BDA
?f of Graham Young(LDSIreland 1881, in
practice until 1925)

APPENDIX 3

EARLIEST DIRECTORY EVIDENCE OF RESIDENT DENTISTS IN THE TOWNS IN THE REGISTER

Abergavenny	1852	Chepstow	1853	Greenwich	1845
Alderney	1852	Chertsey	1855	Guernsey	1839
Aylesbury	1850	Chester	1793	Guildford	1845
Banbury	1848	Chesterfield	1854	Halifax	1816
Barnsley	1828	Chichester	1839	Hanley	1835
Barnstaple	1840	Colchester	1848	Hanwell	1855
Bath	1786	Coventry	1839	Hartlepool	1851
Bedford	1854	Cowes	1839	Hastings	1831
Berwick	1820	Croydon	1845	Henley in Arden	1811
Beverley	1835	Darlington	1847	Hereford	1835
Birkenhead	1843	Dawlish	1852	Hertford	1850
Birmingham	1770	Derby	1828	High Wycombe	1853
Blackburn	1843	Dereham	1853	Huddersfield	1845
Bolton	1836	Devizes	1842	Hull	1792
Boroughbridge	1851	Devonport	1830	Huntingdon	1855
Boston	1826	Dodbrook	1840	Ipswich	1823
Bourn	1849	Doncaster	1851	Kendal	1848
Bradford	1840	Dorchester	1852	King's Lynn	1836
Braintree	1839	Dorking	1855	Kingsbridge	1844
Brampton	1855	Douglas	1837	Kingston on Thames	1845
Brecon	1840	Dover	1831	Lancaster	1848
Bridgewater	1848	Dunstable	1851	Landport	1848
Brighton	1818	Durham	1847	Leamington	1822
Bristol	1787	East Grinstead	1845	Leeds	1809
Bromley	1851	Eastbourne	1845	Leicester	1794
Buckingham	1854	Enfield	1851	Leominster	1794
Burslem	1822	Evesham	1854	Lewes	1845
Burton on Trent	1811	Exeter	1791	Lewisham	1845
Bury	1850	Exmouth	1840	Lichfield	1794
Bury St Edmunds	1823	Fakenham	1850	Lincoln	1826
Camborne	1847	Falmouth	1852	Liskeard	1852
Cambridge	1830	Fenny Stratford	1854	Liverpool	1767
Canterbury	1838	Folkestone	1855	Loughborough	1850
Cardiff	1848	Frome	1852	Louth	1849
Carlisle	1828	Gateshead	1833	Ludlow	1844
Chatham	1838	Gloucester	1841	Lyme Regis	1855
Chelmsford	1855	Gravesend	1842	Macclesfield	1841
Cheltenham	1830	Great Malvern	1850	Maidstone	1839

Manchester	1781	Shepton Mallet	1850	Woolwich	1839
Mansfield	1853	Sherborne	1855	Worcester	1788
Margate	1849	Shipley	1853	Worthing	1849
Melcombe Regis	1855	Shrewsbury	1828	Yarmouth	1839
Monmouth	1850	Sleaford	1855	Yeovil	1840
New Alresford	1848	Southampton	1811	York	1809
Newark	1828	Southsea	1852		
Newbury	1844	South Shields	1851		
Newcastle under Lyme	1854	Spilsby	1849		
Newcastle upon Tyne	1811	St.Helier	1832		
Newport (Isle of Wight)	1848	Stafford	1850		
Newport (Mon)	1852	Stamford	1798		
Northampton	1839	Stockport	1841		
North Shields	1828	Stockton on Tees	1847		
Norwich	1783	Stoke on Trent	1850		
Nottingham	1798	Stonehouse	1814		
Paignton	1852	Stowmarket	1846		
Penrith	1855	Stratford upon Avon	1845		
Penzance	1847	Sunderland	1834		
Plymouth	1822	Swansea	1840		
Poole	1840	Taunton	1830		
Portsea	1823	Tavistock	1844		
Portsmouth	1839	Teignmouth	1840		
Preston	1818	Tetsworth	1854		
Reading	1821	Tipton	1850		
Reigate	1855	Torquay	1844		
Retford	1850	Truro	1847		
Richmond (Surrey)	1848	Tunbridge Wells	1839		
Ripon	1840	Uxbridge	1832		
Rochdale	1838	Wakefield	1851		
Rochester	1851	Warwick	1841		
Romsey	1811	Weymouth	1828		
Ross	1847	Whitchurch	1842		
Runcorn	1846	Whitehaven	1855		
Ryde	1839	Wigan	1841		
Saffron Walden	1855	Wimborne Minster	1848		
Salford	1824	Winchester	1852		
Salisbury	1839	Windsor	1798		
Scarborough	1841	Wisbeach	1850		
Sheffield	1811	Woburn	1850		
Shelton	1846	Wolverhampton	1838		

APPENDIX 4

POSSIBLE FAMILY CONNECTIONS BETWEEN PROVINCIAL AND LONDON DENTISTS BEFORE 1855

*(terminal dates do not necessarily indicate end of practice)

PROVINCIAL			LONDON	
Name	Place	*Dates of Directory entries	Name	*Dates of Directory entries
Ballard, George	Frome	1852	**Ballard**, William	1854-55
Barclay, James	Derby	1854-55	**Barclay**, Henry	1854-55
Barnard, J. F.	Dover etc.	1836-47	**Barnard**, George	1844-55
Barnard, A.	St. Helier	1839-49		
Barrett, John Smith	Bury	1850	**Barrett**, Henry J.	1848-53
Bartlett, Henry Val.	Sheffield	1848	**Bartlett**, George	1835-55
Bartlett, John	Bristol	1793	Bartlett, William	1836-55
Bartlett, H. N.	Foulsham	1853	Bartlett, E. B.	1841-55
			Bartlett, Geo. Bateman	1855
Beacall, Edwin	Sheffield	1852-55	**Beacall**, William	1823-55
Bellis, William Andrew	Douglas	1843-44	**Bellis**, Francis	1853-55
Bishop, T.	Woolwich	1855	**Bishop**, W.	1851-53
Blundell, Walter	Brighton	1845-52	**Blundell**, William	1847
			Blundell, Thomas	1847
Bowden	Bristol	1833	**Bowden**, Frederick	1847-55
Bradley, T. D.	Brighton	1854-55	**Bradley**, R.	1805-42
Bradshaw, Francis J.	Leicester	1835	**Bradshaw**, Richard	1855
Brooks, John	Liverpool	1832-53	**Brooks**, Richard	1853-54
Brooks, Robert Heygate	Banbury	1849-55		
Canton	Richmond	1851	**Canton** (many)	1851
Capper, John Devis	Norwich	1850	**Capper**, Charles	1853-55
Cobb, J. S.	Yarmouth	1853	**Cobb**, Robert	1845-55
Davis, Albert & J.	Birmingham	1852	**Davis**, Albert J.	1851-54
Dick	Sheffield	1845	**Dick**, John	1835-44
Duff, John	Bristol	1850-53	**Duff**, Alex	1846-55
Downing, Richard	Newcastle	1827-55	**Downing**	1811, 22
Fuller, Edward	Hastings	1839	**Fuller**, Edmund	1838
Garner, Edward	Boston	1849	**Garner**, Edward S.	1832-55
Gilbert, George	Portsea	1852, 55	**Gilbert**, Henry	1851-55
			Gilbert, William	1853-55
Hampson, Elijah	Liverpool	1843-47	**Hampson**, James	1836-55
Imrie, Robert Marshall	Manchester	1834-45	**Imrie**, William Henry	1823-55
			Imrie, Marshall	1832
Kyan, J. Howard	Chelmsford	1855	**Kyan**, J. H. jun.	1851
Marsh, Robert Jardine	Birmingham	1849-50	**Jardine**, John	1842, 45
Norman, Richard R. B.	Yarmouth	1850-53	**Norman**, Robert	1843
			Norman, John	1843
Parkinson, Felix	Bath	1829-49	**Parkinson** (7 genera-	1785-
Parkinson, George	Bath	1850-54	tions)	1895
Perfect, G.	Southsea	1855	**Perfect**, Alfred	1843-55
Sheffield, John	Carlisle	1855	**Sheffield**, Isaac	1842-55
Sheffield, Thomas sen.	Carlisle	16.. 48		
Sheffield, Thomas jun.	Exeter	1837-55		
Sherwin	Sheffield	1830	**Sherwin**, Francis	1851-55
Sherwin, James	Sheffield	1855		
Shew (various)		1796-53	**Shew**, Christopher	1822-44
			Shew, William	1845-55
Smale, Charles	Manchester	1848-55	**Smale**, Thomas	1832-42
			Smale, Henry	1838-55
Smartt, T.	Gravesend	1850	**Smartt**, Charles	1851-55
Snell, Harry B.	Stonehouse	1850-52	**Snell**, James	1838-41
Tracy, John	Ipswich etc.	1844-55	**Tracy**, Samuel John	1851-55
Way, Edward	Tunbridge	1849	**Way**, S. A.	1835-42

APPENDIX 5

DENTAL FAMILIES ESTABLISHED IN THE PROVINCES BEFORE 1855

*(terminal dates do not necessarily indicate end of practice)

Name	Place	*Dates of Directory Entries	Name	Place	*Dates of Directory Entries
Alex, J.	Cheltenham Oxford	1830, 35	**Brown**, George	Leamington	1832-54
			Brown, Henry S.	Warwick	1841-54
Alex, Montague	Cheltenham	1839-55	Brown, Samuel	Birmingham	1809
- -				Henley	1811-29
Atkinson, John	Leeds	1817-55	- -		
Atkinson, John H.	Leeds	1845-55	**Buckell**, John W.	Winchester	1852
- -			Buckell, William	Salisbury	1848-55
Ball, Frederick	Newcastle	1847-53	Bucknell, John	Chichester	1839
Balls, W.	Newcastle	1844	- -		
- -			**Cafferata**, Jas. L.	Sunderland	1834-55
Bate, Charles	Plymouth	1840-52	Cafferata, Joseph	Liverpool	1816-29
Bate, Charles S.	Swansea	1844-53	- -		
- -			**Cherriman**, Jno. V.	Brighton	1843-55
Beal, Mary Ann	Sheffield	1854	Cherriman, Reuben	Brighton	1845
Beal, Richard	Sheffield	1849-55	- -		
- -			**Clarke**, E.	Brighton	1850-55
Berend, Louis	Liverpool Manchester	1829-55	Clarke, (son)	Brighton	1850-55
			- -		
Berend, Samuel	Liverpool	1824-55	**Clarke**, Isaiah W.	Nottingham	1828-55
- -			Clarke, (son)	Nottingham	1846-55
Blackmore, Edward	Barnstaple	1840-52	Clarke, James	Nottingham	1841-54
(son of above)	Barnstaple	1850-52	Clarke, Robert	Nottingham	1844
Blackmore, Julia	Taunton	1848-52	- -		
Blackmore, Richard	Taunton	1830-40	**Cogan**, John Dan.	Bath	1840-54
- -			Cogan, Samuel W.	Taunton	1848
Boardman----	Plymouth	1822	- -		
Boardman, Mrs.	Plymouth	1830	**Cooper**, Robert	Liverpool	1845-46
Boardman, William	Exeter	1823	Cooper, S & Co.	Liverpool	1846-55
- -			Cooper, Thomas	Rochdale	1838-41
Bott, George sen.	Nottingham	1798-1819	- -		
Bott, George jun.	Birmingham	1797-1805	**Corey**, Charles	Liverpool	1853-55
Bott, Sophia	Birmingham	1808-47	Corey, Wm.	Brighton	1850
Bott, Parker	Nottingham	1822-25	- -		
- -			**Crawcour**, Barnett	Norwich	1822, 30
Boulnois, Jas. Jos.	Bristol	1803-26	Crawcour, Henry	Norwich	1836
Boulnois, John	Bristol	1826-30	Crawcour, Lindsay	Windsor	1853
- -			Crawcour, M.	Exeter	1816, 22
Brewer, Theodore	Bath	1793-1822	- -		
Brewer, James	Bath	1822-26	**Davies**, Albert	Liverpool	1852
- -			Davies, John	Liverpool	1852
			- -		

Name	Place	*Dates of Directory Entries	Name	Place	*Dates of Directory Entries
De Berry, Sam.	Birmingham	1837, 39	**Faulkner**, Jno. sen.	Manchester	1811-43
De Berry (son)	Birmingham	1837, 39	Faulkner, Jno. jun.	Manchester	1815-38
- - - - - - - - - - - -			Faulkner, Thomas	Manchester	1788-1819
De Loude, Louis	Liverpool	1834-35	Faulkner, Th. John	Manchester	1822-55
	Wolverhampton	1838-51	Faulkner, John	Greenwich	1845-50
De Loude (son)	Wolverhampton	1851	- - - - - - - - - -		
De Loude, Th. C.	Liverpool	1832	**Fay**	Hull	1838, 39
- - - - - - - - - - - -			Fay, Tullius Priest	Liverpool	1839-55
Dixon, John	Leeds	1828-41	- - - - - - - - - -		
Dixon, Ruth	Leeds	1842-46	**Fothergill**, Alex.	Darlington	1851-55
Dixon & Picnot	Leeds	1846-55	Fothergill, Wm.	Darlington	1847-55
- - - - - - - - - - - -			- - - - - - - - - -		
Downing, B.	Newcastle	1853	**Fox**, Chas. Prideaux	Torquay	1844
Downing, Edward	Newcastle	1841-55	Fox, Cornelius W.	Plymouth	1844-47
Downing, Rich. jun.	Newcastle	1839-47	Fox, Geo. Fred.	Gloucester	1849-53
Downing, Richard	Newcastle	1820-55	Fox, Robert Were	Exeter	1828-55
Downing, Wm.	Newcastle	1844	Fox, Rbt. Were jun.	Bristol	1838-55
Downing, M.	Bristol	1853	Fox, Silvanus Bevan	Exeter	1855
- - - - - - - - - - - -			- - - - - - - - - -		
Edwards, Edward	Bath	1846-54	**Fox**, Thomas	Plymouth	1836
Edwards, James	Bath	1848-54	Fox, George	(various)	1839-52
- - - - - - - - - - - -			- - - - - - - - - -		
English, Thomas	Birmingham	1818-47	**Fuller**, Edward	Hastings	1839
English, Th. Rob.	Birmingham	1841-55	Fuller, Francis	Leicester	1835, 41
- - - - - - - - - - - -			- - - - - - - - - -		
Ensor, Silas	Birmingham	1816-22	**Gabriel**, Arnold	Liverpool	1853
Ensor, Wm. Edw.	Liverpool	1837-55	Gabriel, John	Hull	1838-39
- - - - - - - - - - - -			Gabriel, Lyon	Hull, Liverpool	1840-47
Eskell, Abraham	Birmingham	1849-55	Gabriel, --	Croydon	1855
Eskell, Albert	Liverpool	1845-55	- - - - - - - - - -		
Eskell, Francis	Manchester	1848	**Garner**, Edward	Boston	1849
Eskell, Frederick	Manchester	1843-52	Garner, Joseph Sam.	Boston	1849-50
Eskell, Fred A.	Manchester	1851-55	- - - - - - - - - -		
Eskell, Louis	Bradford	1847-55	**Garnett**, Geo. Belk	Huddersfield	1850-55
Eskell, Phillipus	Sheffield	1837-55	Garnett, Henry Wm.	Sheffield	1845-55
Eskell, A.	Doncaster	1851	- - - - - - - - - -		
- - - - - - - - - - - -			**Goldstone**, --	Bath	1793-1809
Evatt, Hy. Royle	Sheffield	1837-46	Goldstone, Alfred	Bristol	1841-49
Evatt, James	Leeds	1849	Goldstone, C.	Bath	1793-96
Evatt, William	Sheffield	1811-41	Goldstone, Edward	Devizes	1842
- - - - - - - - - - - -			Goldstone, George	Bath	1800
Farthing	Taunton	1840	- - - - - - - - - -		
Farthing, John	Southampton	1843-47	**Goodman**, James	Taunton	1852
Farthing, John	Guildford	1845	Goodman, Samuel	Bath	1854
Farthing, John	Exeter	1848-52	- - - - - - - - - -		
Farthing, John	Cardiff	1855	**Groves**, --	Stonehouse	1814
Farthing, Will.	Southampton	1845	Groves, Anthony N.	Exeter	1822-30
- - - - - - - - - - - -			Groves, Edwin	Exeter	1837-55
			Groves, John	Exeter	1827-54

Name	Place	*Dates of Directory Entries	Name	Place	*Dates of Directory Entries
Harrison, Robert	Hull	1848-55	**Jordan**, Henry	Derby	1846-52
Harrison, Rbt. E.	Hull	1848-55	Jordan, Hy. Edward	Reading	1840-55
Hart, --	Bath	1824	**King**, Edward John	Exeter	1848-50
Hart, Hammett	Bristol	1793-1819	King, Norman	Exeter	1843-55
Hart, Mrs.	Bristol	1816-22			
Hart, Joseph	Bristol	1822-55	**Levander**, Joseph	Exeter	1830-55
Hart, A. S.	Bristol/London	1822-49	Levander, John	Teignmouth	1848
Hartley, Francis W.	Halifax	1840-41	**Levason**, Joseph	Cheltenham/	1839-52
Hartley, William	Leeds	1847		Hereford	
			Levason, Lewis	Chester/	1828-53
Hawker, Robert	Devonport	1830		Leamington	
Hawker, Henry	Liverpool	1851-55			
			Lindon, Ann Maria	Manchester	1843
Helsby, Charles	Manchester	1846-55	Lindon, Bracewell	Manchester	1836-38
Helsby, Richard	Manchester	1828-55	Lindon, John	Manchester	1824, 28
			Lindon, William	Manchester	1828-34
Hutchinson, James	Nottingham	1835-50			
Hutchinson, Massey	Huddersfield	1853-55	**Little**, --	Bristol	1850-55
Hutchinson, Matilda	Nottingham	1844	Little, Henry	Plymouth etc.	1830-47
Hutchinson, Thomas	Nottingham	1828-55			
			Lloyd, Richard	Liverpool	1841-55
James, John	Worcester	1840-55	Lloyd, Thomas Bridge	Manchester	1834-46
James, Thomas	Worcester	1840-41	Lloyd, Th. Whitfield	Liverpool	1818-48
Jardine, J.	Bradford	1847	**Lukyn**, Christopher	Coventry	1845-50
Jardine, Marsh Rob.	Birmingham	1849-50	Lukyn, Edward	Leamington	1850
			Lukyn, John	Nottingham	1844-50
			Lukyn, W.	Nottingham	1853-55
Jones, Grenville	Shrewsbury	1834-44	Lukyn, William	Oxford/	1830-50
Jones, Hy. Micholls	Ex/Chester/Shr.	1827-51		Leamington	
Jones, Horatio	Shrewsbury	1850-51			
			Lyon, Henry	Cambridge	1850-55
Jones, Sam. Aaron	Norwich	1842-55	Lyon, William	Cambridge	1855
Jones, Wm.	Norwich	1839	Lyon, Lemuel	Ipswich	1855
Jones, Isaiah	Norwich	1830	Lyon, Leo	Bristol	1798
Jones, Ch. John	Cambridge	1830, 46	**Manne**, Elizabeth	Hull	1851-52
Jones, John	Bury St. Edmunds	1823	Manne, Geo. Arthur	Hull etc.	1798-1852
Jones, John	Cambridge	1839, 50-55			
			Martin, John	Portsmouth	1839-55
Jones, John	Manchester	1824, 28	Martin, Stables	Portsmouth	1852
Jones, John	Liverpool	1851-52			
Jones, Robert	Preston	1851-53	**Moss**, Barnett	Manchester	1836-46
Jones, John	Preston	1851	Moss, Emanuel	Manchester	1828-29
			Moss, Isaac	Bristol	1831
Jordan, Charles	Manchester, Liverpool	1840-49	**Murphy**, Edward	Derby	1828-31
Jordan, John	Manchester	1850-52	Murphy, Jas. Brabazon	Derby	1831-55

Name	Place	*Dates of Directory Entries	Name	Place	*Dates of Directory Entries
Nelson, George	Preston	1854-55	Robertson, Henry	Stoke	1850
Nelson, Nathaniel	Liverpool	1839-55	Robertson, James	Worcester	1847-55
Nelson, W.	Liverpool	1843	Robertson, William	Birmingham	1823-55
Nightingale, Daniel	Newcastle	1827-55	Rose, Donald	Liverpool	1832-41
Nightingale, C.	N. Shields	1855	Rose, Elizabeth	Liverpool	1832-34
Nightingale, Dan. Th.	Newcastle	1855	Rose, James	Liverpool	1823-29
Nightingale, William	Newcastle	1844	Rose, Jas. Edward	Liverpool	1845-55
			Rose, John Fred.	Preston	1851-55
Ormrod, John	Manchester	1794-1802	Rose, Robert	Preston	1837-48
Ormrod, Mary	Manchester	1804, 08			
			Rowland, Smith	Liverpool	1829-48
Parkinson, Sam. M.	Liverpool	1855	Rowland, (son)	Liverpool	1829-37
Parkinson, Solomon	Liverpool	1853	Rowland, Chas. S.	Liverpool	1839-41
Parkinson, Walter	Liverpool	1848			
			Sayles, Fr. Alban	Lincoln	1826-55
Parsons, Robert	York	1837-51	Sayles, Lewis Ch.	Sheffield	1822-54
Parsons, Thomas	York	1855			
			Sedmond, Joseph	Plymouth	1822-44
Patrick, --	Bolton	1836	Sedmond, --	Bristol	1797-98
Patrick (son)	Bolton	1836	Sedmond, Mrs.	Bristol	1797-98
Patrick, Hugh	Chorlton	1843	Sedmond, Richard	Plymouth	1847-52
Patrick, Robert	Bolton	1843-55			
			Sheffield, John	Carlisle	1852, 55
Perry, William	Liverpool	1794-1837	Sheffield, Thomas	Carlisle	1828-52
Perry, Wm. Duncan	Liverpool	1821-39	Sheffield, Th. jun.	Exeter	1829-55
Pilling, Edmund	Blackburn	1843-55	Shew, (son of R)	Bath	1830-41
Pilling, James	Blackburn	1851-55	Shew, Charles	Bristol	1828-55
			Shew, George	Bath	1796-1809
Pratt, --	Chichester	1839	Shew, George	Cheltenham	1830-49
Pratt, (son)	Chichester	1839	Shew, Henry	Bristol	1801-38
			Shew, Robert	Birmingham/Bath	1800-41
Prideaux, Francis	Taunton	1852			
Prideaux, Th. S.	Southampton	1833-49	Simpson, James	Manchester	1846
			Simpson, John	Manchester	1838-41
Quintin, A. U.	Gloucester etc.	1847-53			
Quintin, A. T.	Gloucester	1849-53	Singleton, Jno. A.	Worcester	1830
Quintin, L. C.	Gloucester etc.	1847-53	Singleton, Walter	Worcester	1840
			Singleton, Wm. Rob.	Worcester	1840
Ramsden, George	Bradford	1841			
Ramsden, Henry	Bradford	1845-55	Smith, H.	Newcastle	1855
			Smith, E.	Newcastle	1855
Redward, E.	Ryde	1855	Smith, S. E.	Newcastle	1850
Redward, Wm. C.	Portsea	1839-55			
			Stephens, Jno. H.	Plymouth	1850-52
Richeraud, Ferd.	Manchester	1846	Stephens, Jas. C.	Devonport	1840-52
Richeraud, Morris	Liverpool	1845	Stephens, N. C.	Truro	1847-52

Name	Place	*Dates of Directory Entries	Name	Place	*Dates of Directory Entries
Stewart, Charles	Bristol	1838-55	**Wright**, T. S.	Coventry	1845-50
Stewart, Mark	Bristol	1828-36	Wright, T. S. jun.	Leamington	1842-54
Sutton, Geo. Wm.	Louth	1849			
Sutton, R. C.	Louth	1855			
Sylvester, G. J.	Worcester	1837-55			
Sylvester, John	Worcester	1850			
Tearne, Chas. jun.	Worcester	1788-98			
Tearne, Chas. sen.	Worcester	1788-98			
Tearne, Chas. M.	Worcester	1820-40			
Tearne, T. S.	Worcester	1847-53			
Thomas, Connoly	Liverpool	1824-29			
Thomas, William	Liverpool	1825			
Thompson, John N.	Nottingham	1847			
Thompson, William	Nottingham	1825-53			
Thwaites, J.	Bristol	1853-55			
Thwaites, J. H. B.	Bristol	1848-53			
Tibbs, John	Barnstaple	1850			
Tibbs, John May	Teignmouth etc.	1852			
Tibbs, Somerset	Cheltenham	1839-53			
Tinn, Geo. Tristram	Newcastle	1847-55			
Tinn, T.	Newcastle	1844			
Webster, Thomas	Leeds	1830			
Webster, (son)	Leeds	1830			
Whatford, J. T.	Worthing	1849-55			
Whatford, W. S.	Brighton	1839-55			
Willson, Isaac	Bath	1812-50			
Willson, John	Bath	1841-54			
Wilson, Charles	Sheffield	1837			
Wilson, Edward	Sheffield	1849-54			
Wilson, William	Sheffield	1852-55			
Winckworth, John	Bath	1819-48			
Winckworth, W. D.	Bath	1846-54			
Wright, --	Bristol	1816-18			
Wright, (son)	Bristol	1816-18			

BIBLIOGRAPHY

A General

Boase, F., *Modern English Biography* (London,1892)

Cope, Sir Z.V., *The Royal College of Surgeons of England, a history* (London,1959)

English, B., 'Probate valuations and the Death Duty Registers', *Bull.Inst.Hist.Res.*,57(1985),80-91

Harbury, C.D. and D.M.W.N. Hichens,*Inheritance and wealth inequality in Britain* (London,1979)

Holloway, S.W.F., 'Medical education in England, 1830-1858: a sociological analysis', *History*,49(1964),299-324

Holmes, G., *Augustan England; profession, state and society, 1680-1730* (London,1982)

Loudon, I.S.L., 'The nature of provincial medical practice in eighteenth century England', *Med.Hist.*,29(1985),1-32

O'Brien, P.K., 'British incomes and property in the early nineteenth century', *Ec.Hist.Rev.*,12(1959-60),255-67

Peterson, M.J., 'Gentlemen and medical men: the problem of professional recruitment', *Bull.Hist.Med.*,58(1984),457-73

Porter, R. and D., *In sickness and in health* (London,1988)

Poynter, F.N.L., *The evolution of medical education in Britain*

(London,1966)

Poynter, F.N.L., ed., *Medicine and science in the 1860s* (London,1968)

Woodward, J. and D. Richards, *Health care and popular medicine in nineteenth century England* (London,1977)

Wrigley, E.A. and R.S. Schofield, *The population history of England, 1541-1871* (London,1981)

B **Bibliography of directories**

Austin, R.A., *Catalogue of the Gloucestershire collection in the Gloucester Public Library* (Gloucester,1928)

Birkenhead Public Library, *A finding list of the directories, roll of electors, census returns in the local history collection* (Birkenhead,n.d.)

Bristol Public Library, *Bristol bibliography* (Bristol,n.d.)

Burgess, W.F.and B.R.M. Riddell, *Kent directories located*, 2nd ed. (Maidstone,1978)

Chester Libraries and Museums, *The general reader's guide to 19th century Chester* (Chester,n.d.)

Cornwall County Library, *Local studies* (Redruth,n.d.)

Derbyshire County Library, *A guide to the directories of Derbyshire and surrounding counties, held by Derbyshire County Library and the Derbyshire Record Office* (Derby,1977)

Emery, N. and D.R. Beard, *Staffordshire directories, a union list of directories relating to the geographical county of Stafford* (Hanley,1966)

Farrant, J., *The commercial directories of Gloucestershire, a first list* (Gloucester,1969)

Farrant, J., *Wiltshire directories* (Salisbury,1967)

Hillier, R.W.E., *Catalogue of directories and poll books for Northamptonshire, Huntingdonshire and the city of Peterborough* (Peterborough,1977)

Kent County Libraries, *Kent bibliography* (Maidstone,n.d.)

Norton, J.E., *Guide to the national and provincial directories of England and Wales, excluding London, published before 1856* (London,1950)

Norwich Public Library, *Directories in the local studies department* (Norwich,1981)

Reading Public Library, *Reading local collection* (Reading,n.d.)

Somerset County Library, *Preliminary check list of Somerset directories* (Taunton,n.d.)

Suffolk Record Office, *Suffolk County directories, 1784-1939* (Ipswich,n.d.)

Tupling, G.H., rev., enl., ed. by S. Horrocks, *Lancashire directories* (Preston,1968)

Worcestershire Record Office, *Consolidated chronological list of Worcestershire directories held in or near Worcestershire* (Worcester,1959)

C Works referred to in the main text

1. Primary sources
a. Manuscript

Account books (1830–46) of James Prew (Ms 5208–5214, Wellcome Library)

Account books (1864–70) of James Blair Lloyd (Weaver Museum, School of Dentistry, University of Liverpool)

Calendars of Probate (Principal Probate Registry), 1858–1915 (for grants of probate for individuals)

Calendars of Wills at Bristol, Devon, Gloucester, Lancashire, Leicester and Somerset Record Offices (for wills of individuals)

Enumerators' returns ; 1841 census: Bath, Bristol, Cheltenham, Leeds, Newcastle upon Tyne, York; 1851 census: Bath, Birmingham, Bristol, York (for individuals)

Index to Deaths (Registrar General), 1837–1915 (for deaths of individuals)

Minutes (1862–63) of the College of Dentists (Ms I 105, Royal Society of Medicine)

Odontological Society of Great Britain, autograph letters of original members and other communications concerning its foundation in 1856 (Ms 229, Royal Society of Medicine)

Rate books of Bristol, 1831–46 (Bristol Record Office)

b. Newspapers (including compilations), dental and medical journals systematically searched

Aris's Birmingham Gazette, 1741–99, 1804–06, 1821–22

Bath Chronicle, 1800–10

British Dental Journal, 1903–13

British Journal of Dental Science, 1856–1916

British Quarterly Journal of Dental Surgery, 1843

Cambrian, 1804–06

Cambridge Chronicle, 1794–1802

Cheltenham Free Press and Gloucester Herald, 1834–36, 1839

Cheltenham Journal, 1829

Chester Chronicle, 1797–1818, 1823–24

Dental advertisements, publications/printed matter, 399, archive of
    the British Dental Association

Dental Record, 1881–1906

Dental Review, 1859–67

The Dentist, 1899

Forceps, 1844–45

Journal of the British Dental Association, 1881–1902

Kentish Gazette

Kentish Observer

Lancaster Gazette, 1801–04, 1831

Lancet, 1823–63

Leeds Intelligencer, 1780–84

Leeds Mercury, 1800, 1820, 1840

Leicester Journal, 1769–1811

Leicester and Nottingham Journal

Liverpool Chronicle, 1800–07

Liverpool Courier, 1808–11

Liverpool Mercury, 1811–40

Manchester Mercury, 1793–1802

Manx Sun

Menzies Campbell Collection of Newspaper Advertisements (Royal College of Surgeons of England) [MCC in text]

Monmouthshire Merlin, 1829–31

Monthly Review of Dental Surgery, 1872–80

Nottingham Journal, 1785

Purland, T., *Dental memoranda* [Purland scrapbook in text] (Ms 63518, Wellcome Library)

Quarterly Journal of Dental Science, 1857–59

Reading Journal and Oxford Chronicle, 1800–10

Robinson, E., *Compilation of lectures, advertisements etc. taken from Aris's Gazette in the 18th century* (unpublished compilation, 1972, Birmingham City Library)

Salopian Journal, 1798–1800, 1803–25, 1827–28, 1835, 1840, 1845

Shrewsbury Chronicle, 1797, 1801–02

Transactions of the Odontological Society, 1856-64

Williamson's Liverpool Advertiser, 1788-92

Worcester Herald

Worcester Journal, 1840-41

York Chronicle, 1772-79, 1790-99

York Courant, 1739-47, 1800-10

c. Printed (only those trade directories referred to in the main text
   are included; the complete list is to be found in *appendices 1 and
   2*)

Allen, C., *Operator for the teeth* (York,1685)

Andrews, C.B., ed., *Torrington diaries* (London,1935)

Bate, C.S., 'On the education of dentists', *Lancet* (1846),230-31

Bell, T., *The anatomy, physiology and diseases of the teeth* (London,
   1835)

Bew, C., *Operations on the causes and effects of diseases in the
   teeth and gums* (London,1819)

Billing, M., *Directory and gazetteer of Devonshire* (Birmingham,1857)

Binns, J. and G. Brown, *A directory for....Leeds* (Leeds,1800)

Breham, E., *Treatise on the structure, formation, and various
   diseases of the teeth and gums* , 3rd ed. (Liverpool,1821)

Charlton and Archdeacon, *Directory of Leeds* (Leeds,1849)

Chettle, H., *Kind-Harts Dreame* (London, 1592), in *Early English
   poetry, ballads and popular literature of the middle ages*

(London,1841), Percy Society, V

Colbran, J., *Handbook and directory for Tunbridge Wells* (Tunbridge Wells,1850)

Cooper, W., *Post Office directory of Southampton* (Southampton,1847)

Craven, *Commercial directory of the County of Huntingdon and the town of Cambridge* (Nottingham,1855)

Davenport, J.W., *The mirror of dentistry* (London,1852)

Davies, H., *Cheltenham annuaire* (Cheltenham,1840)

De Loude, L.C., *Surgical, operative and mechanical dentistry* (London, 1840)

Erith, F.N., *Bath annual directory* (Bath,1850)

Fauchard, P., *Le chirurgien-dentiste* (Paris,1728)

Forbes and Knibb, *Post Office directory of Southampton* (Southampton, 1849)

Forbes and Knibb, *Directory of Southampton* (Southampton,1851)

Fox, J., *The natural history and diseases of the human teeth* , 2nd ed. (London,1814)

General Medical Council, *Dentists Register* (London,1879)

Gidney, E., *A treatise on the structure, diseases and management of the teeth* (Utica,1824)

Gore, J., *Liverpool directory* (Liverpool,1775)

Gray, J., *Dental practice* (London,1837)

Guillemeau, J., *Les oeuvres de chirurgie* (Paris,1612)

Harris, C.A., *The dental art, a practical treatise on dental surgery* (Baltimore,1839)

Henstock, A., ed., *Diary of Abigail Gawthorn of Nottingham, 1751-1810* (Thoroton Society,1980)

Hinton, I.T., *The watering places of Great Britain ...* (London,1831)

Hunter, J., *The natural history of the human teeth* (London,1771)

Hunter, J., *A practical treatise on the diseases of the teeth* (London,1778)

Jackson, G., *The Bath archives - diaries and letters* , ed. Lady Jackson (London,1873)

J.B., 'Quack dentists', *Lancet* (1839),383-84

Jordan, H., *Practical observations on the teeth* (London,1851)

Kelly, F., *Post Office London directory* (London,1851)

Large, *Gravesend ... directory* (Gravesend,1851)

Lee, S., *A collection of the names of merchants living in and about the city of London* (London,1677)

Leppard, W., *Brighton and Hove directory* (Brighton,1845)

Levison, J.L., 'Exposure of quackeries in dental surgery', *Lancet* (1831),764

Levison, J.L., *Practical observations on the teeth and gums* (London, 1838)

Levison, J.L., 'Suggestions for a faculty of dental-surgeons', *Lancet* (1840-41),898

London and provincial medical directory (London,1847)

Lukyn, E., *Dental surgery and mechanics* (London,1846)

Lukyn, T., *An essay on the teeth and dental practice* , rev.ed. (London,1853)

Mathews, *Bristol directory* (Bristol,1835)

Mathews, *Bristol directory* (Bristol,1838)

Mathews, *Bristol directory* (Bristol,1839)

McAulay, *Berkshire Almanac* (Reading,1853)

Moncrieff, *Visitors' new guide* (Leamington,1822)

Mortimer, W.H., *Observations on the growth and irregularity of children's teeth* (London,1845)

Mosely, E., *Teeth, their natural history* (London,1862)

Murphy, J.L., *Popular treatise on the structure, diseases and treatment of the human teeth* (London,1837)

'Nemo', 'Professional reminiscences', *Quart.J.dent.Sci.*,1(1857),209

Nicholles, J., *The teeth, in relation to beauty, voice and health* , 2nd ed.(London,1834)

Pharmaceutical Society of Great Britain, *Register of pharmaceutical chemists and chemists and druggists* (London,1869)

Pigot, J., *London ... directory* (London,1836)

Purland, T., 'Dental memoranda', *Quart.J.dent.Sci.*,1(1857),63–65, 201–04,342–46,460–63; 2(1858),121–23,242–43,353–55,490–93

Purland, T., *Practical directions for preserving the teeth; advice to parents* (London,1831)

Raffald, E., *Manchester directory* (Manchester,1772)

Registrar General, *Report of the 1841 census* (London,1841)

Registrar General, *Report of the 1851 census* (London,1851)

Registrar General, *Report of the 1861 census* (London,1861)

Registrar General, *22nd annual report (1861)* (House of Commons Papers,1861,XVIII,545)

Robertson, W., *Practical treatise on the teeth*, 4th ed. (London,1846)

Robinson, J., *The surgical, mechanical and medical treatment of the teeth* (London,1846)

Robson, W., *London commercial directory* (London,1821)

Robson, W., *Classification of trades and street guide* (London,1829)

Rowe, G., *Illustrated Cheltenham guide* (Cheltenham,1845)

Royal College of Surgeons of England, *List of members of the Royal College of Surgeons in London* (London,1805,25,35,45)

Sigmond, J., *A practical and domestic treatise on the diseases and irregularities of the teeth and gums* (Bath,1825)

'Senex', 'A reminiscence of dentistry in the old days; a fortunate dental student, 1855', *Br.J.dent.Sci.*,63(1920),6-12

Silverthorne, H., *Bath directory* (Bath,1841)

Simmons, S.F., *Medical Register* (London,1779,80,83)

Sketchley, J., *Bristol directory* (Bristol,1775)

Slater, I., *Directory ... of ... Lincolnshire* (Manchester,1850)

Slater, I., *Directory ... of Yorkshire and Lincolnshire* (Manchester, 1839)

Smith, J., *Topography of Maidstone and its environs* (Maidstone,1839)

Snape, J., *The physiology of the teeth* , 2nd ed. (London,1851)

Snell, J., *Practical guide to operations on the teeth* (London,1831)

Society of Apothecaries, *A list of persons who have obtained certificates of their fitness and qualification to practise as apothecaries from Aug 1 1815 to July 31 1840* (London,1840)

Society of Apothecaries, *A list of persons who have obtained certificates of their fitness and qualification to practise as apothecaries from Aug 1 1840 to July 31 1852* (London,1852)

'Suaviter et fortiter', 'Quackery and country practice', *Br.J.dent.Sci.*,2(1858),49

Tallis, *A comprehensive gazetteer of Gravesend* (Gravesend,1839)

Waite, G., *An appeal to the Parliament, the medical profession and the public, on the present state of dental surgery* (London, 1841)

Ward, R., *North of England directory* (Newcastle upon Tyne,1853)

Wardroper, W., *Practical treatise on the structure and diseases of the teeth and gums* (London,1835)

White, F., *General directory of Hull* (Sheffield,1846)

White, R., *The management of the teeth* (London,1844)

White, W., *Directory and gazetteer of Leeds and the clothing district of Yorkshire* (Leeds,1853)

Williams, J., *Directory of the principal market towns in Hertfordshire* (London,1850)

Woodcroft, B., *Abridgements of specifications relating to medicine, surgery and dentistry, 1620–1866*, 2nd ed.(London,1872)

Wooffendale, R., *Practical observations on the teeth* (London,1783)

Woodhouse, A.J., 'Reminiscences of fifty-four years in the dental profession', *J.Br.Dent.Assoc.*,18(1897),21-31

Worde, Wynkyn de, *Cocke Lorelles Bote* (c.1515) in *Ancient poetical tracts of the 16th century* (London, 1843), Percy Society, VI

Wright, *Brighton perambulator* (Brighton,1818)

2. Secondary sources

Albert, W., *The turnpike road system in England, 1663-1840* (Cambridge,1972)

Boggis, F.W., 'The Chevalier Ruspini, dental surgeon to George IV', *Br.dent.J.*,42(1921),336-38

Boyes, J., 'Medicine and dentistry in Newcastle upon Tyne in the 18th century', *Proc.R.Soc.Med.*,50(1957),229-35

'Boz' [Charles Dickens], *Memoirs of Joseph Grimaldi* (London,1838)

British Dental Association, *Dental manpower requirements to 2020* (London,1982>)

Brown, P.S., 'Medicines advertised in the 18th century Bath newspapers', *Med.Hist.*,20(1976),152-68

Brown, P.S., 'Notes on advertising dentists in 18th century Bath', *Notes and Queries for Somerset and Dorset* ,30(1977),278-82

Brown, P.S., 'The providers of medical treatment in mid-nineteenth century Bristol', *Med.Hist.*,24(1980),297-314

Burnby, J.G.L., 'A study of the English apothecary from 1660-1760' (unpublished Ph.D. thesis, University of London,1979)

Burnby, J.G.L., *A study of the English apothecary from 1660-1760* (London,1983)

Burnett, J., *A history of the cost of living* (Harmondsworth,1969)

Burnett, J., *Plenty and want* (Harmondsworth,1968)

Bynum, W.F. and R. Porter (ed.), *Medical fringe and medical orthodoxy, 1750-1850* (London,1987)

Campbell, J.M., 'Chevalier Batholomew Ruspini', *Dent.Mag.Oral Topics,* 70(1953),402-22

Campbell, J.M., 'The Crawcours', *Dent.Pract.,*8(1957),108-09

Campbell, J.M., *Dentistry then and now* (Glasgow,1981)

Campbell, J.M., 'Early dental advertisements', *Dent.Items* ,71(1949), 1229-44

Campbell, J.M., 'Early women dentists', *Br.dent.J.,*82(1947),123-24

Campbell, J.M., 'Eleazer Gidney', *Dent.Mag.Oral Topics* ,67(1950),249-64

Campbell, J.M., *From a trade to a profession* (Glasgow,1958)

Campbell, J.M., 'George Fellowes Harrington', *Dent.Mag.Oral Topics* , 72(1955), 225-29

Campbell, J.M., 'Theodosius Purland', *Dent.Mag.Oral Topics* ,78(1961), 201-06

Cohen, R.A., 'Messrs. Wedgwood and porcelain dentures, correspondence 1800-1815', *Br.dent.J.,*139(1975),27-31 and 69-71

Cohen, R.A., 'The Talma family', *Br.dent.J.,*126(1969),319-26

Cohen, R.A., 'Work in progress', *Lindsay Club Newsletter [now Dental Historian]* ,10(1984),11

Cohen, R.A., and J. Chatfield, 'Thomas Bell, zoologist, palaeontologist, dentist', *Lindsay Club Newsletter [now Dental Historian]* ,6(1980),4-6

Cohen, R.A., E.A. Marsland and C. Hillam, 'William Robertson of Birmingham, 1794-1870', *Br.dent.J.*,142(1977),64-69 and 99-102

Cope, Sir Z.V., *Sir John Tomes, pioneer of British dentistry* (London, 1961)

Corbett, M.E., 'An investigation into the pattern of dental caries in a 19th century British urban population' (unpublished DDS thesis, University of Birmingham,1975)

Corbett, M.E. and W.J. Moore, 'The distribution of dental caries in ancient British populations: IV, 19th century', *Caries Res.*, 10(1976),401-14

Cranfield, G.A., *The development of the provincial press, 1700-1760* (Oxford,1962)

De Maar, F.E.R., 'Theodor Picnot en zijn kast', *Tandheelkundige Studenten Almanak* (1976),310-14

Dobson, J., 'The Royal dentists', *Ann.R.Coll.Surg.Eng.*,46(1970),277-91

Dobson, J. and R.M. Walker, *Barbers and barber-surgeons of London* (Oxford,1979)

Dolamore, W.H., 'Some old advertisements', *Br.dent.J.*,45(1924),185-87

Donaldson, J.A., 'Peter de London, toothdrawer', *Br.dent.J.*, 119(1965),147-48

Donaldson, J.A., 'A Rowlandson caricature', *Br.dent.J.*,104(1958),6

Gray, T.C., 'Whatever happened to Felix Yaniewicz?', *Proc.R.Soc.Med.*, 71(1978),292-99

Hardwick, J.L., 'The incidence and distribution of caries throughout the ages in relation to the Englishman's diet', *Br.dent.J.*, 108(1960),9-17

Henry, C.B., 'The Iron Duke's dentures', *Br.dent.J.*,125(1968),354-56

Hill, A., *The history of the reform movement in the dental profession in Great Britain* (London,1877)

Hillam, C., 'James Blair (1747-1817), provincial dentist', *Med.Hist.*, 22(1978),44-70

Hillam, D.G. and C., 'The Bott family of dentists', *Dent.Hist.*, 11(1985),1-10

Hoffmann-Axthelm, W., *History of dentistry* (Chicago,1981)

Holloway, S.W.F., 'The Apothecaries' Act, 1815: a reinterpretation', *Med.Hist.*,10(1966),107-29 and 221-36

Hudson, J.C., *The parents' handbook - or guide to the choice of employments, professions, etc.* (London,1842)

Hughes, S.G., 'The life and work of John Howard Mummery', *Bull.Hist.Dent.*,31(1983),69-81

Lindsay. L., 'The London dentist of the 17th century', *Br.dent.J.*, 80(1946),75-80

Lindsay. L., 'The London dentist of the 18th century', *Dent.Surg.*, 24(1927),179-85 and *Proc.R.Soc.Med.*,20(1927),355-66 [Lindsay 1927a]

Lindsay. L., 'Notes on the history of dentistry in England up to the beginning of the 19th century', *Br.dent.J.*,48(1927),268-74

Lindsay. L., 'Personalities of the past', *Br.dent.J.*,98(1955),28-9, 69-70,99,133-4,176-7,217-8,259,295-6,334-5,363-4,405,455-6; 99(1955),23-4,56-7,86-7,129,164,207,238

Lindsay, L., 'Samuel Lee Rymer and the National Dental Hospital', *National Dental Hospital Gazette*, (March 1937)

Lindsay. L., *A short history of dentistry* (London,1933)

Lindsay. L., 'Thomas Berdmore', *Br.dent.J.*,49(1924),225–238

Loudon, I.S.L., 'A doctor's cash book: the economy of general practice in the 1830s', *Med.Hist.*,249–68

MccKendrick, N., J. Brewer and J.H. Plumb, *The birth of a consumer society* (Bloomington,1982)

Moore, W.J. and M.E. Corbett, 'The distribution of dental caries in ancient British populations: I, Anglo-Saxon period', *Caries Res.*,5(1971),151–68

Moore, W.J. and M.E. Corbett, 'The distribution of dental caries in ancient British populations: II, Iron age, Romano-British and Mediaeval periods', *Caries Res.*,7(1973),139–53

Moore, W.J. and M.E. Corbett, 'The distribution of dental caries in ancient British populations: III, 17th century', *Caries Res.*, 163–75

Musgrove, F., 'Middle-class education and employment in the 19th century', *Ec.Hist.Rev.*,12(1959–60),99–111

Peterson, M.J., *The medical profession in mid-Victorian London* (California,1978)

Phillips, A.D.M. and J.R. Walton, 'The distribution of personal wealth in English towns in the mid-nineteenth century', *Trans.Inst.Brit.Geog.*,64(1975),35–48

Porter, R., *English Society in the 18th century* (Harmondsworth,1982)

Read, D., *Opinion in three English cities* (Leeds,1961)

Richards, N.D., 'Dentistry in the 1840s', *Med.Hist.*,12(1968),137–52

Richards, N.D., 'Destiny or dynasty: the Fox family of doctors and dentists', *Bull.Soc.Soc.Hist.Med.*,16(1975),11-13

Richards, N.D., 'A study of the development of dental health services in the United Kingdom – the profession and treatment services (1840-1921)' (unpublished Ph.D. thesis, University of London, 1978)

Robinson, C., 'Dental manpower ratios: factors influencing dentists' cBoice of practice location' (unpublished M.Sc.(Community Dentistry) dissertation, University of Manchester,1978)

Rubinstein, W.D., *Men of property* (London,1981)

Schiach, G.R., 'James Gordon of Bristol: an echo from the past', *Proc.R.Soc.Med.*,3(1912-13),88-96

Seligman, E.R.A., *The income tax* (New York,1914)

Spencer, E.M., 'Notes on the history of dental dispensaries', *Med.Hist*,26(1982),47-66

Stoy, P.J., 'Early dentistry in Belfast', *Br.dent.J.*,120(1966),253-58,297-300

Townend, B.R., 'Mr. Patence, quack', *Dent.Mag.Oral Topics* ,59(1942), 169-81

Wallis, P.J. and R.V., *18th century medics; subscriptions, licences and apprenticeships* (Newcastle upon Tyne,1985)

Webber, B., *James Orrock, R.I.: painter, connoisseur, collector* (London,1903)

Weinberger, B.W., *History of dentistry* (St. Louis,1948)

Williams, B., *The making of Manchester Jewry* (Manchester,1976)

Wright, D.W., 'London dentists in the 18th century: a listing from the trade directories in the Guildhall Library', *Dent.Hist.*,

12(1986),8-16

Young, S., *Annals of the Barber-Surgeons* (London,1890)

Zwanberg, D. van, 'The training and careers of those apprenticed to apothecaries in Suffolk, 1815-1858', *Med.Hist.*,27(1983),139-50

INDEX

of the main text and the place names mentioned in *appendix 2*

Aberdeen, 57
Abergavenny, 93,176,200
abscesses, 120
account books, 47,60,143,146
acting profession, 131
acute ulcerative gingivitis, 106
advertisements, 4-5,37,47,53,77,
    86-7,89,106,118,121,128,133,
    137-9,141
advertising, 36,132-9
advertising pamphlets, 97
agencies, 138
Albert, Edward, 82
Albucasius, 9
Alderney, 93,172
Aldridge, 55
Alex, 89
Alex, J., 80
Alex, Montague, 7,83,143
Allen, Charles, 12
Alnwick, 91
Alsop, Edward, 18
amalgam, 99
Amboyna toothpowder, 137
America, 23,55-6,79,131
Amsterdam, 79
anaesthesia, 97,103
Anglo-Saxon period, 123
apical abscesses/cysts, 100,103
Apothecaries' Act of 1815,126
apothecaries, 18-9,27,51,55
apprenticeship, 20,22,25-8,30,35,
    83,126

apprenticeship records, 1,6
Aranson, Pasco, 80
Archer, 5
artificial teeth/dentures, 12,
    15-7,54,57,105-6,109-10,115,
    117,121,137,141; bridges, 103;
    by post, 77;clasps, 105;demand
    for, 112; gold bases, 140-1;
    human teeth, 141-2;ivory, 105-
    7,110,139,141; ligatures, 105-
    6,112; partial dentures, 105,
    107-8,112; porcelain, 105,108,
    110,140-2; springs, 105,107
Ash, Claudius, 108,141,148
Ashburn, 130
Ashton-under-Lyne, 143
assembly rooms, 130
assistants, 22,28-30,39,43,47-8,
    61,76,83,92
assizes, 130
aurists, 19
Axminster, 87
Aylesbury, 82,86,93,203-4

Baker, Stephen, 46
Banbury, 92,94,96,166,214,238
barber-surgeons, 12,18
Barber-Surgeons Company, 54
barbers, 9-10,13
Barbers' Company of London, 9
Barnsley, 91-2,130,133,228
Barnstaple, 92,162,241
Barron, William Henry, 28

Bate, Charles Spence, 21,32,57, 146
Bath, 18,28-30,38,40,42,46-8,54, 57,59-60,72-4,78-82,84,87,92, 96,107,116,128,146,158-9,162, 164-5,169,171,177-8,186-7,190-3,201,210-1,213,218-9,223,225, 228,231-4,242-3,247-8
Bavaria, 79
Bayley, William Henry, 81
Bedford, 93,174,244
beeswax, 105-6
Belfast, 40,59
Bell, Thomas, 45,97-8,104,106,
Bellejean, 15
benevolent fund, 48
Berdmore, Thomas, 22-3,48,117
Berend, Louis, 79,94
Berend, Samuel, 8,79,94
Bergamo, 16
Berlin, 79,94
Berwick, 92,202
Beverley, 93,95,208
Bew, Charles, 81,94,131,144
bills of mortality, 120
Bingley, 133
Bird, 55
Birkenhead, 92,196,201-2,236,243,247
Birmingham, 7,17-8,22,25,27-8,37-8,40,42,55,58,63,72,77,81,84-5, 87,91-2,94-5,116-7,128,130,137, 139,156-8,162-3,166,171,174-5,178-9,184,188,193-4,196-200,204,207 8,210,214-8,222-6,229-30,233-5, 238,242-5,247-9
bite planes, 104
Blackburn, 92,96,212-3,222
Blackmore, 55
blacksmiths, 11,14
Blair, James, 18,22,37,41-2,55,

57,59,77,88,109,118,125,128-31 134,145-6
bleeders, 18-9
bleeding, 126
boarding schools, 119
Bolton, 92,157,169,220,227
bone loss, 100
bone setter, 19
Boroughbridge, 93,158,190
Boston, 80,167,171,185,226,244
Bott family, 146
Bott, George sen., 18,22,28,45, 63,88,125
-Bott's Benevolent Society, 63
Bott, George jun., 23,27,41,119, 130
Bott, Sophia, 22,37
Boucher, James, 57
Bourdet, Étienne, 140
Bourn, 225
Bourquin, 94
Bradford, 73,87,90-2,133,166, 177,180,185,188,197,202,209 214.220,224-6,239
Braintree, 70,73,92,155
Brampton, 93,225
branch practices, 72,85-91,132
-provincially based, 88-9
Brecon, 92,201
Breham, Edward, 116,120
Brewer, Thomas, 18
bricklayers, 19
bridges, 103
Bridgewater, 92,197
Bridgman, John Brooks, 59
Bridgman, William Kencely, 59,95
Brighton, 25,40,73,80-3,92,131, 155,157,159,161-2,164,166,168-72,174,178,183,191,198,204, 211,218-9,222,224,235-6,238,

240,244-5,248
Bristol, 18,38,40,42,46-7,51,54,
  57,60,63,72,77-8,82,87,90,92,
  94-5,107,132,142,156,158,163-4,
  166,168-70,172-4,177,184-5,187-
  8,190-5,202,204,207-8,212-4,218-
  20,222-3,229-33,235-8,241,243,
  245-6,249-50
  -doctors, 46
British Dental Association, 26
Bromley, 234
Bromley, Charles, 30,57,93
Brophy, 54
Brown, Samuel, 87
Brown, Thomas, 6
Browne, John Crow, 109
brushes, 108
Brussels, 142
Bryckette, John, 10
Buckell, 55
Buckingham, 93,166
Burch, Moses, 27
Burnley, 133
Burslem, 92,162
Burton on Trent, 72,92,183
Bury, 93,158,223
Bury St. Edmunds, 92,199,230,242,
  244
business intitiative, 134
business involvements, 46
Butler's Restorative Tooth Powder,
  115

Cafferata, James Lewis, 37,41,48
Cafferata, Philip, 41
calculus, 106,122
Camborne, 92,242
Cambridge, 44,54,82,86,92,128,190,
  198-9,207,229,243
Campion, Henry, 56

Canterbury, 25,86,89,92,95,137,
  159,198-9,209,225
Capperon, 16
Cardiff, 92-3,96,164,181,186,214
  235,250
careers in dentistry, 37-40
  -length of career, 37-40
  -short-term dentists, 39
  -survival rates, 67-8
caricatures, 115-6
caries, 97-8,103,121-5
  -incidence of:Anglo-Saxon
  period,123;Iron Age,123;17th
  century,123;19th century,123
  -increase in, 122,124
  -treatment of, 98-100
Carlisle, 24,26,41,83,92,94,96,
  177,206,213-4,230-1
Carlyle, Thomas, 95
Cartwright, 56
Cartwright & Davis, 56
Cartwright, Samuel, 23,29,60
cash books, 46
cauterisation, 15
cement, 109
census, 1-2,7,28,61,77,92
Chard, 87
charities, 51
Charlton, 54
Chatham, 92,221,235
Chelmsford, 93,201
Cheltenham, 7,38,40-1,73-4,80,
  83-4,87,92,155,168,170-1,173,
  178,188,203-4,206,209-10,218
  220-1,223-5,232-3,240-1
chemists and druggists, 19,21,
  23,51,52-4,63
Chepstow, 93,250
Cherriman, John V, 29,95
Chertsey, 93,200

Chester, 42,54,72,77-8,81-2,92,
94,125,128,134,137,198-9,204,
236,240
Chesterfield, 93,130,212
Chichester, 92,167,190,198,223,
248
children, 119,121,137
 -new attitude to, 118
china shop, 117
chiropody, 19,126
Chorlton, 175,177,183,190,217-8,
220,236,244
Church, 55
city dentists, 74
Clapham, 172
Clarence, Duke of, 144
Clark, Andrew, 80
Clark, Dr., 14
Clark, Ebenezer, 82
Clark, J.P., 83
Clarke, 40,95
Clarke, Thomas, 18
clasps, 105
cleaning *see* scaling
Clifton, 173,194
coach travel, 129-30
Cocke Lorelles Bote, 10
Colchester, 10,92,167,210
College of Dentists, 6,33,64,85,
139
Colne, 133
commercial centres, 72,74
Company of Barber-Surgeons, 9
consumer revolution, 116
consumer services, 116
consumer spending, 130
 -explosion of, 125
Cordon, 80
Corey, 55
Cornwall, Augustus, 80

country practice, 74-5
Coventry, 92,195-6,206,249
Cowes, 200,222
Crawcour, 37,79,109,137-8,145
cross-infection, 100,107
crowding, 108
crowns, 100,103,108-9,121
 -gold pivot, 103
Croydon, 81,92,167,183,185,195,
210,229,236
Cullis, George Henry, 7
cuppers, 1,19,29,46
cutler, 57

Da Fonzi, G.,141
Dappe, John, 54
Darlington, 92,96,183,213
Dash, James, 80
Davidson, James Johnston, 54
Dawlish, 93,241
Dawson, Mrs., 13
De Berri, 95,109
De Chémant, Nicholas Dubois,
138,140-1
Delabarre, Antoine Bernasconi,
79
De la Roche, Peter, 14
De Loude, Louis Charles, 24,50,
55,79,123,140-1
De St. Raymond, Mrs., 134,137
demand for treatment, 116
 -change in, 115
Denbigh, 137
dental disease
 -incidence of, 121
 -iatrogenic, 112
 -severe, 122
dental dispensaries/hospitals,
33,94,143
dental literature, 97

dental practice/population ratios, 76-7
dental preparations, 54,96,108, 111,115,144
dental profession, disunity in, 33
dental schools, 1,33
dentifrice, 108
'dentist', 9,117
'dentist and operator', 117
dentistry
  -before 18th century, 9-13
  -factors in spread of, 112-44
  -geographical expansion, 68-72
dentists
  -mobility, 78-85
  -numbers, growth in, 64-66
  -socio-economic standing, 50-3
  -social mobility, 43
  -trade origins, 17-9
Dentists Register, 6,43,54,58
Denton, 211
dentures, *see* artificial teeth
Derby, 91-2,130,158,169-70,200, 212,214-5,223
Dereham, 158
Devizes, 92,158,187,212
Devonport, 92,159,192,204-5,214, 234,237
Dewsbury, 133
diet, change in, 124
Dinsdale, Cuthbert, 79,83
dissecting rooms, 140
Dixon, James Browne, 55
Dixon, Thomas, 141,143
doctors, 134
  -country, 19
Dodbrook, 92,240-1
Doncaster, 93,133,180,200,243
Dorchester, 93,178

Dorking, 93,177
'double row' of teeth, 104,118
Douglas, Isle of Man, 160,173, 186,200,221
Dover, 81,89,92,95,158,178,190, 198,214
Downing, Edward, 59
Downing, Richard, 59
Drake, 96
Dreschfeld, Leopold, 37,79,94
druggists, 18,22,125
Drury, Alexander Rupert, 81
Du Verdière, 16
Dumergue, Charles, 15
Dunsford, 55
Dunstable, 93,96,213
Durham, 93,96,168,177,213-4,216, 240
duty, 119
dynasties, 42-3

East Anglia, 128
East Grinstead, 62,92,202
Eastbourne, 73,92,172
Eden, Thomas, 95
Edinburgh, 27,64,83,93
Edwards, James, 29,57,60,80
Edwards, Messrs., 90
Egyptian mummies, 9
Elland, 133
Ely, 86
empiricism, 33-6,55,112
Enfield, 93,235
Eno, James, 55
enterprise, 89,112,125,127
epidemiological studies, modern, 123
epilepsy, 120
Eskell, Albert, 79,115
Eskell, Frederick, 95

Evatt, James, 41,109,141
Evesham, 93,197
examinations, 1,33
Exeter, 26,28,38,40-1,44,54,63,
  72,77-8,82,84,87,94,96,162,168,
  171,172,178,180-1,183-6,188-9,
  192-3,196-7,199,201,203-4,207,
  209,212,214,230-1,234,241
Exmouth, 93,203
expansion in numbers, 64-6,70
  -delay before, 69
expansion plates, 104
expectations, financial, 127
extraction, 9-11,13,15,57,103-5,
  108-10,115,120-2

fairs, 130
Fakenham, 75,93,222
Falmouth, 93,211
family involvement, 28,40-5,71,
  89,127
Farthing, John, 79-80
fashion, 72,115-6,134
Fauchard, Pierre, 15,117
Faulkner, Thomas, 18,22,37
Featherstone, 29
fees, 108-10,126
  -reduced, 143
Fenny Stratford, 93,185
Ferguson, Ralph Hodgson, 80
Feryer, Richard, 10
Fielding, Frederick William, 81
filing, 15,98,104,108-9
fillings, 15,98-9,108-10,115,121,
  144
  -materials: amalgams,90,99,110;
  cements,109;gold,99,108-9;
  lead,99,109;platinum,99;
  silver,98,108-9;terro-metallic
  cement,99

Finzi, 94
Fisher, Frederick, 82
Flint, Matthew, 10
Flint, Peter, 28
focal sepsis, 120
Folkestone, 93,174
Forceps, 24-5,32,103-4
foreign practitioners, 78-9
Fort, William, 59
Foulsham, 93
Fox, Charles Herbert, 41
Fox, Charles Prideaux, 40,80
Fox, Ernest William, 41
Fox, Frederick Neidhart, 41
Fox, George Anthony, 41
Fox, George Frederick, 28,57,40
Fox, Joseph, 98,122
Fox, Octavius Annesley, 40
Fox, Robert Were sen., 28,40-1,
  44
Fox, Robert Were jun., 40,57
Fox, Sylvanus Bevan, 40
Fox, Walter Henry, 41
Foy, 17,79,117
fractured jaws, 103
France, 54,79,117
franchise system, 24
free treatment, 137
Frome, 93,158
fustian cutter, 18-9

Gabriel, Lyon, 82
Gantherry, 55
Garner, Joseph Samuel, 80
Gason, 16
Gateshead, 92,202
Gedge, William Edward, 80
geographical expansion, 68-72
George, John Durance, 29
Germany, 54,78-9

Gidney, Eleazer, 79
gingivectomy, 107
Gladstone, William Ewart, 51
Glasgow, 23,93
Gloucester, 40,92,184,210,224,241, 243,246
gold, 99,103,108-9,140-1
Goldstone, 18,54-5
Gosling, George, 14
Göttingen, 94
governors of hospitals, 51
Grassington, 133
Gravesend, 92,171,195,211,235,248
graveyards, 140
Gray, John, 20,25,30-3,36,54-5, 57,64,98-9,104-5,112,115,122,127
Greenough's Tincture, 54
Greenwich, 82,92,182,195,210,223
Grimaldi, 79,94,109,116-7,131,137
Guernsey, 92,156,173,196,246,249
Guildford, 92,156,181,208,244
Guillemeau, Jacques, 12

Haarlem, 79
Hair, Quintin Burns, 37,82,87
hairdressers, 18,19,27,117,125
Halifax, 72-3,81,84,167,171,175, 177,180,188,192,217,220,226, 248-9
Hamburg, 94
Hamilton's tincture, 96
Hammersmith, 239
handbill, 134
Hanley, 55,92,176,209,235
Hanover, 79
Hanwell, 93,236
Harborough, 130
Harding, Thomas Henry, 95
Harrington, George Fellowes, 82
Harris, Chapin A., 97,100,103,107, 125-6,141
Hart, Abraham Septimus, 42,82
Hart, Hemet, 54,137
Hart, Joseph, 42
Hartlepool, 93,96,213
Haslam, 8
Haslam, Simeon, 82
Hastings, 91-2,167,185,197,218, 224,235,244
Heath, 144
Heaton Norris, 93,229
Hemet, Jacob, 15
Hemet's Dentifrice, 115
Henley, 87,92
Henley in Arden, 6,166-7
Henry, Mr., 23,55
Hepburn, Duncan, 80
herbalists, 19,52
Hereford, 92,95,204,209,224,240
Hertford, 82,93,192
Hesketh, Birch, 18
Hexham, 91
Hextall, Clay, 5
High Wycombe, 93,202
Highgate, 167
Hill, Alfred, 35,64
Hockliffe, 130
Hopton, 55
Hornor, Benjamin, 29,134
Hoskins, Francis, 82
Huddersfield, 87,92,133,175,186, 194-5,197,229-30
Hugo, 55
Hull, 72,79,82,84,87,91-2,96, 160-1,168,174-5,177-8,182,185, 190-2,204,208-15,217,220, 224-5,228,234,247,249
human teeth, 141
Hunt, William, 81,94
Hunter, John, 111,122,127

Hunter, Mrs., 119
Huntingdon, 93,204

iatrogenic disease, 112
impression materials, 105-6
Imrie, William, 41
income, 45-6,48,126
incompetence, 35-7
indigestion, 120
inducements, 137
industrial towns, 74
infection, 106
inflammation of the pulp, 97
inns, 130
instrument makers, 19,28,57
Ipswich, 43,80,92,169,185,187,202, 207,242
Ireland, 64,134
Iron Age, 123
Isdael, 117
Isle of Man, 5,92-3
Isle of Wight, 92
Italy, 16,54
itinerant toothdrawer, 131
ivory, 105-7,110,139,141
ivory turners, 125

James & Co., Michael [Mallan], 56
Jardine, J., 87
Jarritt, 82
Jeffs, 134
Jersey, 157-60,183,196,201-2,207, 209,223,230,239
jewellers, 18-9,54,117,125
Jewish dentists, 25
Jobson, D.W., 55
Jones, 24-5
Jones & Bell, 82,86,89
Jones, Henry, 56,82,89
Jones, Isaiah, 109

Jordan, Henry, 119,142
Jordan, John, 56,89
Jullion, Paul, 15,94,109

Karran, James, 23
Keighley, 133
Kemble, Elizabeth, 131
Kendal, 92,96,133,188,212
Kent, 23,37,82,89,94
key, 103-4
Kidd, T.D., 83
King, Edward, 23,25,29,94
King, Joseph, 29,59
King, Norman, 63
King, Thomas Edward, 59
King's Lynn, 92,95-6,165,177, 199,201,214,217,228,239,248-9
Kingsbridge, 92,178,184
Kingston, 92,188,244
Knaresborough, 133

Lambert, William, 62
Lancaster, 59,92,133,159,242
Lancet, 32,34,45,50
Landport, 92,227
Landymiey, 15
Landzelle, 94
laudanum, 100
Law, Robert, 54,81
Le Dray, 24-5,89-90,95,96,109
Le Dray & Davis, 89
Le Sec, 5
lead, 99,109
Leamington Spa, 72-3,80,82,84, 87,91,92,95,166-7,174,190,195, 198,203-4,206,212,225,236,249,
leeches, 107
Leeds, 41,72,77,79,84,87,91-2, 115,130,133-4,141,143,156-7, 164,167,169,172-6,179-80,185

190,192,198-9,202,211,214-5,217,
222,224,226,229-30,233,244,246,
248-9
Leek, 130
Leeson, Robert, 14
legislation, 44
Leicester, 5,18,20,22,27,34,41,72,
80,91,94,125,130,134,138,155-6,
162,164,169,170,180,185,190,193,
205,210,212,226,237,245-6
Leigh, 94,137
Leigh, Edward Philip, 80
Lemaire, 15
Lemale, Thomas, 108
Leominster, 72-3,129,164
L'Estrange, [Francis?], 8
Levason, George, 86-7
Levason, Lewis, 82,87
Levison, Jacob Leslie, 32,34,36,
99,110
Lewes, 73,93,169,248
Lewis, 117
Lewisham, 92,202
Licence in Dental Surgery (LDS),
6,33
Licence of the Society of Apothe-
caries (LSA), 20
Lichfield, 18,72-3,243
ligatures, 105-6,112
Lincoln, 87,92,159,171,197,213,
228-9,234,242
Liskeard, 93,215
literary and philosophical socie-
ties, 51
Little, 44
Liverpool, 8,18,23,37-8,40,42,44,
54-5,57,62-3,72,77,79-85,87,89-
90,92-6,125,128,132,139,143,155-
8,160,162,164-6,168-9,172,174-5,
179,182-3,185-6,190,192,194-5,

197-202,204-7,209,211,213-4,
216-7,219-22,224-8,234-6,
238-40,242-7,249-50
Lloyd, James Blair, 42,143
Lloyd, Richard, 28,62
Lloyd, Thomas Bridge, 42
Lloyd, Thomas Whitfield, 42,57,
77,128
local politics, 51
location for dental practices,
72-4,75,93
London, 12,37,45,53,57-8,63,74,
76-83,86-7,89-91,94-5,115-6,
118,128,130,134,137-8,140-1,
160,164,172,175,182,204,207,
210-4,219,222,224,228,239-40
242-4
*London and provincial medical
directory*, 54
London School of Dental Surgery,
6
London trade directories, 92
loose teeth, 16,106
Loughborough, 93,130,240
Louth, 87,92,174,198,208,228,239
Lowe, 82
Lucas, Dr., 16
Ludlow, 92,196
Lukyn, William, 29,80,82,128-9
Lyme Regis, 73,87,93,208
Lyon, 94
Lyon, Henry, 86,109
Lyttleton, Lord, 116

Macclesfield, 70,92,130,179
Maclean, 29
Maidstone, 86,92,95,132,156,159,
161,167-8,171,190,198-9,234
Mallan family, 25,87,89-90,95-6,
139 *see also* James & Co

Mallan & Son, 56
Mallan & Sons, 24
Mallan, James Michael, 56
Mallan, John, 24
Malvern, 73,93
managers, 87,91
Manchester, 16,18,22,37,42,72,77,
   79,82,84-5,90,92,94-5,128,130,
   133,148,155-61,165,168,172,175,
   177,179-82,185-6,188,190-5,197,
   199-200,202,204-6,208,211,214,
   217-9,221-2,225-6,230,234-6,238,
   242,245-6,248-9
Manchester Dental Hospital, 94
Manne, George Arthur, 54,81,87,95
Mannheim, 137
manpower, 92
   -supply of, 125-7
Mansfield, 93,95,130,170
manufacturing towns, 72
Margate, 73,92,223
Martiniani, 15
Mason, William, 87
masonic lodges, 51,63
materials manufacturer, 19
mechanical dentistry, 27
mechanics, 47-8,61,126
Medical Directory, 20
medical electricity, 19,79
medical families, 20-1
medical men, 20,23,48-51,55
Medical Register, 54
medical training, 19
Medwin, Aaron, 82
Meears, 55
Melcombe Regis, 93,201
Membership of the Royal College
   of Surgeons (MRCS), 20
Merryweather, J., 82
Messenger, 55

Michel, Peter, 48,79
Middleton, 55
Middleton, Thomas, 14
Middleton, Thomas Patchett, 82
Midlands, 128
Milpentine, 15
mineral cement, 99
mineral paste, 110
Mineral Succedaneum, 90,99
mineral teeth, 108,141
Mitchell, John William, 95
mobility, 78-85
Moggridge, 24
Monmouth, 93,201,212
Moor, 81,94,116,119
Moore, 87
Morgan, Frederick, 57
Morley [sic], Alexander Mosely,
   96
Mortimer, 139
mortuaries, 140
Mosel[e]y, Abraham, 24,87,90
Mosely family, 89-90
Mosely, Alexander, 41
Mosely, Alfred Isaiah, 41,96
Mosely, Benjamin Ephraim, 41,96
Mosely, Charles, 90-1,96
Mosely, Ephraim, 41,90-1,96,142
Mosely, Lewin, 90-1,96
Mosely, Simeon, 90-1,96
Mouton, Claude, 94
Mummery, John Rigden, 81
Murphy, Joseph Kinnaird, 58

Nailer, William, 18
Nathan, 55
Neibaur, Alexander, 8
Nelson, 55
New Alresford, 73,92,195
new practices, 65,67,71-2

New York, 79
Newark, 93,208,240
Newbury, 93,96,214,226
Newcastle under Lyme, 93,96,177, 212
Newcastle upon Tyne, 16,53,55,59, 79,82-3,87,90,92,96,131,158, 175-7,184,195,202,208,210,212-4, 216-7,220,222-3,235,238-9,244, 246
Newport (Isle of Wight), 155,167, 211,242
Newport (Mon.), 93
Newport Pagnell, 86
newspapers, 2, 4-5 *see also* provincial press
Nicholles, John, 119-20,141
Nightingale, Charles, 87
Nightingale, Messrs. (Daniel), 87
normal schools, 33
Norman, William, 27
Normansell, Thomas, 94
North Holloway, 168
North Shields, 73,87,92,195,210, 216,248
North Wales, 128
Northampton, 80-1,92,94,130,194, 201,238-9,249
Norwich, 34,54,59,72,74,79,81,132, 137,163-5,168,172,174-5,177,189, 194,196,199,216,224-5,230,239, 244-5,248-9
Nottingham, 18,22,28,34,40,45,54, 72,80,82,84,94,125,128,130,137, 159,162-4,169-72,176,183,192, 194-5,197,201,206-8,212,215,217, 224,228,230,236,240-1
novelty, 116,121,126
Nowell, 55
numbers of dentists, 64-8

obituaries, 28,41,43
Odontological Society of London, 6,7,33,139
offshoots of London practices, 42
'operators for the teeth', 11,12 15,117
optics, 126
oral /ygiene, 108
Orme, Mr., 115
Ormrod, John, 18
Orrock, James, 20,27,94
orthodontic treatment, 15,104, 109
–bite planes, 104
–crowding, 108
–expansion plates, 104
Otley, 133
Oxford, 29,54,81-2,92,128,155-6, 161,200-1,206,236,238,243
Oxley, 55

Paignton, 172
Palermo, 16
Palmer, Gasgoigne, 41
Palmer, James Edwin, 41
Palmer, Thomas Gill, 7,41,57,81, 94
para-medical field, 126
Paris, 15-6,79,94-6,116,140-1
Parkinson, Felix, 30
Parkinson, George T., 81
Parma, 16
Parmly, 57
Parsley, Joseph, 18
Parson, Thomas C., 57
Parsons, Joseph Henry, 143
partial dentures, 105,107-8,112
partnerships, 29,89
Pateley, 133

Patence, 138
patent medicine vendors, 18-9,125
patients
  -eminent, 116
  -social élite, 117,124
Payne, Thomas Pibble, 30
Pearsall, Robert, 7
Peart, Henry, 126
Peckham, 160
Peckover, Charles, 40
Peckover, Hugh Douglas, 40
Peckover, Lancelot Eric Charles,
  40
Penrith, 93,96,206,212
Penzance, 92,172,207
Pepys, Mrs. Samuel, 12
perfumers, 18-9,125
periodontal disease, 103,106
  -bone loss, 100
  -calculus, 106,122
  -chronic periodontitis, 106
  -loose teeth, 16,106
  -plaque, 106
  -'scurvy of the gums', 106
  -treatment of, 13,15,79,106,108-
    9,115
Perkins, W., 57
perruke makers, 18-9,125
Perry & Co, 89
Perry, William, 18
Persimore, John, 14
Peter of London, 10
Peterborough, 41,81,94
Pharmaceutical Society of Great
  Britain, 54
pharmacy, 6,19
Phillips, Edward James Montagu,
  42
Phillips, S., 93
physicians, 19,52,55,126

Pilleau, 12,15,94
plaque, 106
platinum, 99
Plattin, Howard, 93
Plymouth, 44,87,92,94,155,158-
  60,162,164,169,171,175,178,
  184-5,190,193,198,204-5,219,
  225,230,237,242,246
Pontefract, 133
Poole, 92,175,190,238
porcelain, 110
  -dentures, 140
  -teeth, 105,108,110,141-2
ports, 72,74
Portsea, 92,186,207,222,224,228
Portsmouth, 82,92,155-6,177,190,
  208
practices
  -length, 37-40
  -sale of, 45
  -exchange of, 46
Preston, 59,92,96,158,172,183,
  199,212-4,216,226-7,246
previous/second trades, 18-9,21
Prew, James, 29-30,42,46-8,60-1,
  87-8,95,107-9,146
Prew, Thomas, 42,60
Prideaux, 40
Prideaux, Thomas Sims, 82
Prince Regent, 131,144
Prior, William, 16
private courses, 23
probate, 40-1,43,48-50,61-2
professional classes, 73
professional education, 21-33
  -brief, 22,30
  -dental institutions, 33
  -lack of supervising body, 26
  -scheme for, 32
  -untrained dentists, 28,39

professional expenses, 47-8
professional societies, 1,33
professionalism, 36
prosthetic cases, 107
prosthetics, 139 *see also* artificial teeth
provincial medical practice, 19, 126
provincial press, 75,132
 -circulation, 133
pulmonary consumption, 120
pupil, 30
 -advertisement for, 28
Purland, Theodosius, 25,119-20

race meetings, 130
Rae, William, 127
Ramsgate, 86,89,95
Raquet Court, 54
Ravizzotti, 94
Read, T. and W., 95
Reading, 80,92,96,161-2,172,193, 200,213-4,223,236-7,244,249
Reale, 29
recurrent costs of treatment, 142
registration, 1,6
Reigate, 93,208
repairs, 107
reputation, 91
resident dentists, 54,92
resorts, 73
Restieaux, Andrew, 34,54,79,118, 137,145
retained roots, 105
Retford, 87,93,229,243
rheumatism, 120
Richeraud, Ferdinand, 79,109
Richmond (Surrey), 92,95,168,171, 190,197,205
Richmond (Yorkshire), 82

Ripon, 92,133,190
Robertson, Henry, 42
Robertson, James (Bath), 30,41, 60,81
Robertson, James (Worcester), 41-2,58,87
Robertson, William, 8,22,25,42, 55,63,97-9,116,121-2,124-5, 137,139
Robinson, James, 6,21,23,25,29-33,57,85,90,97,100,103,110, 126-7,142
Rochdale, 92,133,172,175,206
Rochester, 93,200,210
Rogers, 81
Rogers, Thomas (Leicester), 80-1
Rogers, Thomas (Southampton), 81
Romsey, 72-3,92,211
Rose, James, 8
Rose, John Frederick, 80
Rose, Robert, 80
Ross, 92,171,224
Rotherham, 133
Rothwell, 55
Rowlandson, Thomas, 115-6,141
royal appointments, 12,144
Royal College of Surgeons in London, 11,31-3,45,54,57,62
Royal Masonic Institution for Girls, 63
royal patronage, 116
Runcorn, 92,236
Ruspini, Bartholomew, 15-7,29, 53-4,63,78-9,138,145
Rutter, William, 15,117
Ryde, 82,155,205-6,223-4
Rymer, Samuel Lee, 57,64,81

Saffron Walden, 93,167
Sale, 29

Salford, 162,173-4,182,195,212
Salisbury, 92,167,173
Samuel, H., 94
Saunders, Josiah, 82
Sayles, 55
Sayles, Frederick Alban, 87
scaling, 13,15,106,108-9
Scarborough, 73,93,96,133,166,212,
    214,243
Scardovi, 15,94
scarification, 107
'scurvy of the gums', 106
Sedmon[d], Mr. & Mrs., 54,78,94,
    145
'Senex', 27,56
Settle, 133
Sheffield, 18,27,56,58,77-8,91-2,
    130,133-4,158-9,162,165,168,175,
    177,179-80,186,188,201,207-8,
    210,212,214-6,225,229,231,244,
    247
Sheffield, Isaac, 41,56,82-3
Sheffield, John, 41,56,82
Sheffield, Thomas, 26,41,94
Shelton, 93,176,209
Shepton Mallet, 93,185
Sherborne, 196
Shew, Christopher, 42,82
Shew, George, 7,28,82
Shew, Robert, 27-8
Shipley, 93,224
short-term dentists, 37,39-40
Shrewsbury, 77,92,128,198-9,240
Sigmond, Joseph, 46,54,78
silver, 99,108-9
Simpson, John, 81
Sinclair, 25
Skipton, 133
Sleaford, 92-3,218
Smale, Thomas, 108

small towns, 72
Smartt, Charles, 109
Smith, William, 23
Snell, James, 29
social season, 87
Society of Apothecaries, 54
South Shields, 93,96,195,208,213
Southampton, 30,79-82,84,92,94,
    158,165,180-1,193,196,199,205,
    207,217,220,223-4,226,237,240,
    243
South Newington, 172
Southsea, 93,221,231
spas, 73-4
Spence, 29,127
Spence, Robert, 27
spheres of influence, 77
Spilsby, 75,92,242
springs, 105,107
St. Albans, 130
St. George's Hospital, London,
    27
St. Helier, 92,157-60,113,196,
    201-2,207,209,223,230,239
Stafford, 17,73,93,207
Stamford, 72-3,216-8,224
Stanbury, Nicholas, 80
Steele, Thomas, 16,79
sterilisation, 100
Stockport, 92,130,201,246
Stockton on Tees, 80,92,96,183,
    213
Stockwell Place, 236
Stoke Newington, 172
Stoke on Trent, 73-4,93,207,225
Stonehouse, 72,92,188,198,236,
    240
Stoney Stratford, 86,130
Stowmarket, 92,230
Stratford on Avon, 92,185,221

Stuart, 55
Styer, Abraham, 80
Suffolk, 44
sugar, increased consumption of,
  124
Sunderland, 37,41,48,92,96,168-9,
  176,198,213,216,225-6,240,247-8
surgeon-apothecaries, 126
'surgeon dentist', 117
surgeons, 18-9,52-3,55,134
Swansea, 92,159,167,180

Tadcaster, 133
Talma, Arman, 15,41,54,78,81,131,
  140,148
tartar, removal of, 115
Taunton, 92,162,171,180,187,195,
  208,223
Tavistock, 8,14,74,85,92-3,128,
  225
Taylor, Thomas, 81
Tearne, 18
technical advances, 139-42
Teignmouth, 87,93,203-4,212,241
terro-metallic
  -teeth, 141
  -cement, 99
Tetsworth, 73,93,173
Thame, 86
Therenez, C. Anthony, 94
Thomas, 82
Thomlyn, William, 10
Thompson, C., 5
Threshfield, 133
Tibbs, Somerset, 7,80,87,95
tic douloureux, 120
tincture of myrrh, 111
Tipton, 93,190
Titterington, William, 59

Tomes, John, 25-6,45,64,127,146
Tomlinson, 7
toothache, 16,120
toothdrawing, 1,10-2,13-4,18-9,
  21,117,126
toothworms, 97
Torquay, 80,93,96,172,184,186,
  212,226
Toscan, Annibal, 16
tours, 128-9,134
towns with dentists
  -18th and 19th centuries, 72
toyman, 18,117,125
Tracey, Nathaniel, 43
Tracy, Hugh, 43
Tracy, John, 43
trade directories, 2-5,7-8,17,
  37,58,64-5,83,85-6,88-9,93
  -accuracy, 3-5
  -advertisements, 95
  -dummy entries, 65
  -problems in use of, 3
transplanting, 111,121,137
transport, 128-32
  -improved roads/communication,
  131
travelling as a way of life, 131
travelling theatre company, 130
treatises, dental, 127
treatment, 97-110
  -adequacy of, 97-8
  -change in demand for, 85-6,
  112-21
  -cosmetic appeal of, 116
  -crowns, 100,103
  -demand for, 112,116,118-9,
  121,142
  -extraction, *q.v.*, 103-4
  -fees for, 108-10,126
  -filing, *q.v.*, 98-9

-filling, *q.v.*, 98-9
-free, 137
-high cost of, 142-3
-in a Bath practice, 107-9
-orthodontic, *q.v.*, 104
-periodontal, *q.v.*, 106-7
-prosthetic, 105-6 *see also* artificial teeth
-recurrent costs of, 142
-social attitude towards seeking,
  143-4
Truro, 93,207,211,237
Tunbridge Wells, 37,73,87,92,95,
  159,190,198,222,244,246
Tupholme, Anne, 93
Turner, 81
Turnham Green, 236
turnover in places, 70
-in dentists, 67
Twyford, Thomas, 18,23

unregistered practice, 6
urban culture, 72
Uttoxeter, 59
Uxbridge, 92,211

Valade, Monsieur, 95
Van Butchell, Martin, 15,127
vanity, 115
victualler, 18
Vision of Piers Plowman, 10
visiting dentists, 15,17,77-8,85,
  128,134,137-8,147
Voice, Gamaliel, 15

Wade, Edwin, 63
Wakefield, 93,130,133,168,208,211,
  226,247
Wall, Robert Hall, 109
Waller, 55

Warwick, 93,95,167
watchmakers, 18-9,28,32,54,57,
  126
watering places, 74
'Waterloo teeth', 140
Watts, John, 15,54
Weale, Thomas, 54,81
wealth, 48-50
Webster, James, 8
Wedgwood, Josiah, 148
Weiss, Felix, 83
Wellington, Duke of, 148
Weymouth, 72-3,92,207,240
Whitchurch, 93,156
White, Richard, 57,59,81
Whitehaven, 93,174
Whitlock, Charles, 131
Whitlock, Michael, 16,37,54,117
Wigan, 93,167-8,227
Wilcock, John H., 109,142
Wildsmith, Benjamin, 18
Williams, George Salusbury [sic]
  46
Williamson, William, 27
Wimborne, 93,227
Winchester, 93,167,193.198-9,226
Winckworth, William, 57
Windsor, 55,72-3,158,172,211-2
Winslow, 86
Wisbeach, 93,167,228-9
Woburn, 93,246
Wolverhampton, 17,93,96,174-5,
  177,194,206,210,212,217
Wood, 83
Woodforde, Parson, 14,126
Woodhouse, A.J., 26-7
Wooffendale, Robert, 18,22-3,83,
  134,140
wool-comber/sorter, 18,125
Woolfryes, Henry, 81

Woolwich, 92,162,166,226,237-8

Worcester, 18,41,58,72,87,196-7, 199,202,209,211,224-5,234-5,239-40

Worthing, 93,169,245

Yaniewicz, Felix, 63,83

Yarmouth, 92,171,207-9,217,245

Yeovil, 81,93-4,196

York, 5,16,29,54,59,63,79,91-2, 133-4,166,179,188,195,200-1, 220,242-3